Sports Injuries Information for Teens

Second Edition

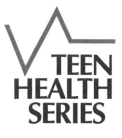

TEEN HEALTH SERIES

Second Edition

Sports Injuries Information for Teens

Health Tips about Acute, Traumatic, and Chronic Injuries in Adolescent Athletes

Including Facts about Sprains, Fractures, and Overuse Injuries, Treatment, Rehabilitation, Sport-Specific Safety Guidelines, Fitness Suggestions, and More

◆

Edited by Karen Bellenir

Omnigraphics

P.O. Box 31-1640, Detroit, MI 48231

Bibliographic Note

Because this page cannot legibly accommodate all the copyright notices, the Bibliographic Note portion of the Preface constitutes an extension of the copyright notice.

Edited by Karen Bellenir

Teen Health Series

Karen Bellenir, *Managing Editor*
David A. Cooke, M.D., *Medical Consultant*
Elizabeth Collins, *Research and Permissions Coordinator*
Cherry Stockdale, *Permissions Assistant*
EdIndex, Services for Publishers, *Indexers*

* * *

Omnigraphics, Inc.
Matthew P. Barbour, *Senior Vice President*
Kevin M. Hayes, *Operations Manager*

* * *

Peter E. Ruffner, *Publisher*

Copyright © 2008 Omnigraphics, Inc.

ISBN 978-0-7808-1011-2

Library of Congress Cataloging-in-Publication Data

Sports injuries information for teens : health tips about acute, traumatic, and chronic injuries in adolescent athletes including facts about sprains, fractures, and overuse injuries, treatment, rehabilitation, sport-specific safety guidelines, fitness suggestions, and more / edited by Karen Bellenir. -- 2nd ed.
    p. cm.
Includes bibliographical references and index.
Summary: "Provides updated basic consumer health information for teens on sports-related injuries, treatment, and rehabilitation, along with safety guidelines and prevention tips. Includes index, and resource information"--Provided by publisher.
    ISBN 978-0-7808-1011-2 (hardcover : alk. paper) 1. Sports injuries. 2. Teenagers--Wounds and injuries--Prevention. 3. Wounds and injuries. I. Bellenir, Karen.
    RD97.S689 2008
    617.1'027--dc22
                                                                          2008009793

∞

Printed in the United States

Table of Contents

Preface ix

Part One: What Student Athletes Need To Know

Chapter 1—Choosing The Right Sport For You 3

Chapter 2—Sports Physicals 9

Chapter 3—Handling Sports Pressure And Competition 15

Chapter 4—Mental Health Issues In Student Athletes 19

Chapter 5—Substance-Related Concerns In Student Athletes 25

Chapter 6—Sports-Related Emotional Injuries 31

Chapter 7—The Female Athlete Triad 35

Chapter 8—Sudden Death In The Young Athlete: Rare And Tragic 41

Chapter 9—Facts About Sports Nutrition 45

Chapter 10—Sports Drinks, Carbohydrate Gels, And Energy Bars 51

Chapter 11—Fitness As A Way Of Life 57

Part Two: Diagnosing And Treating Sports Injuries

Chapter 12—What Are Sports Injuries? 67

Chapter 13—First Aid Tips For Athletes 73

Chapter 14—Emergency Care: What to Expect 79

Chapter 15—Introducing Your Healthcare Team 85

Chapter 16—Questions And Answers About Sprains And Strains 97

Chapter 17—Overuse Injuries In Adolescent Athletes 105

Chapter 18—Facts About Broken Bones 109

Chapter 19—Casts, Splints, And Crutches 121

Chapter 20—Concussions 127

Chapter 21—Facial Sports Injuries 133

Chapter 22—Dental Injuries 139

Chapter 23—Back And Neck Injuries.. 141

Chapter 24—Burners And Stingers 155

Chapter 25—Shoulder Injuries... 159

Chapter 26—Elbow Injuries 173

Chapter 27—Wrist And Hand Injuries 181

Chapter 28—Growth Plate Injuries 193

Chapter 29—Testicular Injuries.. 201

Chapter 30—Knee Injuries 205

Chapter 31—Shin Splints.. 215

Chapter 32—Ankle Sprains 217

Chapter 33—Achilles Tendon Problems 229

Chapter 34—Plantar Fasciitis 239

Chapter 35—Foot Injuries 243

Chapter 36—Guidelines For Returning To Play 255

Part Three: Preventing Sports Injuries

Chapter 37—Getting Hurt Doesn't Have To Happen 261

Chapter 38—Understanding Bones, Muscles, And Joints 267

Chapter 39—Warming Up, Stretching, And Cooling Down 275

Chapter 40—Hard Facts About Helmets 279

Chapter 41—Sports Eye Safety... 285

Chapter 42—Protect Your Teeth With A Mouthguard 289

Chapter 43—Skin Protection Tips For Athletes 293

Chapter 44—Selecting The Right Shoes 301

Chapter 45—Exercise Caution: Be Aware Of Your Surroundings 305

Chapter 46—Protect Yourself From Weather-Related Risks 309

Chapter 47—Safety Tips For Contact Sports 315

Chapter 48—Safety Tips For Non-Contact Team Sports 323

Chapter 49—Safety Tips For Dancing, Gymnastics, And
Other Individual Sports 327

Chapter 50—Safety Tips For Skaters And Skateboarders 331

Chapter 51—Safety Tips For Winter Sports 333

Chapter 52—Safety Tips For Water Sports 343

Chapter 53—Safety Tips For Hiking, Biking, And Other
Recreational Pursuits 353

Part Four: If You Need More Information

Chapter 54—Hazard Screening Reports For Team Sports,
Sports Activities, And Equipment 365

Chapter 55—National Collegiate Athletic Association's
Injury Surveillance System 371

Chapter 56—Resources For More Information About
Traumatic And Chronic Sports-Related Injuries 379

Chapter 57—Resources For More Information About
Fitness And Exercise 387

Index 407

Preface

About This Book

According to the National Institute of Arthritis and Musculoskeletal and Skin Diseases, more than 30 million young people participate in organized sports in the United States. Uncounted others participate in informal sporting and recreational activities. While sports participation offers numerous physical and social benefits, it also carries the risk of injury. In addition to acute injuries—those that happen suddenly—teen athletes are especially vulnerable to overuse or chronic injuries, which develop over time as a result of the repetitive movements associated with coaching drills and early sports specialization. While some sports injuries result from unforeseeable accidents, others result from preventable causes, including poor training practices, improper equipment use, lack of conditioning, or failure to warm up and cool down.

Sports Injuries Information For Teens, Second Edition offers updated information about common acute, traumatic, and chronic injuries. It explains the factors that may put student athletes at risk and describes how most sports injuries can be treated effectively. It discusses symptoms, diagnostic tests, treatments, and rehabilitation strategies for a head-to-toe list of common injuries, including strains, sprains, fractures, and overuse injuries. Sport-specific safety guidelines, the proper use of protective equipment, and suggestions for maintaining fitness are also included along with directories of resources for more information.

How To Use This Book

This book is divided into parts and chapters. Parts focus on broad areas of interest; chapters are devoted to single topics within a part.

Part One: What Student Athletes Need To Know provides information for teens who are interested in participating in sports. It discusses selecting appropriate sports, explains why sports physicals are important, and offers facts about mental and emotional issues sometimes encountered by adolescent athletes. Information about sports nutrition and overall fitness is also included.

Part Two: Diagnosing And Treating Sports Injuries describes different types of injuries related to sports participation. It offers first aid tips, explains typical emergency care procedures, and explains the types of healthcare providers who assist injured athletes. Individual chapters address a head-to-toe list of common injuries, and the part concludes with a chapter on returning to play after rehabilitation.

Part Three: Preventing Sports Injuries describes safe practices, protective gear, and proper equipment that can be used to help keep injuries from occurring. It offers tips about helmets, eye protection, mouth guards, and shoes and lists safety tips for a wide variety of sporting and recreational activities.

Part Four: If You Need More Information provides additional statistical data, and it also includes directories of resources for information about sports injuries and fitness.

Bibliographic Note

This volume contains documents and excerpts from publications issued by the following government agencies: Centers for Disease Control and Prevention (CDC); Consumer Product Safety Commission; National Institute of Arthritis and Musculoskeletal and Skin Diseases; National Institutes of Health; President's Council on Physical Fitness and Sports; and the U.S. Department of Labor.

In addition, this volume contains copyrighted documents and articles produced by the following organizations and individuals: A.D.A.M., Inc.; Ackland Sports Medicine; American Academy of Dermatology; American Academy of Orthopaedic Surgeons; American Academy of Otolaryngology–Head and Neck Surgery; American Board for Certification in Orthotics and Prosthetics and Pedorthics; American College of Emergency Physicians; American College of Sports Medicine; American Council on Exercise; American Dental

Association; American Orthopaedic Foot and Ankle Society; American Physical Therapy Association; American Running Association; American Society for Surgery of the Hand; Baylor College of Medicine; Bicycle Helmet Safety Institute; Center for Orthopaedics and Sports Medicine; Children, Youth and Women's Health Service (South Australia); Cincinnati Children's Hospital Medical Center; Charles Eaton, MD; Jeffrey L. Halbrecht, MD; Hospital for Special Surgery; Hughston Sports Medicine Foundation, Inc.; Institute for Arthroscopy and Sports Medicine; National Athletic Trainers' Association; National Center for Sports Safety; National Collegiate Athletic Association (NCAA); National Safety Council; National Youth Sports Safety Foundation, Inc.; Nemours Foundation; Nicholas Institute For Sports Medicine and Athletic Trauma; Prevent Blindness America; and Sports Injury Clinic.

Full citation information is provided on the first page of each chapter. Every effort has been made to secure all necessary rights to reprint the copyrighted material. If any omissions have been made, please contact Omnigraphics to make corrections for future editions.

The photograph on the front cover is from Stephen Coburn/Shutter stock.com.

Acknowledgements

In addition to the organizations listed above, special thanks are due to Liz Collins, Research and Permissions Coordinator; Cherry Stockdale, Permissions Assistant; and Elizabeth Bellenir and Nicole Salerno, editorial assistants.

About the *Teen Health Series*

At the request of librarians serving today's young adults, the *Teen Health Series* was developed as a specially focused set of volumes within Omnigraphics' *Health Reference Series*. Each volume deals comprehensively with a topic selected according to the needs and interests of people in middle school and high school.

Teens seeking preventive guidance, information about disease warning signs, medical statistics, and risk factors for health problems will find answers to their questions in the *Teen Health Series*. The *Series*, however, is not intended to serve as a tool for diagnosing illness, in prescribing treatments, or as a substitute for the physician/patient relationship. All people concerned about medical symptoms or the possibility of disease are encouraged to seek professional care from an appropriate health care provider.

If there is a topic you would like to see addressed in a future volume of the *Teen Health Series*, please write to:

Editor
Teen Health Series
Omnigraphics, Inc.
P.O. Box 31-1640
Detroit, MI 48231

Locating Information within the *Teen Health Series*

The *Teen Health Series* contains a wealth of information about a wide variety of medical topics. As the Series continues to grow in size and scope, locating the precise information needed by a specific student may become more challenging. To address this concern, information about books within the *Teen Health Series* is included in *A Contents Guide to the Health Reference Series*. The *Contents Guide* presents an extensive list of more than 14,000 diseases, treatments, and other topics of general interest compiled from the Tables of Contents and major index headings from the books of the *Teen Health Series* and *Health Reference Series*. To access *A Contents Guide to the Health Reference Series*, visit www.healthreferenceseries.com.

Our Advisory Board

We would like to thank the following advisory board members for providing guidance to the development of this Series:

Dr. Lynda Baker, Associate Professor of Library and Information Science, Wayne State University, Detroit, MI

Nancy Bulgarelli, William Beaumont Hospital Library, Royal Oak, MI

Karen Imarisio, Bloomfield Township Public Library,
Bloomfield Township, MI

Karen Morgan, Mardigian Library, University of Michigan-Dearborn,
Dearborn, MI

Rosemary Orlando, St. Clair Shores Public Library,
St. Clair Shores, MI

Medical Consultant

Medical consultation services are provided to the Teen Health Series editors by David A. Cooke, M.D. Dr. Cooke is a graduate of Brandeis University, and he received his M.D. degree from the University of Michigan. He completed residency training at the University of Wisconsin Hospital and Clinics. He is board-certified in internal medicine. Dr. Cooke currently works as part of the University of Michigan Health System and practices in Ann Arbor, MI. In his free time, he enjoys writing, science fiction, and spending time with his family.

Part One

What Student Athletes Need to Know

Chapter 1

Choosing The Right Sport For You

Corey and Angie, twin brother and sister, enjoy playing all kinds of outdoor games and sports with their friends. They especially love playing pickup games of basketball and touch football. On particularly nice days, Corey and Angie have been known to kick around the soccer ball, toss around the baseball, or go on long runs.

In just a month the twins will be high school freshmen and neither can figure out which sport to try out for in the fall. Corey is deciding between football, soccer, and cross-country. Angie is debating whether to try her hand at a sport she has never played, like field hockey, or go with one she knows, like soccer or cross-country. They're facing a dilemma a lot of teens face—which sports to play and which sports to give up.

So Many Sports, Only One You!

For some people, choosing which sports to pursue throughout high school is hard because they have never really played an organized sport before and aren't sure what they'll most enjoy. For others it's a tough decision because their friends don't like to play the same sports.

No matter what your sports dilemma is, you have to make the decision that is best for you. If you're great at soccer but would rather play football because you think it's more fun, then give the pigskin a go (just make sure it's cool with mom and dad)!

Sports are meant to be fun. If there is a sport you really enjoy but you aren't sure if you can make the team, try out anyway. What's the worst that can happen? If you get cut you can always try another sport. And sports like cross-country and track don't typically cut participants from the team. You can still participate even if you're not on the meet squad.

Every Now And Then There's An "I" In Team

Some sports, like lacrosse or field hockey, require every person on the field to be on the same page. Sure, certain people stand out more than others but superstars don't necessarily make a good team!

Sports like tennis, track and field, cross-country, swimming, gymnastics, and wrestling are all sports where individual performances are tallied into team scores. Of course there are exceptions, like relays in track and swimming, but for the most part it's possible to win a solo event in these sports and still have your team lose or vice-versa.

♣ It's A Fact!!
When Most Organized Sports Land On The School Calendar

<u>Fall</u>	<u>Winter</u>	<u>Spring</u>
• Cheerleading	• Basketball	• Badminton
• Cross-County	• Cheerleading	• Baseball (boys)
• Dance Team	• Dance	• Golf
• Field Hockey (girls)	• Gymnastics	• Lacrosse
• Football (guys)	• Ice Hockey	• Rugby
• Soccer	• Indoor Track and Field	• Softball (girls)
• Volleyball	• Swimming and Diving	• Tennis
• Water Polo	• Wrestling	• Track and Field

♣ **It's A Fact!!**
You Aren't Under Contract!

If you try a sport for a season and you don't enjoy it, or it's not what you
expected, it's OK to try out for another sport the next year. Don't let parents or
coaches persuade you to stick with something you don't want to—
ultimately it's your decision.

No one knows you better than you do. Maybe you enjoy the spotlight. Maybe
you get annoyed by the way teammates act when they are über-competitive.
Or maybe you just don't like competing with friends for a spot in the starting
lineup. For whatever reason, team sports might not be your thing—and that's
fine. Luckily, there are many individualized sports to choose from.

If Your School Doesn't Have Your Sport

Some schools are limited in resources—a city school may not have a lot
of fields, for example, while a rural school may not have enough students to
make up a team for every sport.

A school's geographic region can also play a role. If you live in a climate
where it snows from the fall to the spring, your school may not be able to
participate in a lot of outdoor sports.

If your school doesn't have your sport, don't let it get you down. You can
always try out for a different sport during the same season or look into whether
your local town has a recreational league that you can join.

If Organized Sports Aren't Your Thing

Many people are attracted to the competition and popularity that can
come with team sports. Others love the camaraderie and unity that are present
in a team atmosphere. But for some people, teams are just frustrating and
another form of cliques. If you're not the biggest fan of organized sports,
where you have to follow someone else's schedule and rules, many other fun
and exciting options are out there for you.

You might already have an exercise routine or activity you like to do in your free time, but if you're looking for something that will both keep you busy and allow you to blow off steam, try some of these activities:

Climb to the top: If you scaled trees and walls when you were younger, then the perfect activity for you is rock climbing. Rock climbing offers participants one of the best all-around workouts possible. As a rock climber, you work your hands, arms, shoulders, back, stomach, legs, and feet—all at once!

✔ **Quick Tip**
If You Don't Have It, Start It!
If you are interested in a sport, and your school doesn't have it, maybe you and some friends can talk to the administration and start a club or intramural team. With enough willing participants and the school's permission, you could have a high school cricket team!

Take a hike (yes, you can bring your bike)! Ever wonder what kinds of cool things are waiting on those nature trails not too far from your house? Why not find out? While you're at it, you'll get a good workout. Hiking and trail biking are two great ways to learn about nature while still getting that heart rate up. Even if you are just going to a local trail, always bring at least one other person along in case something happens. If you're going for an intense multi-day hike, you should bring someone who is experienced and trained in hiking.

Water world ... starring: YOU! The water is the perfect place to give yourself new challenges. There are plenty of water activities for all levels of difficulty and energy. Besides swimming, try canoeing, kayaking, fishing, rowing, sailing, wakeboarding, water skiing, windsurfing, and, if you're feeling particularly daring, surfing.

Find your inner self: Many activities can strengthen you physically and mentally. Workouts like yoga, Pilates, and t'ai chi can be relaxing and taxing all at once.

• Yoga has tons of benefits. It can improve flexibility, strength, balance, and stamina. In addition to the physical benefits, many people who practice yoga say that it reduces anxiety and stress and improves mental clarity.

- Pilates is a body conditioning routine that seeks to build flexibility, strength, endurance, and coordination without adding muscle bulk. Pilates also increases circulation and helps to sculpt the body and strengthen the body's "core" or "powerhouse" (torso). People who do Pilates regularly feel they have better posture, are less prone to injury, and experience better overall health.

- T'ai chi is an ancient Chinese martial art form that is great for improving flexibility and strengthening your legs, abdominal or core muscles, and arms.

♣ It's A Fact!! Benefits Of Strength Training

- Increases endurance and strength for sports and fitness activities

- Improves focus and concentration, which may result in better grades

- Reduces body fat and increases muscle mass

- Helps burn more calories even when not exercising

- May reduce the risk of short-term injuries by protection tendons, bones, and joints

- Helps prevent long-term medical problems such as high cholesterol or osteoporosis (weakening of the bones) when you get older

Make Sure To Take An Off-Season—But Not A Season Off!

Whether you choose one sport or three, make sure you give yourself a break from intense competition with some cross-training activities. Through cross-training you can take a rest from your sport or sports while still getting a workout and staying in shape.

Two examples of cross-training are swimming and cycling. They not only help build cardiovascular strength, but also help in muscle growth. Swimming can really help tone your upper body, while cycling strengthens your upper legs.

You can also try outdoor bike rides and runs on nice days, stopping periodically to do sit-ups and push-ups. These simple exercises can work and tone your core muscles.

That time between seasons is also the perfect opportunity to get into a strength-training routine. Before starting strength training, consult your doctor and school's strength and conditioning coach. Your doc will be able to give you health clearance to participate in the different types of physical activities, and your strength coach can come up with a workout to help you prepare for your specific sports.

Chapter 2

Sports Physicals

You already know that playing sports helps keep you fit. You also know that sports are a fun way to socialize and meet people. But you might not know why the physical you may have to take at the beginning of your sports season is so important.

In the sports medicine field, the sports physical exam is known as a preparticipation physical examination (PPE). The exam helps determine whether it's safe for you to participate in a particular sport. Most states actually require that kids and teens have a sports physical before they can start a new sport or begin a new competitive season. But even if a PPE isn't required, doctors still highly recommend them.

What is a sports physical?

There are two main parts to a sports physical: the medical history and the physical exam.

Medical history: This part of the exam includes questions about:

About This Chapter: "Sports Physicals," July 2006, reprinted with permission from www.kidshealth.org. Copyright © 2006 The Nemours Foundation. This information was provided by KidsHealth, one of the largest resources online for medically reviewed health information written for parents, kids, and teens. For more articles like this one, visit www.KidsHealth.org, or www.TeensHealth.org.

- serious illnesses among other family members

- illnesses that you had when you were younger or may have now, such as asthma, diabetes, or epilepsy

- previous hospitalizations or surgeries

- allergies (to insect bites, for example)

- past injuries (including concussions, sprains, or bone fractures)

- whether you've ever passed out, felt dizzy, had chest pain, or had trouble breathing during exercise

- any medications that you are on (including over-the-counter medications, herbal supplements, and prescription medications)

The medical history questions are usually on a form that you can bring home, so ask your parents to help you fill in the answers. If possible, ask both parents about family medical history.

Looking at patterns of illness in your family is a very good indicator of any potential conditions you may have. Most sports medicine doctors believe the medical history is the most important part of the sports physical exam, so take time to answer the questions carefully. It's unlikely that any health conditions you have will prevent you from playing sports completely.

Physical examination: During the physical part of the exam, the doctor will usually:

- record your height and weight

- take a blood pressure and pulse (heart rate and rhythm) reading

- test your vision

- check your heart, lungs, abdomen, ears, nose, and throat

- evaluate your posture, joints, strength, and flexibility

✎ **What's It Mean?**

Preparticipation Physical Examination (PPE): A physical exam that helps determine whether it's safe for you to participate in a particular sport.

✔ Quick Tip
Answer the questions as well as you can. Try not to guess the answers or give answers you think your doctor wants.

Although most aspects of the exam will be the same for males and females, if a person has started or already gone through puberty, the doctor may ask girls and guys different questions. For example, if a girl is heavily involved in a lot of active sports, the doctor may ask her about her period and diet to make sure she doesn't have something like female athlete triad.

A doctor will also ask questions about use of drugs, alcohol, or dietary supplements, including steroids or other "performance enhancers" and weight-loss supplements, because these can affect a person's health.

Some schools may require that a PPE include an electrocardiogram, or EKG, for all athletes. An EKG, which takes about 10 minutes, measures the electrical activity of a person's heart. EKGs don't hurt—electrodes that measure heart rate and rhythm are placed on the chest, arms, and legs, and a specialist reads the results.

At the end of your exam, the doctor will either fill out and sign a form if everything checks out OK or, in some cases, recommend a follow-up exam, additional tests, or specific treatment for medical problems.

Why is a sports physical important?

A sports physical can help you find out about and deal with health problems that might interfere with your participation in a sport. For example, if you have frequent asthma attacks but are a starting forward in soccer, a doctor might be able to prescribe a different type of inhaler or adjust the dosage so that you can breathe more easily when you run.

Your doctor may even have some good training tips and be able to give you some ideas for avoiding injuries. For example, he or she may recommend specific exercises, like certain stretching or strengthening activities, that help prevent injuries. A doctor can also identify risk factors that are linked to specific sports. Advice like this will make you a better, stronger athlete.

When and where should I go for a sports physical?

Some people go to their own doctor for a sports physical; others have one at school. During school physicals, you may go to half a dozen or so "stations" set up in the gym; each one is staffed by a medical professional who gives you a specific part of the physical exam.

If your school offers the exam, it's convenient to get the exam done there. But even if you have a PPE at school, it's a good idea to see your regular doctor for an exam as well. Your doctor knows you—and your health history—better than anyone you talk to briefly in a gym.

If your state requires sports physicals, you'll probably have to start getting them when you're in ninth grade. Even if PPEs aren't required by your school or state, it's still smart to get them if you participate in school sports. And if you compete regularly in a sport before ninth grade, you should begin getting these exams even earlier.

You should have your physical about six weeks before your sports season begins so there's enough time to follow up on something, if necessary. Neither you nor your doctor will be very happy if your PPE is the day before baseball prac-

> ♣ **It's A Fact!!**
>
> Getting a sports physical once a year is usually adequate. If you're healing from a major injury, like a broken wrist or ankle, however, get checked out after it's healed before you start practicing or playing again.

tice starts and it turns out there's something that needs to be taken of care before you can suit up.

What if there's a problem?

What happens if you don't get the OK from your own doctor and have to see a specialist? Does that mean you won't ever be able to letter in softball or hockey? Don't worry if your doctor asks you to have other tests or go for a follow-up exam—it could be something as simple as rechecking your blood pressure a week or two after the physical.

Your doctor's referral to a specialist may help your athletic performance. For example, if you want to try out for your school's track team but get a slight pain in your knee every time you run, an orthopedist or sports medicine specialist can help you figure out what's going on. Perhaps the pain comes from previous overtraining or poor running technique. Maybe you injured the knee a long time ago and it never totally healed. Or perhaps the problem is as simple as running shoes that don't offer enough support. Chances are, a doctor will be able to help you run without the risk of further injury to the knee by giving you suggestions or treatment before the sports season begins.

It's very unlikely that you'll be disqualified from playing sports. The ultimate goal of the sports physical is to ensure safe participation in sports, not to disqualify the participants. Most of the time, a specialist won't find anything serious enough to prevent you from playing your sport. In fact, fewer than 1% of students have conditions that might limit sports participation, and most of these conditions are known before the PPE takes place.

Do I still have to get a regular physical?

In a word, yes. It may seem like overkill, but a sports physical is different from a standard physical.

The sports physical focuses on your well-being as it relates to playing a sport. It's more limited than a regular physical, but it's a lot more specific about athletic issues. During a regular physical, however, your doctor will address your overall well-being, which may include things that are unrelated to sports. You can ask your doctor to give you both types of exams during one visit; just be aware that you'll need to set aside more time.

Even if your sports physical exam doesn't reveal any problems, it's always a good idea to monitor yourself when you play sports. If you notice changes in your physical condition—even if you think they're small, such as muscle pain or shortness of breath—be sure to mention them to a parent or coach. You should also inform your physical education teacher or coach if your health needs have changed in any way or if you're taking a new medication.

Just as professional sports stars need medical care to keep them playing their best, so do teenage athletes. You can give yourself the same edge as the pros by making sure you have your sports physical.

Chapter 3

Handling Sports Pressure and Competition

Most people play a sport for the thrill of having fun with others who share the same interest, right? But it's not always fun and games. Most student athletes who play competitive sports have had thoughts that go like this at one time or another: "Man, I can't believe I let the ball in the goal, and I know from the look in coach's eyes he wasn't happy."

There can be a ton of pressure in high school sports. A lot of the time it comes from the feeling that a parent or coach expects you to always win. But sometimes it comes from inside, too: Some players are just really hard on themselves. And individual situations can add to the stress: Maybe there's a recruiter from your number one college scouting you on the sidelines. Whatever the cause, the pressure to win can sometimes stress you to the point where you just don't know how to have fun anymore. Perhaps it could even be the reason why you haven't been playing as well lately.

How can stress affect sports performance?

Stress is a feeling that's created when we react to particular events. It's the body's way of rising to a challenge and preparing to meet a tough situation

About This Chapter: "Handling Sports Pressure and Competition," August 2007, reprinted with permission from www.kidshealth.org. Copyright © 2007 The Nemours Foundation. This information was provided by KidsHealth, one of the largest resources online for medically reviewed health information written for parents, kids, and teens. For more articles like this one, visit www.KidsHealth.org, or www.TeensHealth.org.

with focus, strength, stamina, and heightened alertness. A little stress or the right kind of positive stress can help keep you on your toes, ready to rise to a challenge.

The events that provoke stress are called stressors, and they cover a whole range of situations—everything from outright danger to stepping up to take the foul shot that could win the game. Stress can also be a response to change or anticipation of something that's about to happen—good or bad. People can feel stress over positive challenges, like making the varsity team, as well as negative ones.

Distress is a bad type of stress that arises when you must adapt to too many negative demands. Suppose you had a fight with a close friend last night, you forgot your homework this morning, and you're playing in a tennis match this afternoon. You try to get psyched for the game but can't. You've hit stress overload! Continuous struggling with too much stress can exhaust your energy and drive.

Eustress is the good type of stress that stems from the challenge of taking part in something that you enjoy but have to work hard for. Eustress pumps you up, providing a healthy spark for any task you undertake.

What can I do to ease pressure?

When the demands of competition start to get to you, try these relaxation techniques:

Deep breathing: Find a quiet place to sit down. Inhale slowly through your nose, drawing air deep into your lungs. Hold your breath for about 5 seconds, then release it slowly. Repeat the exercise five times.

Muscle relaxation: Contract (flex) a group of muscles tightly. Keep them tensed for about 5 seconds, then release. Repeat the exercise five times, selecting different muscle groups.

Visualization: Close your eyes and picture a peaceful place or an event from your past. Recall the beautiful sights and the happy sounds. Imagine stress flowing away from your body. You can also visualize success. People who advise competitive players often recommend that they imagine themselves

✔ **Quick Tip**

When sports become too stressful, get away from the pressure. Go to a movie or hang out with friends. Put your mind on something completely different.

completing a pass, making a shot, or scoring a goal over and over. Then on game day, you can recall your stored images to help calm nerves and boost self-confidence.

Mindfulness: Watch out for negative thoughts. Whether you're preparing for a competition or coping with a defeat, repeat to yourself: "I learn from my mistakes!" "I'm in control of my feelings!" "I can make this goal!"

How can I keep stress in check?

If sports make you so nervous that you get headaches, become nauseated, or can't concentrate on other things, you're experiencing symptoms of unhealthy, potentially chronic (which means long-lasting and continuous) stress. Don't keep such stress bottled up inside you; suppressing your emotions might mean bigger health troubles for you later on.

Talk about your concerns with a friend. Simply sharing your feelings can ease your anxiety. Sometimes it may help to get an adult's perspective—someone who has dealt with stress over and over like your coach or fitness instructor. Here are some other things you can do to cope with stress:

- Treat your body right. Eat well and get a good night's sleep, especially before games where the pressure's on.

- Learn and practice relaxation techniques, like those described in the previous section.

- Get some type of physical activity other than the sport you're involved in. Take a walk, ride your bike, and get completely away from the sport that's stressing you out.

- Don't try to be perfect—everyone flubs a shot or messes up from time to time (so don't expect your teammates to be perfect either!). Forgive yourself, remind yourself of all your great shots, and move on.

It's possible that some anxiety stems only from uncertainty. Meet privately with your coach or instructor. Ask for clarification if his or her expectations seem vague or inconsistent. Although most instructors do a good job of fostering athletes' physical and mental development, you may need to be the one who opens the lines of communication. You may also want to talk with your parents or another adult family member.

If you're feeling completely overscheduled and out of control, review your options on what you can let go. It's a last resort, but if you're no longer enjoying your sport, it may be time to find one that's less stressful. Chronic stress isn't fun—and fun is what sports are all about.

Recognizing when you need guidance to steer yourself out of a stressful situation doesn't represent weakness; it's a sign of courage and wisdom. Don't stop looking for support until you've found it.

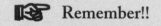 **Remember!!**
Enjoy The Game
Winning is exhilarating! But losing and some amount of stress are part of almost any sports program—as they are in life. Sports are about enhancing self-esteem, building social skills, and developing a sense of community. And above all, sports are about having fun.

Chapter 4

Mental Health Issues In Student Athletes

When you think of a student-athlete's health, you probably are inclined to think primarily of the person's physical/medical condition and what effect an injury will have on athletic performance. A student-athlete's "mental health" might be viewed as secondary to physical health; however, it is every bit as important. It makes little sense to try to separate the "mind" and "body." One affects the other. Medical problems often have psychological or emotional consequences. Psychological problems (for example, eating disorders, substance-related problems, etc.) typically have medical consequences. Student-athletes who suffer from depression after an injury illustrate the relationship between "physical" and "mental" health. At the same time, some depressed student-athletes are at increased risk of injury. Given the interrelationship between the physical and mental, it might be helpful to think of student-athletes with mental health problems as "injured"—just as you would of a student-athlete who has a physical or medical problem. As with physical injuries, mental health problems may, by their severity, affect athletic performance and limit or even preclude training and competition until successfully managed and treated.

About This Chapter: From "Managing Student-Athletes' Mental Health Issues," Developed by Ron A. Thompson, PhD, FAED, and Roberta Trattner Sherman, PhD, FAED, Bloomington Center for Counseling and Human Development, Bloomington, Indiana. © 2007 National Collegiate Athletic Association (www.ncaa.org). Reprinted with permission.

Mood Disorders

Mood disorders sometimes are called affective disorders, but more frequently are simply called "depression." Approximately 10 percent of the American population suffers from a mood disorder during any one-year period, which is the same percentage of depression in college students as reported by the National Mental Health Association. Certainly, most people will feel depressed for short periods from time to time for various reasons. However, when the depression becomes more severe, lasts longer, and occurs more frequently, evaluation and treatment are warranted. Although most mood disorders primarily involve low mood or depression, bipolar disorder consists of episodes of abnormally elevated (high) moods, in addition to the characteristic low moods.

Signs And Symptoms/Identification

Typically, mood disorders (or depression) are characterized by:

- Low or sad moods, often with crying episodes;

- Irritability or anger;

- Feeling worthless, helpless, and hopeless;

- Eating and sleeping disturbance (reflected in an increase or decrease);

- A decrease in energy and activity levels with feelings of fatigue or tiredness;

- Decreases in concentration, interest, and motivation;

- Social withdrawal or avoidance;

- Negative thinking;

- Thoughts of death or suicide;

- In severe cases, intent to commit suicide with a specific plan, followed by one or more suicide attempts.

Effects On Health And Performance

You can tell from these depressive symptom descriptions that most aspects of a person's life are negatively affected by the disorder. Athletic performance is no exception. In fact, poorer performance would be expected. If a student-athlete is not eating or sleeping well and feels tired or fatigued, you would expect performance to decrease from a physiological perspective. Add in emotional and cognitive components of low mood, decreased motivation, poor concentration, and negative thinking, and you could not expect a student-athlete to perform well. Poor sport performance can increase a student-athlete's depression and the pressure to perform better. Depression may also increase a student-athlete's risk of injury.

Depression And Risk Of Injury

A student-athlete may become depressed after an injury, but the relationship between depression and injury may also occur in reverse order. Depression can precede an injury and may increase a student-athlete's risk of injury. Depression in many student-athletes occurs for nonsports related reasons. For such student-athletes, their depression—or more specifically their depressive symptoms—may increase the likelihood of injury primarily through distraction (decreased concentration resulting in being less alert, responding more slowly, or making poor decisions or judgments). A depressed batter might be less able to avoid being hit by a fastball. A diver might more easily lose where she is in space before impacting the water. Additional risk to the student-athlete may increase because the body has been medically compromised from the depressive symptoms of eating and sleep disturbance.

Anxiety Disorders

♣ It's A Fact!!
According to the National Institute of Mental Health, anxiety disorders are the most common type of mental illness in the U.S. Approximately 40 million people over the age of 18 are affected each year.

Everyone from time to time experiences symptoms of anxiety. For individuals with an anxiety disorder, however, these symptoms tend to be bothersome daily and worsen when pressure or stress occur.

The cause of anxiety can vary with the disorder and the individual. Most anxiety disorders are probably due to genetic factors, personality factors, or life experiences.

Signs And Symptoms/Identification

Anxiety symptoms can be general or specific to a particular stressful situation or set of circumstances. They may or may not have an apparent cause. Symptoms can include any of the following:

- Excessive worry, fear or dread

- Sleep disturbances, especially difficulty falling asleep

- Changes in appetite, including either an increased need to eat when anxious or difficulty eating due to anxiety

- Feelings ranging from a general uneasiness to complete immobilization

- Pounding heart, sweating, shaking, or trembling

- Impaired concentration

- A feeling of being out of control

- Fear that one is dying or going crazy

- A disruption of everyday life

Effects On Performance

Not all anxiety is necessarily bad. In fact, a little anxious excitement can facilitate performance if managed properly. Some student-athletes without anxiety disorders may experience anxiety or nervousness when under pressure in an important competition. Often these student-athletes can overcome these problems with instruction in mental skills training that can help them focus, concentrate, and perform. However, student-athletes with an anxiety disorder are less apt to be able to manage their anxiety properly and positively. Depending on the nature of the anxiety disorder, effects can vary. An anxiety disorder can negatively affect concentration, primarily through the student-athlete being distracted by his or her symptoms, which could include physical and psychological symptoms. These difficulties can affect the student-athlete before, during and after competition. During competition, many of these student-athletes will have difficulty focusing; or they will focus on the negative rather than the positive. Before competition, they are inclined to worry that they will not perform well, perhaps setting up their worst fears. After a competition, especially one in which they perceive that their performance was inadequate, they worry that they are "not good enough" and that significant others (that is, coaches, teammates, family, friends, etc.) will be disappointed in them.

Eating Disorders And Disordered Eating

Eating disorders are somewhat of a misnomer. They are not only disorders of eating. They are mental disorders that manifest themselves in a variety of eating and weight-related symptoms. Focus should not only be on eating disorders such as anorexia nervosa, bulimia nervosa, or an eating disorder not otherwise specified; it also should include "disordered eating."

Prevalence, Risk Factors, And Causes

Eating disorders result from a combination of factors that include genetics, personality, sociocultural pressures regarding thinness, social learning, and family issues. Although sport participation for most individuals is a healthy experience, aspects of the sport environment can increase the individual's risk for an eating disorder.

Eating disorders often begin or worsen during transition periods, such as when an individual leaves home to attend college. Because eating disorders usually are triggered by dietary restraint (dieting) for weight loss, they tend to be more prevalent in sports that emphasize a thin body size or a low weight, such as cross country, diving, gymnastics, lightweight rowing, and wrestling. However, eating disorders for many student-athletes are not directly related to their sport. They likely would have the disorder even if they were not student-athletes. For these student-athletes, athletics may simply be another stressor that increases the need for the disorder.

♣ It's A Fact!!

Eating disorders are common among college-age females. They are much less common among males, but it should be remembered that 10 to 25 percent of individuals with eating disorders are male.

Effects On Performance

Of all the disorders discussed in this chapter, performance is probably most affected by eating disorders and disordered eating. In general, healthier student-athletes perform better, and health is greatly affected by nutrition. Because of inadequate nutrition, student-athletes with eating difficulties tend to be malnourished, dehydrated, depressed, anxious, and obsessed (with eating, food, and weight). In addition to their negative effects on a student-athlete's physiology, these problems decrease concentration and the capacity to play with emotion.

Regarding the physical effects of disordered eating, research suggests that intense dieting can negatively affect VO2max and running speed for some student-athletes. Because most individuals with eating problems are restricting their caloric intake, they are likely to ingest inadequate amounts of carbohydrate in part because they often view carbohydrates as being "fattening." Restricting carbohydrates—the best energy source—leads to glycogen depletion sooner. Without adequate carbohydrate ingestion, the body tends to convert protein into a less efficient form of energy. The risk of muscle-related injury and weakness increases with inadequate protein. For a variety of reasons (that is, restriction of carbohydrates, induced vomiting, excessive exercise, etc.), student-athletes with disordered eating are apt to be dehydrated, which negatively affects athletic performance.

Chapter 5

Substance-Related Concerns In Student Athletes

In this chapter, the term "substance" refers to a variety of drugs or chemicals, including those that are legal, illegal, prescribed, over-the-counter (OTC), and performance-enhancing. Primary focus is on substances that appear to be used frequently by college-age individuals, and those that for various reasons may be student-athletes' substance of choice. Although substance use often is associated with terms like "abuse," "dependence" or "addiction" to indicate the severity of use, that part of the identification process is well beyond the scope of this chapter. The focus of this information is to help coaches identify a student-athlete with a possible problem, refer the student-athlete to the appropriate professional who can assess the extent of the problem and arrange necessary treatment. Much of the information in this chapter was drawn from the six National Collegiate Athletic Association (NCAA) studies investigating substance use by student-athletes. Based on the self-reporting of drug use, these data are probably conservative. Actual use is apt to be higher than reported use.

About This Chapter: From "Managing Student-Athletes' Mental Health Issues," Developed by Ron A. Thompson, PhD, FAED, and Roberta Trattner Sherman, PhD, FAED, Bloomington Center for Counseling and Human Development, Bloomington, Indiana. © 2007 National Collegiate Athletic Association (www.ncaa.org). Reprinted with permission.

Substances

Alcohol

Current Usage: Although alcohol consumption decreased among student-athletes from 1989 to 2005, more than three-fourths of the student-athletes surveyed in a 2005 NCAA study reported using alcohol during the previous 12 months. More disturbing was the increase in the number of student-athletes who reported drinking six or more or 10 or more drinks in a sitting.

Effects On Performance: Alcohol is a central nervous system (CNS) depressant. It can decrease concentration, coordination, reaction time, strength, power, and endurance. Alcohol also can inhibit the body's absorption of nutrients. For these reasons, alcohol will negatively affect performance. The extent of the effect depends on the amount and type of alcohol ingested, the weight and health of the individual, and the timing of the alcohol consumption. For "heavy drinkers," the effect can last for days.

Reasons For Use: Most individuals consume alcohol recreationally to "feel good" or "have a good time." Some, however, use it as a means to calm themselves to avoid or manage anxiety. Some will even suggest that alcohol acts as an "ergogenic" that allows them to perform better by helping them to "relax." Some may use alcohol to help them sleep. Others will use alcohol in response to being depressed; however, because it is a CNS depressant, alcohol only serves to further (biochemically) depress them.

Signs And Symptoms: The signs and symptoms of alcohol (ab)use can vary with the type and amount of alcohol consumed and the individual's personality. In general, student-athletes with this problem might be expected to be more irresponsible regarding commitments or responsibilities to school, sport, and relationships.

> ♣ **It's A Fact!!**
> Findings in a recent NCAA survey suggested that many student-athletes do not see alcohol consumption as a problem. Almost 60 percent of student-athletes reported that they did not believe that alcohol affected their athletic performance. However, almost 30 percent admitted that they had performed poorly in practice or a competition because of drinking or drug use.

They might be more likely to drink in situations that could be dangerous to themselves or others. They might show a propensity for getting into trouble when drinking (that is, fighting, legal problems, etc.). These examples are observable signs, but it should be remembered that drinking alone often is a sign of an alcohol problem. Thus, a student-athlete who abuses alcohol may do his or her drinking alone and avoid drawing attention to observable signs.

Stimulant-Type Substances—Amphetamines, Cocaine, Ephedrine, And Medications For Attention Deficit/ Hyperactivity Disorder (ADHD)

In contrast to a CNS depressant like alcohol, substances in this class are CNS stimulants. Whereas CNS depressants slow the nervous system, CNS stimulants speed up the nervous system. Users sometime refer to these drugs as "speed."

Current Usage: The percentage of student-athletes reporting using amphetamines, cocaine, and ephedrine is small (four percent or less). However, amphetamine and cocaine use by student-athletes has been increasing in recent years. Ephedrine use has not increased. This type of drug use often begins before college.

The abuse of medications for ADHD is a relatively new phenomenon, but one that is increasing in prevalence—especially in the college population. These medications, when used by individuals who need them for treatment of their hyperactivity symptoms (that is, distractibility) have a paradoxical effect. Although ADHD medications are stimulants, they decrease the individual's distractibility and facilitate concentration and focus. Some individuals are illegally or illicitly obtaining the medications for their own use or for sale. These medications usually are amphetamines such as Adderall and Dexedrine.

Effects On Performance: Because the drug makes a student-athlete feel more energetic and alert, it is assumed that it will positively affect performance. The drug can make many individuals nervous or jittery, which would negatively affect any skill requiring fine motor coordination and concentration. Performance also can be negatively affected because this type of drug increases heart rate and blood pressure. In addition to these potential problems, drugs like ephedrine can increase body heat production and body temperature. Because these drugs can lead the student-athlete to feel overly energetic, they may lead to overexertion, which could result in injury or even death in extreme cases. It is ironic that many student-athletes may be taking these drugs as an "ergogenic" aid to help them perform better, when in fact these drugs may have more of an "ergolytic" (negative performance) effect.

Reasons For Use: This type of drug usually is used for "energy" or to raise mood. It also may be used for weight control/loss. Amphetamines also may be used to improve performance.

Signs And Symptoms: Common signs and symptoms include shakiness, rapid speech or movements, difficulty sitting still, difficulty concentrating, lack of appetite, sleep disturbance, and irritability.

Marijuana

Current Use: Marijuana is the most widely used illegal drug by the general population. Marijuana appears to be a drug of choice for college students, and it appears to be a popular drug used by student-athletes. Although marijuana use by student-athletes has declined in recent years, a 2005 NCAA study found almost 20 percent of student-athletes reported having used the drug in the past year.

Effects On Performance: The effects of marijuana on sport performance are much like those of alcohol. It can slow reaction time, impair both motor and eye-hand coordination, and affect time perception. Research related to the duration of the effect of this drug is inconclusive, but some researchers believe it can last an entire day or longer.

Reasons For Use: Student-athletes reported that they used marijuana for recreational and social purposes in order to "feel good."

Signs And Symptoms: Signs and symptoms vary depending on the frequency of use. There may be no signs associated with infrequent use. Possible signs could include red eyes, paraphernalia related to marijuana use (that is, papers, pipes, etc.), and scales for weighing the drug. Physical symptoms could include lethargy and increased appetite, especially immediately after smoking the drug.

Anabolic Steroids

Current Usage: Steroid use by student-athletes has been decreasing. Now, less than two percent report using steroids. The majority of users are male. Of those who use steroids, more than half say they use them to enhance performance and that their use began before college.

Effects An Performance: Steroid use typically is associated with an increase in athletic performance. Steroids can increase muscle mass, and as a result may increase strength, power, speed, and endurance.

Reasons For Use: The primary reason reported for steroid use is performance enhancement from an increase in size and strength, and to recover more quickly from an injury.

Signs And Symptoms: Signs and symptoms can include a variety of changes in the student-athlete. Some changes may occur in the size and musculature of the body. There may be personality changes, often with a variety of psychiatric symptoms, including increased anger and aggression, or what has sometimes been referred to as "roid rage." Physical/medical signs can range from acne to reproductive system dysfunction to liver and cardiovascular system problems.

Chapter 6

Sports-Related Emotional Injuries

Desirable Outcomes Of Participation

Ideally, well organized youth sports programs provide a safe, wholesome environment where children can enjoy their spare time and sports experience.

Desirable outcomes of this experience include: having fun; the development of sound character, self esteem, confidence, friendships, trust; and the accomplishment of goals.

Unfortunately, not all children have a positive experience in youth sports programs. Certain behaviors and philosophies have been found to create a destructive environment causing some children to be scarred for life.

Emotional Abuse

Emotions, defined by Richard Lazarus, Professor Emeritus at Cal-Berkeley are as follows: "Negative emotions include: anger, anxiety, fright, sadness, guilt, shame, envy, jealousy, and disgust. Positive emotions we would like developed include: relief, hope, happiness/joy, pride, love, gratitude, and compassion."

Emotional abuse occurs when an individual treats a child in a negative manner which impairs the child's concept of self. This may include a parent/

guardian/caregiver, coach, teacher, brother, sister, or a friend. Emotional abuse is, perhaps, the most difficult abuse to identify and the most common form of maltreatment in youth sports.

Examples include: rejecting; ignoring; isolating; terrorizing; name calling; making fun of someone; putting someone down, saying things that hurt feelings; and/or yelling.

Additional examples of emotional abuse:

• Forcing a child to participate in sports;

• Not speaking to a child after he/she plays poorly in a youth sports game or practice;

• Asking a child why he/she played poorly when it meant so much to you;

• Hitting a child when his/her play disappoints you;

• Yelling at a child for not playing well or for losing;

• Punishing a child for not playing well or for losing;

• Criticizing and/or ridiculing a child for his/her sports performance.

Statements such as: "You're stupid, you're an embarrassment, you're not worth the uniform you play in," are damaging and hurt a young athlete's self esteem and their value as a human being. If said long enough or strong enough these statements or other negative statements may become beliefs of the athlete and may carry forth into their adult life.

Philosophical Abuse

Healthy philosophies foster emotionally healthy children. They are based on sound objectives and nurture the concept that the well-being of a child is more important than his/her performance or winning. The American Sport Education Program suggests, "Athletes First, Winning Second."

Examples of destructive philosophies:

• Win at all cost philosophy—"winning is the only thing";

• Making a child believe his/her self worth relies on wins and losses. The following illustration demonstrates how this belief is established:

the first thing you ask a child when he/she comes home is, "Did you win—what was the score?"

Parental Misconduct At Youth Sports Events

It has been widely reported and well documented that parental rage in youth sports is becoming a commonplace occurrence. Examples of parental misconduct:

• Booing or taunting;

• Physically hitting another parent, official, or player;

• Using profane language or gestures;

• Yelling at or arguing with game officials, parents, or players.

How Common Is Abuse In Youth Sports?

The Minnesota Amateur Sports Commission conducted a survey in 1993 and found the following incidences of abuse in sports in Minnesota:

• 45.3% of males and females surveyed said they have been called names, yelled at, or insulted while participating in sports.

• 17.5% of people surveyed said they have been hit, kicked, or slapped while participating in sports.

• 21% said they have been pressured to play with an injury.

• 8.2% said they have been pressured to intentionally harm others while playing sports.

• 3.4% said they have been pressured into sex or sexual touching.

• 8% of all surveyed said they have been called names with sexual connotations while participating in sports.

What Are The Effects Of Abuse Or Witnessing Parental Misconduct?

Children who have strong reactions to viewing violence or aggression could develop post traumatic stress disorder.

The trauma associated with witnessing violence can adversely affect a child's ability to learn.

Childhood abuse increases the likelihood that the youth will engage in health risk behaviors including suicidal behavior, and delinquent and aggressive behaviors in adolescence.

Abuse in childhood has been linked to a variety of adverse health outcomes in adulthood. These include mood and anxiety disorders and diseases.

Violence is a learned behavior; children are often learning violence from places where they should be learning positive life skills.

Abuse will "turn the child off" to exercise and sports participation and prevent the development of healthy lifestyles that will promote wellness through the lifespan.

> ♣ **It's A Fact!!**
> **Barriers To Prevention**
>
> People may not be clear what behaviors constitute maltreatment or abuse.
>
> Young athletes may not recognize what's happening to them is abusive.

Resources

- National Youth Sports Safety Foundation, 333 Longwood Avenue, Ste. 202, Boston, MA 02115, 617-277-1171, www.nyssf.org
- Ahead In The Game.Com, www.aheadinthegame.com
- Arizona Sports Summit Accord, www.charactercounts.org/sports/accord.htm
- American Sport Education Program (ASEP), Box 5076, Champaign, IL 61825-5076, 800-747-5698
- Minnesota Amateur Sports Commission, 1700 105th Ave. NE, Blaine, MN 55449, 612-785-5630, www.masc.state.mn.us/resources/index.html
- National Institute for Child Centered Coaching, 3160 Pinebrook Road, Park City, UT 84060, 800-748-4843
- National Alliance for Youth Sports, 2050 Vista Parkway, West Palm Beach, FL 33411, 800-729-2057
- Positive Coaching Alliance, c/o Stanford Athletic Department, Stanford, CA 94305, 650-725-0024, www.positivecoach.org
- Lazarus, RS. (2000) How emotions influence performance in competitive sports. *The Sport Psychologist*, 14, 229–252.

Chapter 7

The Female Athlete Triad

With dreams of college scholarships in her mind, Hannah joined the track team her freshman year and trained hard to become a lean, strong sprinter. When her coach told her losing a few pounds would improve her performance, she immediately started counting calories and increased the duration of her workouts. She was too busy with practices and meets to notice that her period had stopped—she was more worried about the stress fracture in her ankle slowing her down.

Although Hannah thinks her intense training and disciplined diet are helping her performance; they may actually be hurting her—and her health.

What is female athlete triad?

Sports and exercise are part of a balanced, healthy lifestyle. Girls who play sports are healthier; get better grades; are less likely to experience depression; and use alcohol, cigarettes, and drugs less frequently than girls who aren't athletes. But for some girls, not balancing the needs of their bodies and their sports can have major consequences.

About This Chapter: "Female Athlete Triad," October 2006, reprinted with permission from www.kidshealth.org. Copyright © 2006 The Nemours Foundation. This information was provided by KidsHealth, one of the largest resources online for medically reviewed health information written for parents, kids, and teens. For more articles like this one, visit www.KidsHealth.org, or www.TeensHealth.org.

Some girls who play sports or exercise intensely are at risk for a problem called female athlete triad. Female athlete triad is a combination of three conditions: disordered eating, amenorrhea, and osteoporosis. A female athlete can have one, two, or all three parts of the triad.

Triad Factor #1: Disordered Eating

Most girls with female athlete triad try to lose weight primarily to improve their athletic performance. The disordered eating that accompanies female athlete triad can range from avoiding certain types of food the athlete thinks are "bad" (such as foods containing fat) to serious eating disorders like anorexia nervosa or bulimia nervosa.

Triad Factor #2: Amenorrhea

Because a girl with female athlete triad is simultaneously exercising intensely and not eating enough calories, when her weight falls too low, she may experience decreases in estrogen, the hormone that helps to regulate the menstrual cycle. As a result, a girl's periods may become irregular or stop altogether. Of course, it is normal for teen girls to occasionally miss periods, especially in their first year of having periods. A missed period does not automatically mean a girl has female athlete triad. A missed period could mean something else is going on, like pregnancy or a medical condition. If you have missed a period and you are sexually active, talk to your doctor.

Some girls who participate intensively in sports may never even get their first period because they've been training so hard. Other girls may have had periods, but once they increase their training and change their eating habits, their periods may stop.

Triad Factor #3: Osteoporosis

Low estrogen levels and poor nutrition, especially low calcium intake, can lead to osteoporosis, the third aspect of the triad. Osteoporosis is a weakening of the bones due to the loss of bone density and improper bone formation. This condition can ruin a female athlete's career because it may lead to stress fractures and other injuries.

Usually, the teen years are a time when girls should be building up their bone mass to their highest levels—called peak bone mass. Not getting enough calcium during the teen years can also have a lasting effect on how strong a girl's bones are later in life.

Who gets female athlete triad?

Most girls have concerns about the size and shape of their bodies, but girls who develop female athlete triad have certain risk factors that set them apart. Being a highly competitive athlete and participating in a sport that requires you to train extra hard is a risk factor.

Girls with female athlete triad often care so much about their sports that they would do almost anything to improve their performance. Martial arts and rowing are examples of sports that classify athletes by weight class, so focusing on weight becomes an important part of the training program and can put a girl at risk for disordered eating.

Participation in sports where a thin appearance is valued can also put a girl at risk for female athlete triad. Sports such as gymnastics, figure skating, diving, and ballet are examples of sports that value a thin, lean body shape. Some girls may even be told by coaches or judges that losing weight would improve their scores.

Even in sports where body size and shape aren't as important, such as distance running and cross-country skiing, girls may be pressured by team-mates, parents, partners, and coaches who mistakenly believe that "losing just a few pounds" could improve their performance.

The truth is, though, that losing those few pounds generally doesn't im-prove performance at all. People who are fit and active enough to compete in sports generally have more muscle than fat, so it's the muscle that gets starved when a girl cuts back on food. Plus, if a girl loses weight when she doesn't need to, it interferes with healthy body processes such as menstruation and bone development.

In addition, for some competitive female athletes, problems such as low self-esteem, a tendency toward perfectionism, and family stress place them at risk for disordered eating.

What are the signs and symptoms?

If a girl has risk factors for female athlete triad, she may already be experiencing some symptoms and signs of the disorder, such as:

- weight loss;

- no periods or irregular periods;

- fatigue and decreased ability to concentrate;

- stress fractures (fractures that occur even if a person hasn't had a significant injury);

- muscle injuries.

Girls with female athlete triad often have signs and symptoms of eating disorders, such as:

- continued dieting in spite of weight loss;

- preoccupation with food and weight;

- frequent trips to the bathroom during and after meals;

- using laxatives;

- brittle hair or nails;

- dental cavities because in girls with bulimia tooth enamel is worn away by frequent vomiting;

- sensitivity to cold;

- low heart rate and blood pressure;

- heart irregularities and chest pain.

How do doctors help?

An extensive physical examination is a crucial part of diagnosing female athlete triad. A doctor who thinks a girl has female athlete triad will probably ask questions about her periods, her nutrition and exercise habits, any medications she takes, and her feelings about her body. This is called the medical history.

Poor nutrition can also affect the body in many ways, so a doctor might order blood tests to check for anemia and other problems associated with the triad.

The doctor also will check for medical reasons why a girl may be losing weight and missing her periods. Because osteoporosis can put a girl at higher risk for bone fractures, the doctor may also request tests to measure bone density.

Doctors don't work alone to help a girl with female athlete triad. Coaches, parents, physical therapists, pediatricians and adolescent medicine specialists, nutritionists and dietitians, and mental health specialists can all work together to treat the physical and emotional problems that a girl with female athlete triad faces.

It might be tempting for a girl with female athlete triad to shrug off several months of missed periods, but getting help right away is important. In the short term, she may have muscle weakness, stress fractures, and reduced physical performance. Over the long term, she may suffer from bone weakness, long-term effects on her reproductive system, and heart problems.

A girl who is recovering from female athlete triad may work with a dietitian to help get to and maintain a healthy weight and ensure she's eating enough calories and nutrients for health and good athletic performance. Depending on how much the girl is exercising, she may have to reduce the length of her workouts. Talking to a psychologist or therapist can help a girl deal with depression, pressure from coaches or family members, or low self-esteem and can help her find ways to deal with her problems other than restricting her food intake or exercising excessively.

Some girls with female athlete triad may need to take hormones to supply their bodies with estrogen so they can get their periods started again. In such cases, birth control pills are often used to regulate the menstrual cycle. Calcium and vitamin D supplementation is also common for a girl who has suffered bone loss as the result of female athlete triad.

What if I think someone I know has it?

A girl with female athlete triad may try to hide it, but she can't just ignore the disorder and hope it goes away. She needs to get help from a doctor and other health professionals. If a friend, sister, or teammate has signs and symptoms of female athlete triad, discuss your concerns with her and encourage her to seek treatment. If she refuses to seek treatment, you may need to mention your concern to a parent, coach, teacher, or school nurse.

You may worry about being nosy when you ask questions about a friend's health, but you're not: Your concern is a sign that you're a caring friend. Lending an ear may be just what your friend needs.

✔ **Quick Tip**

Tips For Female Athletes

Here are a few tips to help teen athletes stay on top of their physical condition:

- **Keep track of your periods.** It's easy to forget when you had your last visit from Aunt Flo, so keep a calendar in your gym bag and mark down when your period starts and stops and if the bleeding is particularly heavy or light. That way, if you start missing periods, you'll know right away and you'll have accurate information to give to your doctor.

- **Don't skip meals or snacks.** Girls who are constantly on the go between school, practice, and competitions may be tempted to skip meals and snacks to save time. But eating now will improve performance later, so stock your locker or bag with quick and easy favorites such as bagels, string cheese, unsalted nuts and seeds, raw vegetables, granola bars, and fruit.

- **Visit a dietitian or nutritionist who works with teen athletes.** He or she can help you get your dietary game plan into gear and determine if you're getting enough key nutrients such as iron, calcium, and protein. And if you need supplements, a nutritionist can recommend the best choices.

- **Do it for you.** Pressure from teammates, parents, or coaches can turn a fun activity into a nightmare. If you're not enjoying your sport, make a change. Remember: It's your body and your life. You—not your coach or teammates—will have to live with any damage you do to your body now.

Chapter 8

Sudden Death In The Young Athlete: Rare And Tragic

Sudden death in the young athlete is rare, estimated at one out of 100,000 to 300,000 per year. The occurrence is approximately 12 per year in high school athletes, with a male predominance. An underlying cardiovascular disease that is usually asymptomatic and undiagnosed is responsible for most of these tragic events.

The majority of sudden deaths are due to congenital cardiac malformations. Hypertrophic cardiomyopathy (HCM) is the most common cause of sudden, unexpected cardiac death among 12–32 year olds on the athletic field. The risk of sudden death increases until the third decade of life. Unfortunately, there are usually no symptoms prior to sudden death. Diagnosis is difficult because heart-related changes due to HCM might not be present and identifiable until adolescence.

The second most common cause of sudden death is congenital coronary artery anomalies. These arteries supply blood to the heart. Sudden death may be the first sign of this condition and is usually precipitated by exercise. Approximately 25 percent may experience symptoms in the form of palpitations (heart flutter) and/or syncope (passing out).

About This Chapter: "Heart Disease in the Young Athlete," by Michele D. Pescasio, M.D. © 2007 National Center for Sports Safety (www.SportsSafety.org). All Rights Reserved.

Other causes of sudden death include:

- **Myocarditis:** An inflammation of the heart.

- **Mitral valve prolapse (MVP):** Very common. Risk factors are family history, recurrent syncopal or passing out episodes, prolonged QT interval on EKG, marked physical changes in the mitral valve and moderate-to-severe mitral regurgitation (leaky valve), and history of embolic events (throwing blood clots).

- **Wolff-Parkinson-White syndrome:** A pre-excitation syndrome where individuals are susceptible to fast, irregular heart beats.

- **Arrhythmogenic right ventricular dysplasia:** A rare muscle disorder of the right ventricle of the heart.

- **Marfan syndrome:** A disorder affecting the connective tissues, marked by abnormalities in skeletal muscle, eyes, heart, and great vessels.

- **Long QT syndrome:** Is predominantly a hereditary disorder diagnosed by EKG changes. It usually occurs in patients with a history of recurrent syncope.

♣ It's A Fact!!

Up to 450,000 Americans each year, including 7,000 children, lose their lives to sudden cardiac arrest (SCA), reports the American Heart Association (AHA). Without warning, SCA is caused by ventricular fibrillation, an abnormal heart rhythm. Young people suffer the highest incidence of SCA while playing sports. Without defibrillation (a pulse of electricity delivered to the heart) within 3–5 minutes, very few people can survive. Thanks to the availability of small, portable devices known as automated external defibrillators (AEDs), survival rates can jump from less than 5 percent to nearly 70 percent.

Because AEDs have been proven to be so successful in saving lives, The National Athletic Trainers' Association (NATA) has issued an official statement to its 30,000 members encouraging their use.

Source: Excerpted from "National Athletic Trainer's Association Cites Urgent Need for Automated External Defibrillators (AEDS) to Be Available in Secondary Schools," February 27, 2007. © National Athletic Trainers' Association (NATA). All rights reserved. Reprinted with permission.

- **Undiagnosed sudden death:** This condition requires comprehensive cardiovascular testing to exclude structural cardiac diseases that can lead to sudden death.

The athlete's personal and family history is of critical importance. Detection of some of the conditions known to cause sudden death in athletes is very difficult. Frequently, the family history is the only risk factor. Factors that would place an athlete at an increased risk for sudden death are a family history of premature death, significant health problems from cardiovascular disease in close relatives younger than 50 years of age, or if anyone in the family had these conditions. Parents should be responsible for completing the history forms for young athletes.

The personal history should include prior occurrences of chest pain on exertion, passing out during physical activity, and excessive shortness of breath or fatigue during exercise. A personal history of congenital or acquired heart disease, hypertension, murmurs, or palpitations should be noted.

The cardiovascular exam should include, but is not limited to, blood pressure measurements, listening to the heart in at least two positions (sitting/lying or sitting/standing), assessing the femoral artery, and recognizing the physical signs of Marfan syndrome.

The American Heart Association recommends that both a history and a physical exam be performed before participation in organized high school and collegiate sports. It is also recommended that athletic screening be performed by a healthcare worker with the requisite training, medical skills, and background to reliably obtain a detailed cardiovascular history, perform a physical examination, and recognize heart disease. When cardiovascular abnormalities are identified or suspected, the athlete should be referred to a cardiovascular specialist for further evaluation or confirmation.

Finally, despite all of the precautions to prevent sudden cardiac death in young athletes, there are limitations to preparticipation screening. Due to the rarity of these conditions, mass screening is neither practical nor cost-effective. In conclusion, it is virtually impossible to achieve a zero-risk circumstance in competitive sports.

♣ It's A Fact!!
Commotio Cordis—A Blunt Force Injury To The Heart

Since 1998, over 130 athletes have died from commotio cordis, reports the U.S. Commotio Cordis Registry. A medical term for a rare disruption of the heart's electrical system, commotio cordis is caused by a blow to the chest directly over the heart, which occurs between heart contractions, leading to sudden cardiac arrest. It most often occurs in healthy young athletes, due to the pliability of their chest walls.

The National Athletic Trainers' Association (NATA)'s which addresses issues specific to youth and senior athletes, recommends doing the following:

- Encourage all coaches and officials to become trained in cardiopulmonary resuscitation (CPR), automatic external defibrillator (AED) use, and first aid.

- Establish an emergency action plan at all athletic venues. Parents, coaches, officials should be involved in these plans. (NATA's Position Statement on Emergency Planning in Athletics is a useful resource: http://www.nata.org/publicinformation/files/emergencyplanning.pdf). It's important that a certified athletic trainer or other emergency medical professional is on-site in the event of injury.

- Use all-purpose sports chest protectors during practices and games.

- Ensure all protective equipment fits properly and is used as intended by the manufacturer.

- Teach athletes how to protect themselves against chest injuries. Coaches should work with athletes to ensure proper playing and position techniques.

- Maintain an even and clean playing surface.

To view the official statement, please visit www.nata.org/publicinformation/files/ASTFstmt.pdf.

Chapter 9

Facts About Sports Nutrition

Winning Nutrition For Athletes

Whether it's playing football, swimming, or jogging, athletes need to eat a nutritious, balanced diet to fuel their body. Good nutrition, like any sporting event, has basic ground rules. Following these rules and getting plenty of practice will help athletes feel great and score those winning points!

What diet is best for athletes?

All athletes need a diet that provides enough energy in the form of carbohydrates and fats as well as essential protein, vitamins, and minerals. This means a diet containing 55–60 percent of calories from carbohydrates (10 to 15 percent from sugars and the rest from starches), no more than 30 percent of calories from fat, and the remaining (about 10–15 percent) from protein.

That translates into eating a variety of foods every day—grains, vegetables, fruits, beans, lean meats, and low fat dairy products. The base of the diet should come from carbohydrates in the form of starches and sugars. Fluids, especially water, are also important to the winning combination. Dehydration can stop even the finest athlete from playing his or her best game.

About This Chapter: This chapter includes "Winning Nutrition for Athletes," and "Fast Facts about Sports Nutrition." Both are undated documents produced by the President's Council on Physical Fitness and Sports (http://www.fitness.gov), accessed July 2007.

Are carbohydrates important for athletes?

When starches or sugars are eaten, the body changes them all to glucose, the only form of carbohydrate used directly by muscles for energy. Whether carbohydrates are in the form of starches (in vegetables and grains), sucrose (table sugar), fructose (found in fruits and juices), or lactose (milk sugar), carbohydrates are digested and ultimately changed to glucose.

The body uses this glucose in the blood for energy. Most glucose is stored as glycogen in the liver and muscles. During exercise glycogen is broken down in the muscles and provides energy. Usually there is enough glycogen in muscles to provide fuel for 90–120 minutes of exercise.

Most exercise and sport games do not use up glycogen stores so eating carbohydrates during the activity usually isn't needed. But for some athletes, eating or drinking carbohydrates during exercise helps maintain their blood glucose and energy levels.

Most athletes need not be concerned with "carbohydrate loading," the special technique of eating a lot of carbohydrates for several days before an endurance event. Instead, focus on getting enough carbohydrates everyday.

♣ It's A Fact!!
Do athletes need extra protein or
protein supplements to build muscles?

No. Muscles develop from training and exercise. A certain amount of protein is needed to help build the muscles but a nutritious, balanced diet that includes two or three servings from the meat/bean/egg group (6–7 ounces total) and two to three servings of dairy daily will supply all of the protein that the muscles need.

Extra servings of protein in foods or protein supplements do not assist in muscle development. Unlike carbohydrates, protein cannot be stored in the body and any excess will be burned for energy or stored as body fat.

Source: "Winning Nutrition for Athletes," President's Council on Physical Fitness and Sports.

The best way to ensure plenty of energy for exercise is to eat a nutritious, balanced diet that is high in carbohydrates and low in fat with lots of different foods.

What should an athlete eat before, during, and after exercise?

The most important thing is to concentrate on eating a nutritious, balanced diet every day. This provides plenty of energy to grow and exercise. Here are a few tips about eating before, during, and after exercise.

Before

- Have some high carbohydrate foods like bananas, bagels, or fruit juices. These foods are broken down quickly and provide glucose to the muscles.

- The timing of this meal depends on athletes' preference for eating before exercise, but researchers have found that eating something from one to four hours before exercise helps keep plenty of blood glucose available for working muscles.

- It is also critical to drink plenty of cool water before exercise to keep muscles hydrated.

During

- Perspiration and exertion deplete the body of fluids necessary for an optimal performance and lead to dehydration. It is important to drink plenty of cool water, at least a half a cup of water every 20 minutes of exercise. Adding a teaspoon of sugar, a little fruit juice, or a small amount of powdered drink mix flavors plain water and may encourage fluid intake.

- Usually there is no need to worry about replacing carbohydrates unless the exercise lasts over 90 minutes and is hard and continuous. When this happens, drinking a sports drink or other beverage with some sugar in it will fuel and water to the muscles being exercised.

- Make a homemade sports drink by mixing no more than 4 teaspoon of sugar, ¼ teaspoon of salt, and some flavoring (like a teaspoon of lemon juice) in 8 ounces of water.

After

If the exercise was strenuous and lasted a long time, glycogen stores may need refueling. Consuming foods and beverages high in carbohydrates right after exercise will replenish glycogen stores if they are low after exercising.

No matter the intensity of the exercise, it's important to drink plenty of water and eat a nutritious, balanced meal that has lots of carbohydrate rich foods such as grains, pastas, potatoes, vegetables and fruits. A teaspoon of sugar, at only 15 calories per teaspoon, adds flavor to these foods and may increase taste appeal.

More Facts About Sports Nutrition

Water, Water Everywhere

You can survive for a month without food, but only a few days without water.

- Water is the most important nutrient for active people.

- When you sweat, you lose water, which must be replaced. Drink fluids before, during, and after workouts.

- Water is a fine choice for most workouts. However, during continuous workouts of greater than 90 minutes, your body may benefit from a sports drink.

- Sports drinks have two very important ingredients—electrolytes and carbohydrates.

- Sports drinks replace electrolytes lost through sweat during workouts lasting several hours.

- Carbohydrates in sports drinks provide extra energy. The most effective sports drinks contain 15 to 18 grams of carbohydrate in every 8 ounces of fluid.

Rev Up Your Engine With Carbohydrates

Carbohydrates are your body's main source of energy.

- Carbohydrates are sugars and starches, and they are found in foods such as breads, cereals, fruits, vegetables, pasta, milk, honey, syrups, and table sugar.

- Sugars and starches are broken down by your body into glucose, which is used by your muscles for energy.

- For health and peak performance, more than half your daily calories should come from carbohydrates.

- Sugars and starches have 4 calories per gram, while fat has 9 calories per gram. In other words, carbohydrates have less than half the calories of fat.

- If you regularly eat a carbohydrate-rich diet you probably have enough carbohydrate stored to fuel activity. Even so, be sure to eat a pre-competition meal for fluid and additional energy. What you eat as well as when you eat your pre-competition meal will be entirely individual.

Score With Vitamins And Minerals

Eating a varied diet will give you all the vitamins and minerals you need for health and peak performance.

- Exceptions include active people who follow strict vegetarian diets, avoid an entire group of foods, or eat less than 1800 calories a day. If you fall into any of these categories, a multivitamin and mineral pill may provide the vitamins and minerals missing in your diet.

♣ **It's A Fact!!**
Flexing Your Options To Build Bigger Muscles

It is a myth that eating lots of protein or taking protein supplements and exercising vigorously will definitely turn you into a big, muscular person.

- Building muscle depends on your genes, how hard you train, and whether you get enough calories.

- The average American diet has more than enough protein for muscle building. Extra protein is eliminated from the body or stored as fat.

Source: "Fast Facts About Sports Nutrition," President's Council on Physical Fitness and Sports.

- Taking large doses of vitamins and minerals will not help your perfor-mance and may be bad for your health. Vitamins and minerals do not supply the body with energy; and, therefore, are not a substitute for carbohydrates.

Popeye And All That Spinach

Iron supplies working muscles with oxygen.

- If your iron level is low, you may tire easily and not have enough stamina for activity.

- The best sources of iron are animal products, but plant foods such as fortified breads, cereals, beans, and green leafy vegetables also contain iron.

- Iron supplements may have side effects, so take them only if your doc-tor tells you to.

No Bones About It, You Need Calcium Everyday

Many people do not get enough of the calcium needed for strong bones and proper muscle function.

- Lack of calcium can contribute to stress fractures and the bone dis-ease, osteoporosis.

- The best sources of calcium are dairy products, but many other foods such as salmon with bones, sardines, collard greens, and okra also con-tain calcium. Additionally, some brands of bread, tofu, and orange juice are fortified with calcium.

A Weighty Matter

Your calorie needs depend on your age, body size, sport, and training program.

- The best way to make sure you are not getting too many or too few calories is to check your weight from time to time.

- If you're keeping within your ideal weight range, you're probably get-ting the right amount of calories.

Chapter 10

Sports Drinks, Carbohydrate Gels, And Energy Bars

Staying Active Pays Off!

Those who are physically active tend to live longer, healthier lives. Research shows that even moderate physical activity—such as 30 minutes a day of brisk walking—significantly contributes to longevity. A physically active person with such risk factors as high blood pressure, diabetes, or even a smoking habit can get real benefits from regular physical activity as part of daily life.

As many dieters have found, exercise can help you stay on a diet and lose weight. What's more, regular exercise can help lower blood pressure, control blood sugar, improve cholesterol levels, and build stronger, denser bones.

The First Step

Before you begin an exercise program, take a fitness test, or substantially increase your level of activity, make sure to answer the following questions. This physical activity readiness questionnaire (PAR-Q) will help determine your suitability for beginning an exercise routine or program.

About This Chapter: "Selecting and Effectively Using Sports Drinks, Carbohydrate Gels, and Energy Bars," reprinted with permission of the American College of Sports Medicine. Copyright © 2005 American College of Sports Medicine. This brochure is a product of ACSM's Consumer Products Committee.

- Has your doctor ever said that you have a heart condition or that you should participate in physical activity only as recommended by a doctor?

- Do you feel pain in your chest during physical activity?

- In the past month, have you had chest pain when you were not doing physical activity?

- Do you lose your balance because of dizziness? Do you ever lose consciousness?

- Do you have a bone or joint problem that could be made worse by a change in your physical activity?

- Is your doctor currently prescribing drugs for your blood pressure or a heart condition?

- Do you know of any reason you should not participate in physical activity?

If you answered yes to one or more questions, if you are over 40 years of age and have been inactive, or if you are concerned about your health, consult a physician before taking a fitness test or substantially increasing your physical activity. If you answered no to each question, then it's likely that you can safely begin fitness testing and training.

Selecting And Effectively Using Sports Drinks, Gels, And Bars

Fatigue Factors

Depending upon the length of your workout or competition, performance, and endurance are primarily limited by three factors:

- **Loss of body fluids:** According to a large body of research, losing more than two percent of your weight as sweat during prolonged exercise or sports activities can hamper performance.

- **Drop in the levels of blood sugar:** Your brain uses a steady supply of sugar in the blood (blood glucose) for fuel. During exercise or sports performance, you drain glucose levels in your blood. This can give you a lightheaded, sometimes woozy feeling.

- **Depletion of muscle carbohydrate stores:** As you exercise, muscles also use stored carbohydrate (glycogen) as fuel. Depending upon the intensity and duration of your workout or sports participation, your muscles can also lose carbohydrate.

Sports Drinks

Mixtures of water and carbohydrate, sports drinks make an excellent fueling and hydration choice. Years of research clearly shows that for exercise lasting anywhere from 60 minutes to several hours, drinking these carbohydrate beverages significantly boosts endurance performance compared to drinking plain water. According to some research, you can expect an improvement in endurance of about a 20 percent or more in workouts lasting over 90 minutes.

Most sports drinks offer a blend of carbohydrate sources such as the sugars sucrose, glucose, fructose, and galactose. A few beverages may also add maltodextrin, a complex carbohydrate made of several glucose units. Some research suggests that sports drinks that offer a blend of carbohydrates such as glucose and sucrose, rather than a single carbohydrate source, may improve the amount of carbohydrate that eventually gets to the muscles as fuel. By offering your intestinal tract different sugars, the rate of carbohydrate absorption is improved since different sugars are absorbed by different routes. This, in turn, means more "carbs" make it to your muscles as fuel for exercise or sports performance.

Sports drinks also come with added electrolytes. Sodium, the electrolyte lost in the greatest amount in your sweat, helps maintain fluid balance in the body and also promotes the uptake of fluid in your intestines and improves hydration.

What to look for and how to use: Most commercial sports drinks supply a blend of sugars at the right amount: four to nine percent solution or about 13 to 19 grams of carbs per eight ounces. Drinking one and a half to four cups per hour (more if you have heavy sweat losses) will provide you with both the fluid and carbs you need for endurance. Choose a beverage flavor you enjoy as this may encourage you to drink more. "Fitness waters," while tasty, don't provide enough carbohydrate to boost endurance but certainly can keep you hydrated. Drinking prior to exercise and after exercise are also important factors in maintaining proper hydration levels.

Carbohydrate Gels

Pudding-like in texture, carbohydrate gels come in small, single-serve packets much like a sample of shampoo, making them portable fuel that you can easily put in your waistband pocket. Simply tear off the packet top at the perforation and squeeze the gel into your mouth—easily done on the run.

Gels consist of sugars and maltodextrins (the same as sports drinks but without the water), which are easily digested. Many gels come with added electrolytes that, as with sports drinks, help maintain fluid balance. Some gels also have added extras such as ginseng and other herbs, amino acids, vitamins, and co-enzyme-Q10 (a nonessential substance found in the body). Research does not support that these ingredients have any performance benefit, but they probably are present in amounts that are too small to present any risk.

Some gels also contain caffeine in varying amounts. Check the label and consult the manufacturer's website for specific content as some gels have as much caffeine as a half cup of coffee, which may cause nervousness in those not accustom to this stimulant.

What to look for and how to use: Most carb gel packs contain 100 calories or 25 grams of carbohydrate. Try to consume one to three packets for every hour of exercise depending on the intensity and duration. Since gels come in a variety of flavors, from vanilla and chocolate to sonic strawberry and cherry bomb, find one or two you enjoy and remember to swallow them down with about 4 to 8 ounces of water.

Energy Bars

Many types of energy bars are now available. From high protein bars to those that are marketed specifically for women, the energy bar scene is anything but simple. Some label reading is a must when it comes to choosing the right bar for fueling. High-carbohydrate bars make great choices for carbohydrate fueling both before and during a long workout. These bars typically provide about 70 percent of their calories from carbohydrate as sugars (brown rice syrup, sucrose) and grains (oats and rice crisps).

How quickly these carbohydrates get into the circulation is referred to as the glycemic index. Eating a high glycemic index bar means rapid release of carbohydrate into the blood stream, giving the muscles a quick "shot" of fuel, which is ideal during a workout. Eating a low glycemic index bar results in a slower release of sugar into the circulation and thus, sustained energy, which is best before exercise.

Many bar manufactures claim that their profile of carbohydrates sources (such as oats and other complex carbohydrates) are best for a sustained and lasting release of carbohydrate fuel into the circulation. It's true that carbohydrates are digested and appear in the circulation at different rates. Predicting the glycemic index of a bar based on its ingredients is challenging, as carbohydrate types digest at different rates and the protein and fat content of the bar also affect absorption. Most bars have high glycemic index despite their use of various grains and other complex carbohydrates as major ingredients.

What to look for and how to use: Select a bar with about 25–40 grams of carbohydrate and less than 15 grams of protein, which is not a crucial fuel source during exercise. Also, check the label for fat content as some bars can pack a hefty dose, which slows digestion and is not helpful during exercise or sports. Eat one bar about an hour prior to a long workout, and if you're exercising for more than an hour eat one high-carb bar per hour of exercise along with ample water.

Fruits (Orange Slices, Bananas, Dried Fruit)

"Real food" can also be used for fueling a workout. Fruit, whether dried or fresh, supplies a shot of carbohydrate that is well digested. Dried fruit is easily transported, can withstand extreme weather conditions, and is durable enough to survive some shaking and jarring.

What to look for and how to use: Most fruits provide about 15 grams of carbohydrate per serving—about the size of a tennis ball. A serving of dried fruit equals about ¼ cup or the equivalent of dried fresh fruit (two nectarine halves, or four dried plums). Aim for one to two servings before a workout and two to three fruit servings every hour of running. Be sure to consume with ample water to stay hydrated.

✤ It's A Fact!!
A Complete Physical Activity Program

A rounded program of physical activity includes aerobic exercise, strength training exercise, and flexibility training—but not necessarily in the same session. Create a pattern that you'll stick to and that fits into your schedule. Commitment to regular physical activity is more important than the intensity of the workouts. Choose exercises you are likely to enjoy. ACSM's Position Stand "The Recommended Quantity and Quality of Exercise for… Healthy Adults" ©1998 states that aerobic training should be performed three to five days per week for a minimum of 20 minutes per day. Remember, it's better to exercise for a shorter period of time than not at all. Typical aerobic exercises include walking and running (or treadmills), stair climbing, cycling on a stationary or moving bike, rowing, cross-country skiing, and swimming. Many devices offer a combination of these motions. Generally, strength training should be done two to three times per week, using flexible rubber resistance, free weights, or weight machines. For general training, do two to three upper-body and lower-body exercises. Abdominal exercises are an important part of strength training. Flexibility training is important and frequently neglected, resulting in increased tightness as we age and become less active. Stretch with sustained gradual movements lasting at least 15 seconds per stretch. At a minimum, try to stretch everyday.

Chapter 11

Fitness As A Way Of Life

What Is Being "Fit"?

We would all like to be physically fit, but how many of us know what "fit" really means? Does playing softball twice a week make us fit? Or swimming at the neighborhood pool? Or walking to and from work? What amount of activity is enough to keep us fit? Do we all need to follow the same fitness program or are we all different?

Physical therapists answer these kinds of questions all the time. Realizing that each individual is unique, physical therapists have developed specific methods to determine how fit you are and what types of activities promote your optimum level of fitness.

While each individual is unique, physical therapists support the Surgeon General's statement that everyone may substantially improve their health and quality of life by doing moderate-intensity physical exercise for at least 30 minutes every day. Physical therapists encourage people of all ages to begin a program of daily regular exercise to help prevent cardiovascular disease and musculoskeletal disorders.

About This Chapter: "Fitness: A Way of Life," reprinted from http://www.apta.org with permission of the American Physical Therapy Association, © 2007.

Physical therapists are uniquely qualified to develop personalized conditioning programs that, if followed properly, will help prevent injury and promote fitness. Physical therapists would be the first to say they would rather see you before you embark on a fitness program than after you have sustained a painful injury.

This information is designed to increase your understanding of fitness from a total body perspective—the approach used by physical therapists. Total fitness is achieved by matching your body and lifestyle to a fitness program that you will enjoy, a fitness program that can become a way of life.

✎ What's It Mean?

Fitness: Fitness as defined by physical therapists is an ongoing state of health whereby all systems of the body are conditioned to withstand physical stress and are able to perform at an optimum level without injury. A person who is physically fit has a properly aligned body structure, flexible and strong muscles, an efficient heart and healthy lungs, a good ratio of body fat to lean body mass, and good balance.

Note that the above definition does not say, "A person who is fit can run X amount of miles in X minutes." Being fit is just that—a state of being. What activities you choose to perform to achieve and maintain a state of fitness are really up to you!

And, as an added bonus, physical fitness also contributes to mental fitness. There's nothing like being in tip-top shape to give you a positive outlook on life.

Six Elements Of Fitness

The American Physical Therapy Association wants you to understand the total body approach to fitness by looking at the six elements of fitness:

1. Aerobic Capacity
2. Body Structure
3. Body Composition
4. Body Balance
5. Muscular Flexibility
6. Muscular Strength

We'll now look at each of these elements from the physical therapist's perspective, see how a therapist evaluates your body in terms of these elements, and find out how that evaluation can help you achieve overall fitness.

Aerobic Capacity

Aerobic capacity is an index of your cardiovascular system's ability to transport oxygen to working muscles, where the oxygen is used as fuel to produce energy for movement.

You can improve your aerobic capacity by achieving what is called an aerobic response. Although the level necessary to achieve an aerobic response varies with each individual, it is usually reached by exercising at 60 to 80 percent of your maximum heart rate. This ideal rate for exercise (60–80 percent of maximum) is called your target heart rate. Exercising at your target heart rate should be maintained for 20 to 30 minutes and occur at least three times a week for you to attain aerobic fitness.

There are many different types of activities that can generate an aerobic response. Walking can be an excellent activity that is a particularly good aerobic exercise. Some other aerobic activities include jumping rope, swimming, running, cross-country skiing, hiking, aerobic dancing, and bicycling.

Target Heart Rate: To estimate your target heart rate, you must first determine your maximum heart rate. This is done by subtracting your age from 220. If a check-up by your physician indicates no problems, your target heart rate is 60 to 80 percent of your maximum rate. For example: If you are 20 years old, your maximum heart rate is 200. Your target heart rate is 60 to 80 percent of 200, or 120 to 160 beats per minute.

You can monitor your target heart rate by finding your pulse—either lay your fingertips on the palm side of your wrist or lightly against the side of your voice box—and count the pulse for 15 seconds; then multiply this number by four to get your pulse rate in beats per minute.

As you continue to exercise regularly, you will find that it takes more effort to reach your target heart rate. This is a good sign and means that your heart and lungs are getting stronger and that your aerobic capacity is improving.

Resting Heart Rate: Another clear indicator of improved aerobic fitness is your resting heart rate. Take your pulse first thing in the morning, while you are still lying in bed. As your aerobic fitness level improves, your resting heart rate should decrease. This occurs because as your heart becomes a better pump, it can pump more blood with each beat, supplying your muscles with more of the oxygen they need. (Resting heart rates rarely go below 50 beats per minute and are usually between 60 to 100 beats per minute.)

Body Structure

A physical therapist evaluates your body structure by looking for structural malalignments in upper and lower extremities (arms and legs), the head, neck, and trunk. The therapist will check your overall posture by looking at your head, neck, shoulders, spine, pelvis, knees, and feet, from front, side, and back views.

Even a small imbalance in the way you stand—too much weight on one foot, your shoulders "slouched" forward—may lead to pain and injury when you start exercising. If any problems are identified in the evaluation, the physical therapist may give you some exercises to strengthen weak muscles or improve the flexibility of tight muscles, teach you to become more aware of your posture while standing and walking, or recommend specific footwear.

Body Composition

Body composition is the ratio of body fat to lean body mass (bones and muscles). You cannot determine your body composition simply by weighing yourself on a standard scale. In fact, body composition measurements tend to be a much better indicator of your current fitness level than your body weight. Some people who weigh a lot are not fat; they just may be muscular and muscles weigh more than fat. Conversely, a person who maintains a seemingly "ideal" weight may actually be carrying too much fat.

Your physical therapist can determine your body composition by taking fat measurements at various places on your body. Although ideal body fat levels vary with each individual, it is generally accepted that the ideal range of body fat is approximately 10 to 15 percent of total body mass for males and 15 to 22 percent for females; seasoned athletes often have much less. It is at the ideal fat-to-lean ratio that your body is its most efficient. An excessive fat-to-lean body composition puts unnecessary weight on your skeletal structure during exercise without helping you perform your task. Muscles at least work for you; fat just weights you down. (On the other hand, insufficient body fat isn't good for your health either and is common among some athletes and adolescents.)

Body Balance

A physical therapist will check your balance by having you stand, with your eyes closed, on one leg for a brief period of time, then on the other. Although this seems a simple test, it may indicate if you have a neurological (nervous system) problem. Neurological testing evaluates the balance controlled by your brain.

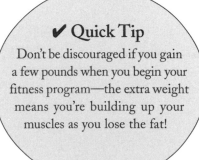

✔ **Quick Tip**

Don't be discouraged if you gain a few pounds when you begin your fitness program—the extra weight means you're building up your muscles as you lose the fat!

Even a minor balance problem may place you at risk for possible injury. If a problem is identified, your therapist may give you some exercise tips that will help to improve your balance.

Muscular Flexibility

Your muscles should be flexible to allow for the full range of motion required by life's many activities, such as stretching, lifting, reaching, and bending. Muscles should be able to lengthen without too much effort, allowing your body and limbs to move efficiently in many different ways.

Just as muscles can be stretched, due to their elastic nature, they can also become shortened when adapting to long periods of inactivity. A shortened or inflexible muscle may be more susceptible to stress and injury.

A physical therapist can determine your flexibility by measuring how far you can move your arms, legs, and torso. The therapist will notice if you have any specific areas of "tightness" and will suggest some gentle exercises to increase flexibility.

Muscular Strength

In addition to being flexible, your muscles should be able to exert force and control movement. For example, flexible muscles will help you bend over to pick up a box, but it's your muscular strength that enables you to lift it.

The physical therapist will determine the strength of your major muscle groups by having you perform weight-resistance exercises and tests.

If your muscles need strengthening, you may embark on a strength-training program designed by your therapist. Usually these exercises do not require heavy lifting or strenuous exercise. You may only need to work with hand weights to strengthen one arm or do strengthening exercises to bring muscles on one side of your body in balance with the other.

Strengthening exercises should condition those muscles that will be used to perform the activity of your choice. If you want to be a long-distance runner, you should condition your leg muscles to withstand stress for long periods of time.

Additional Factors That Affect Fitness

It is important to be aware of, and tell your physical therapist about, any aspects of your lifestyle that may be considered risk factors to your fitness.

Do you:

- Smoke cigarettes?
- Eat "junk" food regularly?
- Take stimulants (drugs, caffeine, even vitamins)?
- Drink alcohol excessively?
- Have a stressful job?
- Feel depressed, lack motivation?
- Have a family health history that includes heart disease, diabetes, or high blood pressure?

Although some of these factors may seem unrelated to your fitness, they may have an effect on your general state of well-being, and may pose risks that should be considered when developing your fitness program.

Starting Your Fitness Way Of Life

1. Decide what sports and activities you most enjoy. Do you play tennis? Swim? Jog? Do you enjoy walking? Make a list of your favorite activities, then list next to these activities a time when you feel you could perform them during an average week.

2. Consult a physical therapist who specializes in sports and orthopaedic physical therapy. To find an appropriate physical therapist near you, look in the yellow pages of your phone book, ask your physician or local hospital, or contact the local chapter of the American Physical Therapy Association. You'll be surprised how many physical therapists are ready to serve you right in your own area.

3. Ask your physical therapist to give you a fitness evaluation. This will determine your present level of fitness, based on the six elements of fitness as described in this chapter. The therapist will check your aerobic capacity, body structure, body composition, body balance, muscular flexibility, and muscular strength. The therapist will tell you what you need to do to improve your present condition.

4. Share the list you developed in Step 1 with your physical therapist. Together, you can choose activities for a balanced fitness program. Your choices should be based on your favorite activities and lifestyle, and on how much time during each week you want to commit to being fit.

♣ **It's A Fact!!**

Fitness For People With Disabilities

There are many ways in which a physical therapist can tailor-make a fitness program for people with disabilities.

The goal of anyone involved in a fitness program is to be at a level appropriate for his or her unique capacity. Your physical therapist is eager to help you meet your challenge and benefit from a fitness program that will keep you fit for life.

5. Begin your fitness program, monitoring your progress based on the suggestions in this chapter, and the advice of your physical therapist. If you suffer an injury, no matter how minor you think it is, tell your physical therapist. It may be helpful in deciding what activities are best for you.

6. Although you may emphasize one area of conditioning as you develop your individualized fitness program, remember that total fitness requires a total body approach. Balance your program with activities that concentrate on the six elements of fitness: aerobic capacity, body structure, body composition, body balance, muscular flexibility, and muscular strength.

Achieving and maintaining fitness is a lifelong commitment. Perhaps you are currently active in sports; but what will you be doing 20 years from now? Your state of fitness need not lessen with age. Just because you may become less active as you grow older, you needn't resign yourself to being less fit.

As you become comfortable with your fitness program—enjoy yourself! Notice how much better you move, breathe and feel. You were meant to be fit! It's just a matter of knowing where to start, and how to get to where you want to be. Remember—fitness is a way of life!

Part Two

Diagnosing And Treating Sports Injuries

Chapter 12

What Are Sports Injuries?

In recent years, increasing numbers of people of all ages have been heeding their health professionals' advice to get active for all of the health benefits exercise has to offer. But for some people—particularly those who overdo or who don't properly train or warm up—these benefits can come at a price: sports injuries.

Fortunately, most sports injuries can be treated effectively, and most people who suffer injuries can return to a satisfying level of physical activity after an injury. Even better, many sports injuries can be prevented if people take the proper precautions.

What are sports injuries?

The term sports injury, in the broadest sense, refers to the kinds of injuries that most commonly occur during sports or exercise. Some sports injuries result from accidents; others are due to poor training practices, improper equipment, lack of conditioning, or insufficient warmup and stretching.

Although virtually any part of your body can be injured during sports or exercise, the term is usually reserved for injuries that involve the musculoskeletal system, which includes the muscles, bones, and associated tissues

About This Chapter: This chapter includes excerpts from "Handout on Health: Sports Injuries," National Institute of Arthritis and Musculoskeletal and Skin Diseases, NIH Pub. 04-5278, April 2004.

> ### ♣ It's A Fact!!
> While playing sports can improve children's fitness, self-esteem, coordination, and self-discipline, it can also put them at risk for sports injuries: some minor, some serious, and still others that may result in lifelong medical problems.
>
> Young athletes are not small adults. Their bones, muscles, tendons, and ligaments are still growing and that makes them more prone to injury. Growth plates—the areas of developing cartilage where bone growth occurs in growing children—are weaker than the nearby ligaments and tendons. As a result, what is often a bruise or sprain in an adult can be a potentially serious growth-plate injury in a child. Also, a trauma that would tear a muscle or ligament in an adult would be far more likely to break a child's bone.

like cartilage. Traumatic brain and spinal cord injuries, (relatively rare during sports or exercise) and bruises are considered briefly. Following are some of the most common sports injuries.

Sprains And Strains: A sprain is a stretch or tear of a ligament, the band of connective tissues that joins the end of one bone with another. Sprains are caused by trauma such as a fall or blow to the body that knocks a joint out of position and, in the worst case, ruptures the supporting ligaments. Sprains can range from first degree (minimally stretched ligament) to third degree (a complete tear). Areas of the body most vulnerable to sprains are ankles, knees, and wrists. Signs of a sprain include varying degrees of tenderness or pain; bruising; inflammation; swelling; inability to move a limb or joint; or joint looseness, laxity, or instability.

A strain is a twist, pull, or tear of a muscle or tendon, a cord of tissue connecting muscle to bone. It is an acute, noncontact injury that results from overstretching or overcontraction. Symptoms of a strain include pain, muscle spasm, and loss of strength. While it's hard to tell the difference between mild and moderate strains, severe strains not treated professionally can cause damage and loss of function.

Knee Injuries: Because of its complex structure and weight-bearing capacity, the knee is the most commonly injured joint. Each year, more than 5.5 million people visit orthopaedic surgeons for knee problems.

Knee injuries can range from mild to severe. Some of the less severe, yet still painful and functionally limiting, knee problems are runner's knee (pain or tenderness close to or under the knee cap at the front or side of the knee), iliotibial band syndrome (pain on the outer side of the knee), and tendonitis, also called tendinosis (marked by degeneration within a tendon, usually where it joins the bone).

More severe injuries include bone bruises or damage to the cartilage or ligaments. There are two types of cartilage in the knee. One is the meniscus, a crescent-shaped disc that absorbs shock between the thigh (femur) and lower leg bones (tibia and fibula). The other is a surface-coating (or articular) cartilage. It covers the ends of the bones where they meet, allowing them to glide against one another. The four major ligaments that support the knee are the anterior cruciate ligament (ACL), the posterior cruciate ligament (PCL), the medial collateral ligament (MCL), and the lateral collateral ligament (LCL).

Knee injuries can result from a blow to or twist of the knee; from improper landing after a jump; or from running too hard, too much, or without proper warmup.

Compartment Syndrome: In many parts of the body, muscles (along with the nerves and blood vessels that run alongside and through them) are enclosed in a "compartment" formed of a tough membrane called fascia. When muscles become swollen, they can fill the compartment to capacity, causing interference with nerves and blood vessels as well as damage to the muscles themselves. The resulting painful condition is referred to as compartment syndrome.

Compartment syndrome may be caused by a one-time traumatic injury (acute compartment syndrome), such as a fractured bone or a hard blow to the thigh, by repeated hard blows (depending upon the sport), or by ongoing overuse (chronic exertional compartment syndrome), which may occur, for example, in long-distance running.

Shin Splints: While the term "shin splints" has been widely used to describe any sort of leg pain associated with exercise, the term actually refers to pain along the tibia or shin bone, the large bone in the front of the lower leg. This pain can occur at the front outside part of the lower leg, including the foot and ankle (anterior shin splints) or at the inner edge of the bone where it meets the calf muscles (medial shin splints).

Shin splints are primarily seen in runners, particularly those just starting a running program. Risk factors for shin splints include overuse or incorrect use of the lower leg; improper stretching, warmup, or exercise technique; overtraining; running or jumping on hard surfaces; and running in shoes that don't have enough support. These injuries are often associated with flat (overpronated) feet.

Achilles Tendon Injuries: A stretch, tear, or irritation to the tendon connecting the calf muscle to the back of the heel, Achilles tendon injuries can be so sudden and agonizing that they have been known to bring down charging professional football players in shocking fashion.

The most common cause of Achilles tendon tears is a problem called tendinitis, a degenerative condition caused by aging or overuse. When a tendon is weakened, trauma can cause it to rupture.

Achilles tendon injuries are common in middle-aged "weekend warriors" who may not exercise regularly or take time to stretch properly before an activity. Among professional athletes, most Achilles injuries seem to occur in quick-acceleration, jumping sports like football and basketball, and almost always end the season's competition for the athlete.

Fractures: A fracture is a break in the bone that can occur from either a quick, one-time injury to the bone (acute fracture) or from repeated stress to the bone over time (stress fracture).

- *Acute fractures:* Acute fractures can be simple (a clean break with little damage to the surrounding tissue) or compound (a break in which the bone pierces the skin with little damage to the surrounding tissue). Most acute fractures are emergencies. One that breaks the skin is especially dangerous because there is a high risk of infection.

- *Stress fractures:* Stress fractures occur largely in the feet and legs and are common in sports that require repetitive impact, primarily running/ jumping sports such as gymnastics or track and field. Running creates forces two to three times a person's body weight on the lower limbs.

The most common symptom of a stress fracture is pain at the site that worsens with weight-bearing activity. Tenderness and swelling often accompany the pain.

Dislocations: When the two bones that come together to form a joint become separated, the joint is described as being dislocated. Contact sports such as football and basketball, as well as high-impact sports and sports that can result in excessive stretching or falling, cause the majority of dislocations. A dislocated joint is an emergency situation that requires medical treatment.

The joints most likely to be dislocated are some of the hand joints. Aside from these joints, the joint most frequently dislocated is the shoulder. Dislocations of the knees, hips, and elbows are uncommon.

Traumatic Brain And Spinal Cord Injuries: Traumatic brain injury (TBI) occurs when a sudden physical assault on the head causes damage to the brain. A closed injury occurs when the head suddenly and violently hits an object, but the object does not break through the skull. A penetrating injury occurs when an object pierces the skull and enters the brain tissue.

Several types of traumatic injuries can affect the head and brain. A skull fracture occurs when the bone of the skull cracks or breaks. A depressed skull fracture occurs when pieces of the broken skull press into the tissue of the brain. This can cause bruising of the brain tissue, called a contusion. A contusion can also occur in response to shaking of the brain within the confines of the skull. Damage to a major blood vessel within the head can cause a hematoma, or heavy bleeding into or around the brain. The severity of a TBI can range from a mild concussion to the extremes of coma or even death.

Spinal cord injury (SCI) occurs when a traumatic event results in damage to cells in the spinal cord or severs the nerve tracts that relay signals up and down the spinal cord. The most common types of SCI include contusion (bruising of the spinal cord) and compression (caused by pressure on the spinal cord). Other types include lacerations (severing or tearing of nerve fibers) and central cord syndrome (specific damage to the cervical region of the spinal cord).

Bruises: A bruise, or muscle contusion, can result from a fall or from contact with a hard surface, a piece of equipment, or another player while participating in sports. A bruise results when muscle fiber and connective tissue are crushed; torn blood vessels may cause a bluish appearance. Most bruises are minor, but some can cause more extensive damage and complications.

What's the difference between acute and chronic injuries?

Regardless of the specific structure affected, sports injuries can generally be classified in one of two ways: acute or chronic.

Acute Injuries: Acute injuries, such as a sprained ankle, strained back, or fractured hand, occur suddenly during activity. Signs of an acute injury include the following:

- Sudden, severe pain

- Swelling

- Inability to place weight on a lower limb

- Extreme tenderness in an upper limb

- Inability to move a joint through its full range of motion

- Extreme limb weakness

- Visible dislocation or break of a bone

♣ It's A Fact!!

Contact sports have inherent dangers that put young athletes at special risk for severe injuries. Even with rigorous training and proper safety equipment, youngsters are still at risk for severe injuries to the neck, spinal cord, and growth plates. Evaluating potential sports injuries on the field in very young children can involve its own special issues for concerned parents and coaches.

Chronic Injuries: Chronic injuries usually result from overusing one area of the body while playing a sport or exercising over a long period. The following are signs of a chronic injury:

- Pain when performing an activity

- A dull ache when at rest

- Swelling

Chapter 13

First Aid Tips For Athletes

If you play a sport then you know that injuries can happen. If you play in an organized team, then your coach will have some level of first aid training—but here is some information that anyone playing sports needs to know.

Any injury should be treated properly to prevent any further harm.

- This means looking after the injury by thinking 'RICE' immediately after the injury happens.

- It also means letting the injury completely heal before returning to play. Use 'MSA' to help you remember what to do.

It is important to treat any injury as soon as possible. If it is obvious that a bone is broken, if the injured area swells rapidly, or if the area below the injury goes white, cold, or numb, you need to seek medical treatment immediately.

Less severe injuries including minor sprains and strains should be treated straight away, using the R.I.C.E method of treatment.

About This Chapter: "Sporting Injuries—Treating Them," reprinted with permission. © 2006 Children, Youth and Women's Health Service, Government of South Australia (www.cyh.com).

✎ What's It Mean?

Fracture (Broken Bone): Broken bones are usually the result of some kind of impact. This could include being hit or kicked by an opponent, or be caused by a combination of momentum (the force caused by movement) and your own body weight during a fall.

Sprain: The word 'sprain' is used to describe an injury to the muscles, tendons, and ligaments surrounding a 'joint' such as an ankle or wrist. This type of injury can be caused by an awkward fall or landing, where the joint is 'forced' past its usual range of movement. Part of the muscle, tendon, or ligaments is torn and the injury takes longer than a strain to heal.

Strain: A 'strain' is the word used to describe an injury that happens when a muscle is damaged by being 'over stretched'. You have probably heard of football players who miss games because of 'hamstring' or 'groin' injuries. These are usually 'strain' injuries caused by a movement or action that stretched a particular muscle further than it was able to go without being damaged.

Stress Fracture: Stress fractures are tiny cracks or weak spots in bones, often in the feet or lower legs. Stress fractures are most common in people who perform 'high impact' sporting activities that involve a lot of running or jumping on hard surfaces. Your muscles usually absorb 'shock' when you move, like shock absorbers on a car. If you run, jump or exercise for too long or too often, your muscles become tired and are unable to absorb as much impact. This exposes the bones to increased stress, and fine cracks begin to appear in the surface of the bone.

R.I.C.E.

R: Rest

Rest from the activity. You might have to take the weight off your foot or leg or support your arm or shoulder in a sling, depending on the injury. Keep the weight off an injured joint for at least 24–48 hours.

I: Ice

Put ice or a cold pack on the bruise (20 minutes on and 20 minutes off). Wrap the ice in a damp cloth rather than putting it straight onto your skin or it might stick to you! (Frozen peas in a plastic bag make a good ice pack). Do not apply heat to a fresh injury. This would increase swelling.

C: Compression

Firmly wrap the injured area, using an elastic bandage. This will support the joint and also help to reduce any swelling.

- Don't wrap the bandage too tight.

- Don't try to use the injured area just because it is bandaged. The injury will need rest for one to two days.

E: Elevation

Try to keep the injured area elevated above the level of the heart when ever you are sitting or lying down.

If an injury is still painful, you should see a doctor to make sure that the injury is not more serious than you first thought. Your doctor may need to prescribe anti-inflammatory medication or want to send you for x-rays to find out the extent of the damage.

✔ Quick Tip
First Aid Training

Have you done any basic first aid training? As a teenager you have more freedom to move around outside the home and away from adults, so it is a good idea for you to know what to do if you or one of your friends is hurt when you are out and about.

Maybe you could ask at your sports club, school or college for information on when and where you could train.

The Red Cross (www.redcross.org) or St. John's (www.stjohn.org.au) websites both give information on training courses, or you may be able to do a first aid course at school.

M.S.A.

After a joint or muscle group has had time to heal, you need to help it recover fully.

M: Movement

After one to two days of rest, begin moving the injured joint (without putting weight on it). If the movement really hurts, the joint will require more rest. Moving the joint as soon as possible will prevent scar tissue from building up around the joint, which would make it harder to move freely later on.

S: Strength

Once the injury has healed and a full range of motion is possible, you may need to do some special exercises to strengthen the muscles that have been weakened by the injury and resting. Your doctor, physiotherapist, trainer, or coach should be able to advise you about what is needed.

A: Alternate Activities

Having an injury doesn't mean an end to your exercise program. It is possible to work 'around' an injury so that you can maintain overall fitness while still allowing the injury time to heal. For example, if you have injured a knee or ankle, you could do upper body work in the gym, or even swimming. If you have injured an arm or shoulder, you could still ride an exercise bike, walk, or do weight training for the lower body.

Concussion

Concussion is when a person loses consciousness after a blow to the head. The brain is able to move a small amount inside the skull, and a blow to the head can cause bruising as the soft brain hits the hard skull. If the person is unconscious for a few minutes or more, that person usually needs care in a hospital. There may be other problems such as a skull fracture as well as concussion. Even for a 'mild' concussion you should be seen by a doctor.

Mild head injuries causing unconsciousness for a few seconds usually do not leave any lasting problems, but for a while after the injury (hours to days), the person can have a bad headache. You may not cope well with school work or other tasks which require good concentration for a few days.

More severe concussion can cause dizziness, confusion, difficulty with remembering things, and restlessness that can last weeks or more. There can also be a long lasting headache. If any of these happen, it is important to check with a doctor. Extra help may be needed, including time off work or school.

Anyone who has a concussion needs to rest, and should not play on.

Your doctor will be able to give advice about how long you should rest before playing sport or exercising again.

The 'Blood Rule'

The 'blood rule' is being used in sports to protect other players against hepatitis B and hepatitis C. Any player who is bleeding from an injury must come off, have the injury cleaned (gloves are worn by the person cleaning the injury), and then a waterproof dressing is applied before the player can return. This also protects other players against HIV, but HIV is not as likely to be transmitted as hepatitis B or hepatitis C.

> ✔ **Quick Tip**
>
> In some sports, someone may encourage you to try steroids to help your injury heal faster. Steroids are dangerous and can cause heart failure and damage to other organs. Do not allow anyone to talk you into using steroids for any reason.

Chapter 14

Emergency Care: What To Expect

Emergency Medicine Is A Specialty

Emergency medicine has come a very long way in a very short time. It got its start back in the late 1950s when doctors realized that battlefield procedures used on American soldiers in the Korean and Vietnam wars could save thousands of lives in hospitals here at home.

By the early 1960s, things were still pretty primitive. Hospitals treated people in poorly equipped emergency "rooms." Interns, residents, or on-call physicians were pressed into E.R. duty. Critically ill patients often were transported in hearses, the only vehicles in which patients could lie flat. Treatment often didn't begin until a patient got to the hospital.

That's hardly the case today. Emergency medicine has developed into a fully recognized specialty. The old emergency rooms now have grown into sophisticated emergency departments, staffed by highly trained emergency medicine specialists.

Over the past 30 years, emergency medicine has become a technologically advanced, board-certified, accredited medical specialty. Today's emergency physicians are specialists just like cardiologists, surgeons, and pediatricians. But compared to other medical specialties, emergency medicine is relatively new. The American Medical Association and the American Board of Medical Specialties officially recognized it as the 23rd medical specialty in 1979.

How To Prevent And Respond To An Emergency

Try to stay calm and make a decision to act. The first minutes after an injury often are the most important. Doctors advise four key steps:

1. **Prevent Emergencies:** Regular exercise and medical check-ups will help protect your health. Follow your doctor's advice to reduce risk factors, such as quitting smoking.

2. **Prepare For Emergencies:** Keep first-aid kits at home, work, and in your car. Recognize emergency warning signs. Keep a list of medications taken by you and your family; note allergies. Take a first-aid class. Post emergency numbers near the telephone.

3. **Recognize Life-Threatening Emergencies:** Not every cut or burn requires a trip to the emergency department. Get help fast, though, when the following warning signs are present:

    • Chest pain lasting two minutes or more

    • Uncontrolled bleeding

    • Sudden or severe pain

    • Coughing or vomiting blood

    • Difficulty breathing, shortness of breath

    • Sudden dizziness, weakness, or change in vision

    • Severe or persistent vomiting or diarrhea

    • Change in mental status, such as difficulty arousing

4. **Act:** Action can mean anything from calling paramedics, applying direct pressure on a wound, performing CPR, or splinting an injury. Never perform a procedure if unsure how to do it.

- Don't move anyone involved in a motor vehicle crash or serious fall or found unconscious, unless the person is in immediate danger of further injury.

- Don't give the victim anything to eat or drink and keep the person covered.

- Apply a clean cloth or sterile bandage if the victim is bleeding. If possible, elevate the injury and apply direct pressure on the wound.

- Begin rescue breathing or CPR if the victim is not breathing or does not have a pulse.

Who Takes Care Of You In An Emergency?

Emergency Physicians

Emergency physicians are medicine's frontline heroes. They treat the toughest cases from all medical specialties. Open 24/7, hospital emergency departments are hectic, crowded places, where doctors often juggle 60 different patients during their long shifts. An emergency physician might deliver a baby or stitch a young boy's deep gash or comfort a teenager after a suicide attempt. These doctors see it all—from gunshot wounds to car-wreck injuries to drug overdoses. It's stressful, but rewarding. Day in, day out, they are saving lives.

There's a good chance you might find yourself in a hospital emergency department some day. More than 114 million people—including more than 40 million children—seek care in the nation's 4,000 hospital emergency departments every year. These patients come from all backgrounds—rich and poor, young and old, insured and uninsured. If you have a medical emergency, you can expect to be cared for by a highly trained emergency specialist.

> ♣ **It's A Fact!!**
> You've probably watched an episode of the long-running TV show, "ER" as dedicated doctors rush a young child from an ambulance or scramble to resuscitate an elderly man whose heart has stopped. It's Hollywood's version of life in an emergency department. Intense, fast-paced, and dramatic—and actually, not all that different from real-life emergency medicine.

Emergency physicians are highly educated and have training that crosses different medical specialties to meet demanding challenges. They work with state-of-the-art diagnostic equipment. They are assisted by well-trained physician assistants and emergency nurses. They conduct innovative research. They follow high standards and stay current with dramatic advances in technology.

They also are governed by a code of ethics and a federal law that requires hospital emergency departments to offer care to all patients, regardless of their ability to pay. That makes emergency physicians a vital part of America's health safety net. They advocate for their patients and try to ensure the best care for people, especially the most vulnerable, who often have nowhere else to go for treatment.

Most emergency physicians practice in hospitals—whether it's a small community hospital or a sprawling academic medical center. But you'll also find some emergency doctors on cruise ships or on military battlefields. Some work with emergency management organizations, such as the Federal Emergency Management Agency, to help communities respond when disasters strike. Others specialize in caring for athletes injured during games. Still other emergency doctors man the nation's poison control centers.

Board Certification

In 1968, a group of eight physicians dedicated to improving emergency care formed the American College of Emergency Physicians, which has pushed to develop the practice as a specialty by setting standards and creating a board certification process. Today, the organization of more than 23,000 members is a voice for emergency physicians and their patients.

Like all doctors, emergency physicians go through four years of college and four years of medical school. After that, they train for three to four more years in a residency program at an accredited teaching hospital. During an emergency medicine residency program, residents care for patients while supervised by physician faculty. They also participate in educational and research activities. They are trained to treat both adults and children in a host of emergencies, such as medical, surgical, trauma, cardiac, orthopedic, and obstetric. They also learn skills for dealing with social problems, such as family violence and substance abuse. As of June 1998, 136 emergency medicine residency programs in the United States were approved by the Accreditation Council for Graduate Medical Education. These programs graduate more than 950 residents a year.

After graduating from residency programs, physicians are eligible to take their rigorous board certification examinations. These are national, extensive assessments of the doctor's ability to provide emergency care. Board-certified emergency physicians receive advanced training in quickly recognizing, evaluating, stabilizing, and treating the emergency symptoms of all medical and traumatic conditions. After completing their board certification exams, emergency physicians then can practice independently. Nearly two-thirds of the estimated 32,000 emergency room physicians are board-certified. Emergency physicians also earn continuing medical education credits—typically 50 hours a year—to keep their medical licenses.

Some emergency physicians pursue additional specialized training after their residency programs, such as in pediatric emergency medicine. Fellowships are usually a year or two long. They can be accredited or non-accredited. An accredited fellowship, however, offers the required training for physicians to receive board certification in a subspecialty, such as toxicology, sports medicine, and pediatric emergency medicine.

If You Visit The Emergency Department, Here's What To Expect

If you arrive by ambulance or are unconscious, you will be assigned to a patient bed immediately and be treated.

If someone else drives you to the emergency department, you will enter the waiting room, where your medical condition will be assessed. No one will be turned away from an emergency department, even if they can't pay.

Triage

When you first arrive, a triage nurse will determine how serious your condition is, based on your symptoms. The nurse may check your vital signs, including temperature, heart rate, and blood pressure. Someone will collect your name, address, and medical history.

Examination

After the initial assessment, you will be placed in an examination area, where an emergency physician will examine you and possibly order tests, such as x-rays, blood, and electrocardiogram. Your vital signs will be monitored. Nurses and other medical staff will assist you.

Treatment

If you are critically ill or require intravenous medications or fluids, you may be admitted to the hospital. If you are not seriously ill, an emergency physician will discuss your diagnosis and treatment plan with you before you are discharged. You may receive written instructions regarding medications, restrictions, or symptoms that may require a follow-up visit.

Why Is The Wait So Long?

Across the United States, emergency departments, are extremely overcrowded. Part of this is due to a lack of capacity. Hundreds of emergency departments have closed in the past decade. At the same time, more people are going.

You may be in the emergency department for hours, especially if your health problem is complicated. Determining why you are sick may require many tests. The doctor may need to talk with another specialist to find out how to help you feel better. It also may take several hours for doctors to stabilize you so that your condition is not life-threatening. If you have a serious injury and need to be admitted to the hospital, you may have to wait in the emergency department until a hospital bed becomes available. This process, known as "boarding," may take hours or even a few days. This practice can cause further delays in an emergency department because other patients must wait even longer for care.

✔ Quick Tip
How can I learn more about emergency medicine?

For more information, go to the American College of Emergency Physicians' website at http://www.acep.org.

Chapter 15

Introducing Your Healthcare Team

Orthopaedics

Orthopaedic Surgery: The Subspecialty

Orthopaedics is a medical specialty concerned with the diagnosis, care, and treatment of patients with musculoskeletal disorders. The physicians who specialize in treating injuries and diseases of the musculoskeletal system are called orthopaedic surgeons or orthopaedists.

Although orthopaedists may perform surgery to restore function lost as a result of injury or disease of bones, joints, muscles, tendons, ligaments, nerves, or skin, they are involved in all aspects of health care pertaining to the musculoskeletal system. They employ medical, physical, and rehabilitative methods as well as surgical methods. Typically, as much as 50 percent of the orthopaedist's practice is devoted to non-surgical or medical management of injuries or disease and 50 percent to surgical management.

About This Chapter: Portions of this text were provided by the American Board for Certification in Orthotics, Prosthetics and Pedorthics; American Physical Therapy Association; Center for Orthopaedics and Sports Medicine; National Athletic Trainers' Association; and the U.S. Department of Labor. Complete citations are given within the text of the chapter.

The orthopaedist also works closely with other health care professionals and often serves as a consultant to other physicians. Orthopaedists, in particular, play an important role in the organization and delivery of emergency care and work as a team player in the management of complex multi-system trauma.

The Scope Of Orthopaedics

Orthopaedics is a specialty of immense breadth and variety. Orthopaedists treat a wide variety of diseases and conditions, including such common injuries

---

✎ What's It Mean?
What is a certified orthotist?

Certified orthotists provide a wide range of services within the sports rehab world, whether they are working with professional and collegiate teams or performing patient care services to the average weekend warrior. When working with sports teams, a certified orthotist (designated by the CO suffix) often serves as the specialist for complex cases involving the use of orthotic products, including knee braces, custom orthotic footwear, or protective elbow braces for baseball players.

For serious sports injuries, including ligament tears and cervical (neck) issues, a CO serves as part of the rehabilitation team that answers to the lead physician. In many instances you'll see the CO working side by side with a patient's therapists, with the CO serving as the technical adviser for the orthotic devices that aid in the recovery of both professional and non-professional athletes.

Here are some terms that may help you better understand the work done by COs.

Custom Fabricated Orthosis: Orthosis which is individually made for a specific patient. Created using an impression generally by means of plaster or fiber cast, a digital image using computer-aided design–computer-aided manufacture (CAD-CAM) systems software, or direct form to patient. Also referred to as molded-to-patient model.

Orthosis: Custom-fabricated or custom-fitted brace or support designed to align, correct, or prevent neuromuscular or musculoskeletal dysfunction, disease, injury, or deformity. Note: this does not include supports or devices carried in as fractures, torn ligaments, dislocations, sprains, tendon injuries, pulled muscles, and ruptured discs. They also treat conditions such as low back pain, sciatica, scoliosis, knock knees or bow legs, bunions, and hammer toes. More recently great advances have occurred in the surgical management of degenerative joint disease with the replacement of the diseased joint by a prosthetic device (total joint replacement). Similarly, the application of visualizing instruments to assist in the diagnosis and surgical treatment of internal joint diseases (arthroscopy) has opened new horizons of therapy.

stock and sold by drug and other stores, corset shops, or surgical supply facilities (for example, fabric and elastic supports, corsets, arch supports, trusses, elastic hose, canes, crutches, cervical collars, or dental appliances).

Orthotics: The science and practice of evaluating, measuring, designing, fabricating, assembling, fitting, adjusting, or servicing an orthosis under a prescription from a licensed physician, chiropractor, or podiatrist to correct or alleviate neuromuscular or musculoskeletal dysfunction, disease, injury, or deformity.

Orthotist: Person who measures, designs, fabricates, fits, or services orthoses as prescribed by a licensed physician, and who assists in the formulation of an orthosis to support or correct disabilities.

Prefabricated Orthosis: Orthosis which is manufactured in quantity without a specific patient in mind which may be trimmed, bent, molded, or otherwise modified for use by a specific patient (custom fitted). A preformed orthosis is considered prefabricated even if it requires the attachment of straps and/or the addition of a lining and/or other finishing work or is assembled from prefabricated components is considered prefabricated. Any orthosis that does not meet the definition of a custom fabricated orthosis is considered prefabricated. Also referred to as custom-fitted.

Source: "What Is a Certified Orthotist?" provided courtesy of Tom Derrick, Director of Public Relations, American Board for Certification in Orthotics, Prosthetics and Pedorthics; remaining text reprinted with permission from www.oandpcare.org, the public information website of the American Board for Certification in Orthotics, Prosthetics and Pedorthics. © 2007. All rights reserved.

The Greek roots of orthopaedics are "ortho" (straight) and "pais" (child), and much of the early work in orthopaedics involved treating children who had spine or limb deformities. Orthopaedists continue to treat children with bone tumors and neuromuscular problems such as muscular dystrophy and cerebral palsy, as well as to correct birth abnormalities such as club foot, hip dislocation, and abnormalities of fingers and toes and growth abnormalities such as unequal leg length. Orthopaedists also treat diseases prevalent in the elderly, such as osteoporosis, as well as arthritis and bursitis.

Some orthopaedists confine their practice to specific areas of the musculo-skeletal system, such as the spine, hip, foot, or hand, knee, sports medicine, or arthroscopy. However, 41 percent of orthopaedic surgeons designate themselves as general orthopaedic surgeons, 36 percent consider themselves as general orthopaedic surgeons with specialty interest, while 23 percent consider themselves as specialists within orthopaedic surgery. Many generalists may have a special interest in a specific area, but still treat most injuries or diseases of the musculoskeletal system.

Arthroscopy: What Is It?

"Knee Arthroscopy," reprinted with permission from the Center for Orthopaedics and Sports Medicine (www.arthroscopy.com). © 2003. All rights reserved. This material does not constitute medical advice. It is intended for informational purposes only. Please consult a physician for specific treatment recommendations.

Arthroscopy is a surgical procedure in which a small fiberoptic telescope (arthroscope) is inserted into a joint. Fluid is then inserted into the joint to distend the joint and to allow for the visualization of the structures within that joint. Usually the surgery is viewed on a monitor so that the whole operating team is aware of the type of surgical procedure that is being performed.

Arthroscopes are approximately 5 mm in diameter, so the incisions are very small (approximately 1/8 inch). During the procedure, which is conducted under anesthesia, the inside of the joint is examined for damaged tissue. The most common types of arthroscopic surgery include removal or repair of a torn meniscus (cartilage), ligament reconstruction, removal of loose debris, and trimming damaged cartilage.

Arthroscopy is much less traumatic to the muscles, ligaments, and tissues than the traditional method of surgically opening the knee with long incisions (arthrotomy). The benefits of arthroscopy involve smaller incisions, faster healing, a more rapid recovery, and less scarring. Arthroscopic surgical procedures are often performed on an outpatient basis and the patient is able to return home on the same day.

While an arthroscope is used in many different types of surgical procedures, the recovery time and outcome of the procedure is related to the type of injury and the type of arthroscopic surgical procedure performed. For example, an arthroscopic surgical ligament reconstruction will take longer to heal and the recovery time will be longer then the patient who has an arthroscopic removal of a loose body.

The Physical Therapist

Excerpted from "APTA Background Sheet 2007," reprinted from http://www.apta.org with permission of the American Physical Therapy Association, © 2007.

Physical therapists (PTs) are health care professionals who diagnose and treat individuals of all ages, from newborns to the very oldest, who have medical problems or other health-related conditions that limit their abilities to move and perform functional activities in their daily lives.

PTs examine each individual and develop a plan using treatment techniques to promote the ability to move, reduce pain, restore function, and prevent disability. In addition, PTs work with individuals to prevent the loss of mobility before it occurs by developing fitness- and wellness-oriented programs for healthier and more active lifestyles.

Physical therapists provide care for people in a variety of settings, including hospitals, private practices, outpatient clinics, home health agencies, schools, sports and fitness facilities, work settings, and nursing homes. State licensure is required in each state in which a physical therapist practices.

All PTs must receive a graduate degree from an accredited physical therapist program before taking the national licensure examination that allows them to practice. The majority of programs offer the doctor of physical therapy (DPT) degree.

Discovering Physical Therapy

"Discovering Physical Therapy," reprinted from http://www.apta.org with permission of the American Physical Therapy Association, © 2007.

What is physical therapy? It's an important question, and the answer will help you understand how a physical therapist can improve your ability to move and function, while also benefiting your general fitness and health.

Physical therapists are experts in "the science of healing and the art of caring." This is what that means:

The Science Of Healing

Patients and physicians are demanding the talents of physical therapists for conservative management of a wide variety of conditions. In many cases, patients are being sent to physical therapy instead of surgery.

Physical therapists help people with orthopedic conditions such as low back pain or osteoporosis; joint and soft tissue injuries such as fractures and dislocations; neurologic conditions such as stroke, traumatic brain injury, or Parkinson disease; connective tissue injuries such as burns or wounds; cardiopulmonary and circulatory conditions such as congestive heart failure and chronic obstructive pulmonary disease; and workplace injuries including repetitive stress disorders and sports injuries.

Physical therapists practice in a variety of settings, including hospitals, private practices, outpatient clinics, home health agencies, schools, sports and fitness facilities, work settings, and nursing homes.

Some physical therapists seek advanced certification in a clinical specialty, such as orthopedic, neurologic, cardiovascular and pulmonary, pediatric, geriatric, sports physical therapy, or electrophysiological testing and measurement.

The Art Of Caring

The individualized, "hands on" approach that characterizes physical therapist care is highly valued by patients. When a physical therapist sees a patient for the first time, he or she examines that individual and develops a plan of care that promotes the ability to move, reduces pain, restores function, and prevents disability. The physical therapist and the patient then work side-by-side to make sure that the goals of the treatment plan are met.

Therapeutic exercise and functional training are the cornerstones of physical therapist treatment. Depending on the particular needs of a patient, physical therapists may "manipulate" a joint (that is, perform certain types of passive movements at the end of the patient's range of motion) or massage a muscle to promote proper movement and function. Physical therapists may use other techniques such as electrotherapy, ultrasound (high-frequency waves that produce heat), hot packs, and ice in addition to other treatments when appropriate.

Physical therapists will also work with individuals to prevent loss of mobility by developing fitness- and wellness-oriented programs for healthier and more active lifestyles.

It is important to know that physical therapy can be provided only by qualified physical therapists or by physical therapist assistants working under the supervision of a physical therapist.

Athletic Trainers

Excerpted from Occupational Outlook Handbook, *U.S. Department of Labor, Bureau of Labor Statistics, 2006.*

Athletic trainers help prevent and treat injuries for people of all ages. Their clients include everyone from professional athletes to industrial workers. Recognized by the American Medical Association as allied health professionals, athletic trainers specialize in the prevention, assessment, treatment, and rehabilitation of musculoskeletal injuries. Athletic trainers are often one of the first healthcare providers on the scene when injuries occur, and therefore must be able to recognize, evaluate, and assess injuries and provide immediate care when needed. They are also heavily involved in the rehabilitation and reconditioning of injuries.

Athletic trainers often help prevent injuries by advising on the proper use of equipment and applying protective or injury-preventive devices such as tape, bandages, and braces. Injury prevention also often includes educating people on what they should do to avoid putting themselves at risk for injuries. Athletic trainers should not be confused with fitness trainers or personal trainers, who are not healthcare workers, but rather train people to become physically fit.

Athletic trainers work under the supervision of a licensed physician, and in cooperation with other healthcare providers. The level of medical supervision varies, depending upon the setting. Some athletic trainers meet with the team physician or consulting physician once or twice a week; others interact with a physician every day. The extent of the supervision ranges from discussing specific injuries and treatment options with a physician to performing evaluations and treatments as directed by a physician.

Facts About Certified Athletic Trainers

From "The FACTS about Certified Athletic Trainers and the National Athletic Trainers' Association," May 21, 2004. © National Athletic Trainers' Association (NATA). All rights reserved. Reprinted with permission.

FACT: All athletic trainers have a bachelor's degree from an accredited college or university. Athletic trainers are health care professionals similar to physical, occupational, speech, language, and other therapists.

All certified or licensed athletic trainers must have a bachelor's or master's degree from an accredited college or university. Degrees are complementary to accredited athletic training majors and include established academic curricula. Athletic trainers' bachelor's degrees are in pre-medical sciences, kinesiology, exercise physiology, biology, exercise science, or physical education. Academic programs are accredited through an independent process by the Commission on Accreditation of Athletic Training Education (CAATE) via the Joint Review Committee on Educational Programs in Athletic Training (JRCAT).

FACT: 70 percent of athletic trainers have a master's degree or doctorate.

Certified athletic trainers are highly educated. Seventy (70) percent of AT credential holders have a master's degree or more advanced degree. Reflective of the broad base of skills valued by the athletic training profession, these master's degrees may be in athletic training (clinical), education, exercise physiology, counseling or health care administration or promotion. This great majority of practitioners who hold advance degrees is comparable to other allied health care professionals.

♣ It's A Fact!!
What's the difference between a
certified athletic trainer and a personal trainer?

Certified Athletic Trainer

An athletic trainer is a person who meets the qualifications set by a state regulatory board and/or the Board of Certification, Inc., and practices athletic training under the direction of a physician.

Certified athletic trainers must have at least a bachelor's degree in athletic training, which is an allied health profession; must pass a three-part exam before earning the ATC credential; must keep their skills current by participating in continuing education; and must adhere to practice guidelines set by one national certifying agency.

Daily duties: Provide physical medicine and rehabilitation services; prevent, assess, and treat injuries (acute and chronic); coordinate care with physicians and other allied health providers; work in schools, colleges, professional sports, clinics, hospitals, corporations, industry, and the military.

Personal Trainer

A personal trainer is a person who prescribes, monitors, and changes an individual's specific exercise program in a fitness or sport setting.

Personal trainers may or may not have higher education in health sciences; may or may not be required to obtain certification; may or may not participate in continuing education; may become certified by any one of numerous agencies that set varying education and practice requirements.

Daily duties: Assess fitness needs and design appropriate exercise regimens; work with clients to achieve fitness goals; help educate the public about the importance of physical activity; work in health clubs, wellness centers, and various other locations where fitness activities take place.

FACT: Athletic trainers know and practice the medical arts at the highest professional standards.

Athletic trainers specialize in injury and illness prevention, assessment, treatment and rehabilitation for all physically active people, including the general public.

FACT: Athletic trainers are regulated and licensed health care workers.

While practice act oversight varies by state, the athletic trainer practices under state statutes recognizing them as health care professionals similar to physical therapists, occupational therapists, and other health care professionals. Athletic training licensure/regulation exists in 44 states, with aggressive efforts underway to pursue licensure in the remaining states. Athletic trainers practice under the direction of physicians.

FACT: An independent national board certifies athletic trainers.

The independent Board of Certification Inc. (BOC) nationally certifies athletic trainers. Athletic trainers must pass an examination and hold a bachelor's degree to become an Athletic Trainer, Certified (ATC). To retain certification, credential holders must obtain 80 hours of medically related continuing education credits every three years and adhere to Membership Standards. The BOC is accredited by the National Commission for Certifying Agencies.

FACT: Athletic trainers are recognized allied health care professionals.

ATs are highly qualified, multi-skilled allied health care professionals and have been part of the American Medical Association's Health Professions Career and Education Directory for more than a decade. Additionally, the American Academy of Family Physicians, American Academy of Pediatrics, and American Orthopaedic Society for Sports Medicine—among others—are all strong clinical and academic supporters of athletic trainers.

FACT: ATs improve patient functional and physical outcomes.

Results from a nationwide Medical Outcomes Survey conducted 1996–1998 demonstrate that care provided by ATs effects a significant change in all outcomes variables measured, with the greatest change in functional outcomes and physical outcomes. The investigation indicates that care provided by ATs generates a change in health-related quality of life patient outcomes. (ref: Albohm MJ, Wilkerson GB. An outcomes assessment of care provided by certified athletic trainers. *J Rehabil. Outcomes Meas.* 1999; 3(3):51-56.)

FACT: ATs specialize in patient education to prevent injury and re-injury and reduce rehabilitative and other health care costs.

Recent studies, reports, outcomes measures surveys, total joint replacement studies, and many other case studies demonstrate how the services of ATs save money for employers and improve quality of life for patients. For each $1 invested in preventive care, employers gained up to a $7 return on investment according to one NATA survey. The use of certified athletic trainers supports a consumer-driven health care economy that increases competition in order to reduce patient and disease costs. Through the use of proper rehabilitation and evaluation, athletic trainers prevent re-injury. The patient's standard of care is enhanced, not sacrificed, with ATs.

Chapter 16

Questions And Answers About Sprains And Strains

This chapter contains general information about sprains and strains, which are both very common injuries. Individual sections describe what sprains and strains are, where they usually occur, what their signs and symptoms are, how they are treated, and how they can be prevented. If you have further questions, you may wish to discuss them with your health care provider.

What is the difference between a sprain and a strain?

A sprain is a stretch or tear of a ligament (a band of fibrous tissue that connects two or more bones at a joint). One or more ligaments can be injured at the same time. The severity of the injury will depend on the extent of injury (whether a tear is partial or complete) and the number of ligaments involved.

A strain is an injury to either a muscle or a tendon (fibrous cords of tissue that connect muscle to bone). Depending on the severity of the injury, a strain may be a simple overstretch of the muscle or tendon, or it can result from a partial or complete tear.

About This Chapter: From "Questions and Answers About Sprains and Strains," National Institute of Arthritis and Musculoskeletal and Skin Diseases (www.niams.nih.gov), May 2004.

Sports Injuries Information For Teens, Second Edition

What causes a sprain?

A sprain can result from a fall, a sudden twist, or a blow to the body that forces a joint out of its normal position and stretches or tears the ligament supporting that joint. Typically, sprains occur when people fall and land on an outstretched arm, slide into a baseball base, land on the side of their foot, or twist a knee with the foot planted firmly on the ground.

Where do sprains usually occur?

Although sprains can occur in both the upper and lower parts of the body, the most common site is the ankle. More than 25,000 individuals sprain an ankle each day in the United States.

The ankle joint is supported by several lateral (outside) ligaments and medial (inside) ligaments. Most ankle sprains happen when the foot turns inward as a person runs, turns, falls, or lands on the ankle after a jump. This

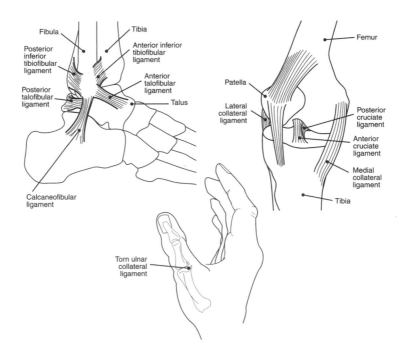

Figure 16.1: Common sites for sprains. Lateral views of the ankle, knee, and thumb (clockwise from upper left).

type of sprain is called an inversion injury. The knee is another common site for a sprain. A blow to the knee or a fall is often the cause; sudden twisting can also result in a sprain.

Sprains frequently occur at the wrist, typically when people fall and land on an outstretched hand. A sprain to the thumb is common in skiing and other sports. This injury often occurs when a ligament near the base of the thumb (the ulnar collateral ligament of the metacarpophalangeal joint) is torn.

What are the signs and symptoms of a sprain?

The usual signs and symptoms include pain, swelling, bruising, instability, and loss of the ability to move and use the joint (called functional ability). However, these signs and symptoms can vary in intensity, depending on the severity of the sprain. Sometimes people feel a pop or tear when the injury happens.

Doctors closely observe an injured site and ask questions to obtain information to diagnose the severity of a sprain. In general, a grade I or mild sprain is caused by overstretching or slight tearing of the ligaments with no

---

♣ It's A Fact!!
When To See A Doctor For A Sprain

- You have severe pain and cannot put any weight on the injured joint.
- The injured area looks crooked or has lumps and bumps (other than swelling) that you do not see on the uninjured joint.
- You cannot move the injured joint.
- You cannot walk more than four steps without significant pain.
- Your limb buckles or gives way when you try to use the joint.
- You have numbness in any part of the injured area.
- You see redness or red streaks spreading out from the injury.
- You injure an area that has been injured several times before.
- You have pain, swelling, or redness over a bony part of your foot.
- You are in doubt about the seriousness of the injury or how to care for it.

joint instability. A person with a mild sprain usually experiences minimal pain, swelling, and little or no loss of functional ability. Bruising is absent or slight, and the person is usually able to put weight on the affected joint.

A grade II or moderate sprain is caused by further, but still incomplete, tearing of the ligament and is characterized by bruising, moderate pain, and swelling. A person with a moderate sprain usually has more difficulty putting weight on the affected joint and experiences some loss of function. An x-ray may be needed to help the health care provider determine if a fracture is causing the pain and swelling. Magnetic resonance imaging is occasionally used to help differentiate between a significant partial injury and a complete tear in a ligament, or can be recommended to rule out other injuries.

People who sustain a grade III or severe sprain completely tear or rupture a ligament. Pain, swelling, and bruising are usually severe, and the patient is unable to put weight on the joint. An x-ray is usually taken to rule out a broken bone. When diagnosing any sprain, the provider will ask the patient to explain how the injury happened. He or she will examine the affected area and check its stability and its ability to move and bear weight.

What causes a strain?

A strain is caused by twisting or pulling a muscle or tendon. Strains can be acute or chronic. An acute strain is associated with a recent trauma or injury; it also can occur after improperly lifting heavy objects or overstressing the muscles. Chronic strains are usually the result of overuse: prolonged, repetitive movement of the muscles and tendons.

Where do strains usually occur?

Two common sites for a strain are the back and the hamstring muscle (located in the back of the thigh). Contact sports such as soccer, football, hockey, boxing, and wrestling put people at risk for strains. Gymnastics, tennis, rowing, golf, and other sports that require extensive gripping can increase the risk of hand and forearm strains. Elbow strains sometimes occur in people who participate in racquet sports, throwing, and contact sports.

What are the signs and symptoms of a strain?

Typically, people with a strain experience pain, limited motion, muscle spasms, and possibly muscle weakness. They can also have localized swelling, cramping, or inflammation and, with a minor or moderate strain, usually some loss of muscle function. Patients typically have pain in the injured area and general weakness of the muscle when they attempt to move it. Severe strains that partially or completely tear the muscle or tendon are often very painful and disabling.

How are sprains and strains treated?

Reduce Swelling And Pain: Treatments for sprains and strains are similar and can be thought of as having two stages. The goal during the first stage is to reduce swelling and pain. At this stage, health care providers usually advise patients to follow a formula of rest, ice, compression, and elevation (RICE) for the first 24 to 48 hours after the injury. The provider may also recommend an

---

✎ What's It Mean?

RICE Therapy

- **Rest:** Reduce regular exercise or activities of daily living as needed. Your health care provider may advise you to put no weight on an injured area for 48 hours. If you cannot put weight on an ankle or knee, crutches may help. If you use a cane or one crutch for an ankle injury, use it on the uninjured side to help you lean away and relieve weight on the injured ankle.

- **Ice:** Apply an ice pack to the injured area for 20 minutes at a time, 4 to 8 times a day. A cold pack, ice bag, or plastic bag filled with crushed ice and wrapped in a towel can be used. To avoid cold injury and frostbite, do not apply the ice for more than 20 minutes.

- **Compression:** Compression of an injured ankle, knee, or wrist may help reduce swelling. Examples of compression bandages are elastic wraps, special boots, air casts, and splints. Ask your provider for advice on which one to use, and how tight to safely apply the bandage.

- **Elevation:** If possible, keep the injured ankle, knee, elbow, or wrist elevated on a pillow, above the level of the heart, to help decrease swelling.

over-the-counter or prescription nonsteroidal anti-inflammatory drug, such as aspirin or ibuprofen, to help decrease pain and inflammation.

For people with a moderate or severe sprain, particularly of the ankle, a hard cast may be applied. This often occurs after the initial swelling has subsided. Severe sprains and strains may require surgery to repair the torn ligaments, muscle, or tendons. Surgery is usually performed by an orthopaedic surgeon.

It is important that moderate and severe sprains and strains be evaluated by a health care provider to allow prompt, appropriate treatment to begin. A person who has any concerns about the seriousness of a sprain or strain should always contact a provider for advice.

Begin Rehabilitation: The second stage of treating a sprain or strain is rehabilitation, whose overall goal is to improve the condition of the injured area and restore its function. The health care provider will prescribe an exercise program designed to prevent stiffness, improve range of motion, and restore the joint's normal flexibility and strength. Some patients may need physical therapy during this stage. When the acute pain and swelling have diminished, the provider will instruct the patient to do a series of exercises several times a day. These are very important because they help reduce swelling, prevent stiffness, and restore normal, pain-free range of motion. The provider can recommend many different types of exercises, depending on the injury. A patient with an injured knee or foot will work on weight-bearing and balancing exercises. The duration of the program depends on the extent of the injury, but the regimen commonly lasts for several weeks.

Another goal of rehabilitation is to increase strength and regain flexibility. Depending on the patient's rate of recovery, this process begins about the second week after the injury. The provider will instruct the patient to do a series of exercises designed to meet these goals. During this phase of rehabilitation, patients progress to more demanding exercises as pain decreases and function improves.

The final goal is the return to full daily activities, including sports when appropriate. Patients must work closely with their health care provider or physical therapist to determine their readiness to return to full activity. Sometimes people are tempted to resume full activity or play sports despite pain or muscle soreness. Returning to full activity before regaining normal range of motion, flexibility, and strength increases the chance of reinjury and may lead to a chronic problem.

The amount of rehabilitation and the time needed for full recovery after a sprain or strain depend on the severity of the injury and individual rates of healing. For example, a mild ankle sprain may require up to three to six weeks of rehabilitation; a moderate sprain could require two to three months. With a severe sprain, it can take up to eight to twelve months to return to full activities. Extra care should be taken to avoid reinjury.

Can sprains and strains be prevented?

There are many things people can do to help lower their risk of sprains and strains:

- Avoid exercising or playing sports when tired or in pain.

- Maintain a healthy, well-balanced diet to keep muscles strong.

- Maintain a healthy weight.

- Practice safety measures to help prevent falls (for example, keep stairways, walkways, yards, and driveways free of clutter; anchor scatter rugs; and salt or sand icy patches in the winter).

- Wear shoes that fit properly.

- Replace athletic shoes as soon as the tread wears out or the heel wears down on one side.

- Do stretching exercises daily.

- Be in proper physical condition to play a sport.

- Warm up and stretch before participating in any sports or exercise.

- Wear protective equipment when playing.

- Run on even surfaces.

Chapter 17

Overuse Injuries In Adolescent Athletes

What is an overuse injury?

An overuse injury is caused by "doing too much." The continual stress placed on the body during physical exertion causes the breakdown of tissue, whether it be bone or tendon. When athletes' demands on their bodies surpass their physical ability, overuse injuries arise, such as stress fractures, tendonitis, and bursitis.

What is a stress fracture?

A stress fracture is a microfracture in the cortex (outside layer) of bone that is a result of repeated physical stress placed on the skeleton that exceeds its capability to remodel for support. Stress fractures differ from regular fractures because they develop over time rather than from one trauma. They often occur in the weightbearing bones of the lower leg and foot. Stress fractures are the most serious type of overuse injury.

How do these injuries develop?

Often stress fractures occur when muscles become exhausted from excessive force and begin to transfer weight onto the bone. This leads to weak sites in the bone that with repetitive activity will become a stress fracture. This can occur as the result of a sudden increase in the intensity of training, which suddenly demands too much from bones that are not used to repetitive stress. A change in equipment, such as footwear, or in playing surfaces, such as from grass to turf, can serve as the variable that also causes stress fractures.

What are the symptoms of overuse injuries?

Athletes with stress fractures usually complain of pain that seems to worsen over time. This is the first signal that the bone cannot withstand the physical stress to which it is being subjected. This pain is often felt at the time of impact. Pressing on the sight of a stress fracture will elicit great pain and there may be swelling around the affected area. As activity is modified to eliminate discomfort, the pain associated with a stress fracture should subside.

Who is most susceptible to stress fractures?

Medical studies have shown that female athletes are more susceptible to stress fractures. This is attributed to the more frequent occurrence of reduced bone density, eating disorders, and infrequent menstrual cycle in women. Athletes who participate in running sports and repetitive loading sports, such as ballet and figure skating, have a greater risk of developing stress fractures because the repetitive stress of the landing on a hard surface can cause injury.

Adolescents are especially susceptible to stress fractures because their bones are expected to support more weight while participating in more rigorous activity. In addition, growth plates, regions of developing cartilage in children's bones that act as centers of the rapid cell production, are especially susceptible to stress fractures, increasing the risk of injury in young athletes. Although all of these factors increase the risk of injury, conditioned athletes can also suffer stress fractures.

What do I do if I develop a stress fracture?

If a stress fracture is suspected, a physician should be consulted to rule out the possibility of more serious injury through physical examination or diagnostic imaging. Like other overuse injuries, the basic treatment of stress fractures involves relative rest and avoidance of all activities that aggravated the injury while maintaining fitness by engaging in pain-free activity. The amount of recovery time depends on the seriousness of the injury, but most stress fractures heal within six weeks. Recognizing the risk factors and modifying behavior accordingly is key in the healing of an overuse injury. Resuming full participation in athletics should be a very gradual process so that the bone can properly adapt to the increased load. During this process applying ice, elevating the injured area, and applying compressive wraps will reduce discomfort and inflammation.

How can these injuries be prevented?

Overuse injuries can be avoided by following safe training procedures. This can be achieved by exercising according to the guidelines below:

- **Gradually increase the intensity of training.** Many overuse injuries occur as a result of a sudden increase in the intensity in training. Effective muscle strength increases at a faster rate than bone strength, which can create an imbalance that causes injury if exercise is increased too rapidly. Athletes should focus on allowing their body to adjust to more strenuous activity to prevent exceeded their physical capability.

- **Use proper equipment.** Wearing equipment that will add support to your body during activity is very important. Runners should make sure to wear sneakers that are not worn so that they have adequate shock absorption that will protect their bones from overuse injuries.

- **Include calcium in your diet.** It is important to keep bones strong and capable of withstanding the pressures placed on it.

- **Maintain appropriate muscle strength.** Proper conditioning will provide muscular stability to the bone during activity. Imbalance in muscle strength can lead to overuse injuries, so uniform strengthening of all muscle groups should be practiced.

☞ **Remember!!**
Athletes should pay close attention to the physical limitations of their bodies by quickly responding to pain and allowing rest when needed. It is important to recognize injuries at their earliest stages and to treat them appropriately so that play is not impeded.

Chapter 18

Facts About Broken Bones

The harder kids play, the harder they fall. The fact is, broken bones, or fractures, are common in childhood and often happen when kids are playing or participating in sports. Most fractures occur in the upper extremities: the wrist, the forearm, and above the elbow. Why? When children fall, it's a natural instinct for them to throw their hands out in an attempt to stop it.

Although many kids will have one at some point, a broken bone can be scary. To help make things a little easier when your next spill results in a fracture, here's the lowdown on what you can expect.

How do I know if it's broken?

Falls are a common part of childhood, but not every fall will result in a broken bone. The classic signs of a fracture are: pain, swelling, and deformity. However if the break isn't displaced (see "What are the different types of fractures?" below), it may be harder to tell.

✔ Quick Tip
What can I do to protect my bones?

Some of the most important things you can do are to follow a diet rich in calcium and vitamin D, maintain an adequate daily intake of protein, monitor your sodium intake, and get plenty of exercise.

Calcium is needed to maintain healthy, strong bones throughout your life. Unfortunately, most Americans do not get enough calcium from their diets. Dairy products like milk, cheese, and yogurt are an excellent source of calcium, and some nondairy foods like broccoli, almonds, and sardines, to name a few, can provide smaller amounts. In addition, many foods that you may already enjoy—juices, breads, cereals—can now be found fortified with calcium. Although food is the best source of calcium because it also provides other essential nutrients, calcium supplements can fill the gap if you're not getting enough from your diet.

Vitamin D plays a significant role in helping your body absorb calcium. The relationship between calcium and vitamin D is similar to that of a locked door and a key. Vitamin D is the key that unlocks the door, allowing calcium to enter your bloodstream. The recommended daily intake for vitamin D is 400 to 800 international units (IU). Many people get this amount through natural exposure to sunlight, which our bodies use to make vitamin D, and by consuming vitamin D-fortified foods like milk. In addition, many calcium supplements are fortified with vitamin D.

Sodium, a main component of table salt, affects our need for calcium by increasing the amount of it we excrete in urine. As a result, people with diets high in sodium, or table salt, appear to need more calcium than people with low-sodium diets in order to ensure that, on balance, they retain enough calcium for their bones.

Protein in excess amounts also increases the amount of calcium we excrete in urine, but it provides benefits for bone health as well. For example, protein is needed for fracture healing.

Source: Excerpted from "Once Is Enough: A Guide to Preventing Future Fractures," National Institute of Arthritis and Musculoskeletal and Skin Diseases (NIAMS), May 2006.

Some telltale signs that your bone is broken are:

- You heard a snap or a grinding noise during the injury.

- There's swelling, bruising, or tenderness around the injured part.

- It's painful for you to bear weight on the injury, touch it, press on it, or move it.

- The injured part looks deformed. In severe breaks, the broken bone may be poking through the skin.

What do I do?

If you suspect that you have a fracture, you should seek medical care immediately.

Do not move—and call for emergency care—if:

- you may have seriously injured your head, neck, or back;

- the broken bone comes through the skin (Apply constant pressure with a clean gauze pad or thick cloth, and keep lying down until help arrives. Don't wash the wound or push in any part of the bone that's sticking out.)

For less serious injuries, it's a good idea to stabilize the injury as soon as it happens by following these quick steps:

1. Remove clothing from the injured part. Don't force a limb out of your clothing, though. You may need to cut clothing off with scissors to prevent causing any unnecessary additional pain.

2. Apply a cold compress or ice pack wrapped in cloth.

3. Place a makeshift splint on the injured part by:

    - keeping the injured limb in the position you find it;

    - placing soft padding around the injured part;

    - placing something firm (like a board or rolled-up newspapers) next to the injured part, making sure it's long enough to go past the joints above and below the injury;

• keeping the splint in place with first-aid tape.

4.   Seek medical care, and don't eat, in case surgery is needed.

What are the different types of fractures?

By simply looking at the injured area, a doctor may be able to tell whether your bone is broken. But he or she will order an x-ray to confirm that you do, indeed, have a fracture and to determine what kind it is.

With a little patience and cooperation, getting an x-ray to look at the broken bone won't take long. Then, you will be well on the way to getting a cool—maybe even colorful—cast that every friend can sign.

X-rays don't hurt. Doctors use a special machine to take a picture to look at the inside of your body. When the picture comes out, it won't look like the ones in your photo album, but doctors have learned how to look at these pictures to see things like broken bones.

A fracture through the growing part of a child's bone (called the growth plate) may not show up on x-ray. If the doctor suspects that you have this type of fracture, he or she will treat it even if the x-ray doesn't show a break.

Children's bones are more likely to bend than break completely because they're softer. Fracture types that are more common in children include:

• **buckle or torus fracture:** one side of the bone bends, raising a little buckle, without breaking the other side;

• **greenstick fracture:** a partial fracture in which one side of the bone is broken and the other side bends (This fracture resembles what would happen if you tried to break a green stick.)

Mature bones are more likely to break completely. A stronger force will also result in a complete fracture of younger bones. A complete fracture may be a:

• **closed fracture:** a fracture that doesn't break the skin;

• **open (or compound) fracture:** a fracture in which the ends of the broken bone break through the skin (these types of fractures have an increased risk of infection);

- **non-displaced fracture:** a fracture in which the pieces on either side of the break line up;

- **displaced fracture:** a fracture in which the pieces on either side of the break are out of line (displaced fractures may require surgery to make sure the bones are properly aligned before casting).

Other common fracture terms include:

- **hairline fracture:** a thin break in the bone;

- **single fracture:** the bone is broken in one place;

- **segmental:** the bone is broken in two or more places in the same bone;

- **comminuted fracture:** the bone is broken into more than two pieces or crushed.

What's involved in getting a splint or cast?

Your doctor may decide that a splint is all that's needed to keep the bone from moving so it can heal. Whereas a cast encircles the entire broken area and will be removed by the doctor when the bone is healed, a splint usually supports the broken bone on one side. It is kept in place with Velcro or it may be wrapped with gauze or a bandage.

When the doctor puts on a splint, a layer of cotton goes on first. Next, the splint is placed over the cotton. A splint may be made of stiff pieces of plastic or metal or can be molded out of plaster or fiberglass to fit the injured area comfortably. Then cloth or straps (which usually have Velcro) are used to keep the splint in place. The doctor might need to readjust the splint later, or you might get instructions on how to do it at home. You might be allowed to remove it carefully to take a bath.

However, most broken bones will need a cast.

A cast, which keeps your bone from moving so it can heal, is essentially a big bandage that has two layers—a soft cotton layer that rests against the skin and a hard outer layer that prevents the broken bone from moving.

These days, casts are made of either:

- **plaster of paris:** a heavy white powder that forms a thick paste that hardens quickly when mixed with water. Plaster of paris casts are heavier than fiberglass casts and don't hold up as well in water.

- **synthetic (fiberglass) material:** made out of fiberglass, a kind of moldable plastic, these casts come in many bright colors and are lighter and cooler. The covering (fiberglass) on synthetic casts is water-resistant, but the padding underneath is not. You can, however, get a waterproof liner. The doctor putting on your cast will decide if you should get a fiberglass cast with a waterproof lining.

Although some kids might find casts cool when they're finally on their broken parts, actually getting them put there can be a scary concept, especially for a person in pain. Knowing what happens in the cast room might help alleviate some worry.

For displaced fractures (in which the pieces on either side of the break are out of line), the bone will need to be set before putting on a cast. To set the bone, the doctor will put the pieces of your broken bone in the right position so they can grow back together into one bone (this is called a closed reduction). During a closed reduction, the doctor will realign the broken bone so that it heals in a straighter position. You will be given medicine, usually through an IV, when this is done to help keep the bone from hurting. A cast is then put on to keep the bone in position.

So how is a cast actually put on? First, several layers of soft cotton are wrapped around the injured area. Next, the plaster or fiberglass outer layer is soaked in water. The doctor wraps the plaster or fiberglass around the soft first layer. The outer layer is wet but will dry to a hard, protective covering. Doctors sometimes make tiny cuts in the sides of a cast to allow room for swelling.

Once the cast is on, the doctor will probably recommend that you prop the splinted or casted area on a pillow or stool for a few days to reduce swelling. And if you have a cast on the foot or leg (called a walking cast), you shouldn't walk on it until it's dry (this takes about one hour for a fiberglass cast and two or three days for a plaster cast).

If the cast or splint is on your arm, the doctor might give you a sling to help support it. A sling is made of cloth and a strap that loops around the back of your neck and acts like a special sleeve to keep your arm comfortable and in place. If you have a broken leg, you will probably get crutches to make it a little easier to get around.

Some pain is expected for the first few days after getting a cast, but it usually isn't severe. Your doctor may recommend acetaminophen or ibuprofen. However, if you seem to be in a lot of pain, call your doctor.

If the cast is causing your fingers or toes to turn white, purple, or blue, the cast may be too tight and you should call your doctor right away. Also be sure to call your doctor if the skin around the edges of the cast gets red or raw—that's typically a sign that the cast is wet inside from sweat or water. Also, you shouldn't pick at or remove the padding from the edges of fiberglass casts because the fiberglass edges can rub on the skin and cause irritation.

What happens in more serious breaks?

Although most broken bones simply need a cast to heal, other more serious fractures (such as compound fractures) may require surgery to be properly aligned and to ensure the bones stay together during the healing process. Open fractures need to be cleaned thoroughly in the sterile environment of the operating room before they're set because the bone's exposure to the air poses a risk of infection.

With breaks in larger bones or when the bone breaks into more than two pieces, your doctor may put a metal pin in the bone to help set it before placing a cast. Don't worry, though— as with any surgery, you will be given medicine so that you won't feel a thing. And when your bone has healed, the doctor will remove the pin.

When will my broken bone heal?

Fractures heal at different rates, depending upon the age of the child and the type of fracture. For example, young children may heal in as little

♣ It's A Fact!!
Surgical Procedures For Bone Fracture Repair

Bone fracture repair is surgery to fix a broken bone using plates, nails, screws, or pins. Bone grafts may be used to allow for proper healing or to speed the healing process.

While the patient is pain-free, using general or local anesthesia, an incision is made over the fractured bone. The bone is placed in proper position, and screws, pins, or plates are attached to or placed in the bone temporarily or permanently. Alternatively, long bones may be fixed with nails placed in the bone cavity.

Any disrupted blood vessels are tied off or burned (cauterized). If examination of the fracture shows that a quantity of bone has been lost as a result of the fracture, especially if there is a gap between the broken bone ends, the surgeon may decide that a bone graft is essential to avoid delayed healing. Bone grafting may be performed using the patient's own bone, usually taken from the hip, or using bone from a donor.

If bone grafting is not necessary, the fracture can be repaired by the following methods:

- One or more screws may be inserted across the break to hold it
- A steel plate held by screws may be drilled into the bone
- A long, thick metal pin (sometimes called a rod or nail) with holes in it, may be driven down the shaft of the bone from one end, with screws then passed through the bone and through a hole in the pin

In some cases, after this stabilization, the microsurgical repair of blood vessels and nerves is necessary. The skin incision is then closed. If the broken

as three weeks, although it may take six weeks for the same kind of fracture to heal in teens.

It's important for you to wait to play games or sports that might use the injured part until your doctor says it's OK.

bone has pierced the skin, the bone ends need to be washed with sterile fluid in the operating room as an emergency procedure to prevent infection. The washing process may need to be repeated if the wound becomes infected.

Indications: Surgical repair is recommended for complicated fractures that are not able to be realigned (reduced) by external, nonsurgical methods. This is especially true of fractures that involve joints, as misalignment of joint surfaces may contribute to the development of arthritis.

Risks: Risks for any anesthesia include the following:

• Reactions to medications

• Problems breathing

Risks for surgery include bleeding and infection.

Expectations: Surgery often allows a person to regain movement and heal faster than nonsurgical treatment. A patient's long-term outlook depends on the severity of the fracture. It is usually not necessary to remove an internal fixation device unless it causes problems.

Convalescence: The length of the hospital stay depends on factors such as the condition of the bone, the presence of infection, the state of the blood and nerve supply, and presence of other injuries. Most fractures heal by six to twelve weeks. Children's bones heal rapidly, usually in six weeks.

Source: "Bone Fracture Repair," © 2007 A.D.A.M., Inc. Reprinted with permission.

Can broken bones be prevented?

Although fractures are a common part of childhood for many kids, some children are more likely to have broken bones than others. For example, children with an inherited condition known as osteogenesis imperfecta have bones that are brittle and more susceptible to breaking.

✔ Quick Tip

I don't want to risk breaking another bone. Should I spend more time "on the sidelines" from now on?

It is perfectly understandable that you want to avoid another fracture. No one who has broken a bone wants to revisit that pain and loss of independence. However, living your life "on the sidelines" is not an effective way to protect your bones. Remaining physically active reduces your risk of heart disease, colon cancer, and type 2 diabetes. It may also protect you against prostate and breast cancer, high blood pressure, obesity, and mood disorders such as depression and anxiety. If that isn't enough to convince you to stay active, consider this: exercise is one of the best ways to preserve your bone density and prevent falls as you age.

What type of exercise is best to reduce my risk of another fracture?

Exercise can reduce your risk of fracturing in two ways: by helping you build and maintain bone density; and by enhancing your balance, flexibility, and strength, all of which reduce your chance of falling.

Building and maintaining bone density: Bone is a living tissue that responds to exercise by becoming stronger. Just as a muscle gets stronger and bigger with use, a bone becomes stronger and denser when it is called upon to bear weight. Two types of exercise are important for building and maintaining bone density: weight-bearing and resistance. Weight-bearing exercises are those in which your bones and muscles work against gravity. Examples include walking, climbing stairs, dancing, and playing tennis. Resistance exercises are those that use muscular strength to improve muscle mass and strengthen bone. The best example of a resistance exercise is weight lifting, with either free weights or weight machines.

Source: Excerpted from "Once Is Enough: A Guide to Preventing Future Fractures," National Institute of Arthritis and Musculoskeletal and Skin Diseases (NIAMS), May 2006.

Be sure you are getting enough calcium to decrease the risk of developing osteoporosis (a condition that also causes the bones to be more fragile and likely to break) later down the line. Also, don't forget to get involved in regular physical activities and exercise, which are very important to bone health. Weight-bearing exercises such as jumping rope, jogging, and walking can also help develop and maintain strong bones.

Although it's impossible to keep out of harm's way all the time, you can help to prevent some injuries by taking simple safety precautions. You can minimize injuries by making sure you always wear helmets and safety gear when participating in sports and using seat belts.

If you do get a broken bone, remember that even though it can be frightening, a fracture is a common, treatable injury that many people experience at one time or another. With a little patience, you will be back to playing and running around before you know it.

♣ It's A Fact!!
Youth Overweight Increases Risk Of Bone Fractures, Muscle And Joint Pain

Children and adolescents who are overweight are more likely than their normal weight counterparts to suffer bone fractures and have joint and muscle pains, according to a study conducted at the National Institutes of Health. The study appears in the June 2006 *Pediatrics*.

The researchers found that the overweight youth were more likely to experience bone fractures and muscle and joint pain than were the non-overweight group. The most common self-reported joint complaint was knee pain, with 21.4 percent of overweight youth reporting knee pain and 16.7 percent of non-overweight youth reporting knee pain. The overweight youth were also more likely to report impaired mobility than the non-overweight youth. Dual energy x-ray absorptiometry (DXA) scans showed that overweight youth were more likely to experience changes in how the bones of the thigh and leg meet at their knees, than were non-overweight youth.

Source: Excerpted from an NIH News Release, National Institute of Child Health and Human Development (NICHD), June 6, 2006.

Chapter 19

Casts, Splints, and Crutches

General Information

Splints and casts support and protect injured bones and soft tissue, reducing pain, swelling, and muscle spasm. In some cases, splints and casts are applied following surgery.

Casts are custom-made and applied by your doctor or an assistant. Casts are often made of plaster or fiberglass. Splints or half casts also can be custom-made, especially if an exact fit is necessary. Other times, a ready-made splint will be used. These off-the-shelf splints are made in a variety of shapes and sizes, and are much easier and faster to use. They have Velcro straps which make the splints easy to adjust and easier to put on and take off. Unfortunately, splints offer less support and protection than a cast and may not be a treatment option in all circumstances.

Fiberglass or plaster materials form the hard supportive layer in splints and casts. Fiberglass is lighter in weight, longer wearing, and "breathes" better than plaster. Both materials come in strips or rolls which are dipped in water and applied over a layer of cotton or synthetic padding covering the injured area. Both fiberglass and plaster splints and casts use padding, usually cotton, as a protective layer next to the skin. When cotton padding, synthetic padding, or plaster is used in the making of a cast, the cast must be kept dry. If these materials become wet significant problems may develop. When a plaster cast gets wet, the cast becomes soft, loses strength, and may no longer adequately immobilize the injured area. As a result, broken bones may heal in the incorrect position if the cast is not replaced. When the cotton or synthetic padding gets wet, it is very difficult to dry. As a result, the wet skin under the wet padding may develop rashes, infections, or become macerated. All of these conditions, require further treatment. To keep these types of casts dry, it is necessary to wear plastic shower bags which are commercially available.

Recently, Gortex cast padding has been developed. This padding is completely waterproof and allows a patient to completely immerse the cast in water without requiring the protection of a plastic bag. With this type of cast padding, coupled with the application of a fiberglass cast, patients may do activities such as showering and swimming without worrying about keeping the injured extremity dry. However, there are some clinical circumstances when this type of cast padding may not be applied.

The splint or cast must fit the shape of the injured arm or leg correctly to provide the best possible support. Sometimes, it may be necessary to replace a cast as swelling decreases and the cast "gets too big." Often as a fracture heals, a splint may be applied again to allow easy removal for therapy.

Cast Care Tips

If your treatment is to be successful, you must follow your doctor's instructions carefully. The following information provides general guidelines only, and is not a substitute for your doctor's advice.

Dos Of Cast Care

1. Swelling due to your injury may cause pressure in your splint or cast for the first 48 to 72 hours. This may cause your injured arm or leg to feel snug or tight in the splint or cast. To reduce the swelling:

✔ Quick Tip

Going Up The Stairs With Crutches

1. Hold the railing with one hand and the crutches together in the other hand.

2. Step up with the "good" or uninvolved leg.

3. Bring the crutches up with the "bad" or injured leg.

Going Down The Stairs With Crutches

1. Stand close to edge and put crutches down to step with the involved leg.

2. Step down with the "good" leg.

To Stand Up With Crutches

1. Hold both crutches in one hand by the hand grips.

2. Put other hand on chair arm and stand.

3. When you are standing, take one crutch and put it under the opposite arm.

Guidelines For Crutch Use

1. Stand straight, shoulders, relaxed.

2. Top of crutch should lie against the ribs, two to three finger widths from the armpit.

3. Hand grips should be positioned so that there is a slight bend in the elbows.

4. Crutch tips should also be about 6 inches from each foot and out to the side.

5. Never hang or press down on the underarm pads. All weight should be on the hands.

Source: "Crutch Use Instructions," reprinted with permission from the Center for Orthopaedics and Sports Medicine www.arthroscopy.com). © 2003. All rights reserved. This material does not constitute medical advice. It is intended for informational purposes only. Please consult a physician for specific treatment recommendations.

- Elevate your injured arm or leg above your heart by propping it up on pillows or some other support. You will have to recline if the splint or cast is on your leg. Elevation allows clear fluid and blood to drain "downhill" to your heart.

- Exercise the fingers or toes to decrease swelling and prevent stiffness and to increase circulation.

- Apply ice to the splint or cast. Place the ice in a dry plastic bag or ice pack and loosely wrap it around the splint or cast at the level of the injury. Ice that is packed in a rigid container and touches the cast at only one point will not be effective.

2. Keep your cast dry if it has a cotton or synthetic lining or if it is a plaster cast. Use a shower bag for bathing.

3. If you have a Gortex cast, you may shower or swim, but rinse well with tap water afterwards.

4. File down any rough spots with an emery board.

5. To ease any discomfort from itching, you may blow cool air inside the cast with a hair dryer.

6. Check circulation by pressing on the nail bed. The nail should turn pale when pressed, but normal color should return immediately when the pressure on the nail is removed. If this does not happen, contact your physician.

7. Inspect the skin around the cast. If your skin becomes red or raw around the cast, contact your doctor.

8. Inspect the cast regularly. If it becomes cracked or develops soft spots, contact your doctor.

9. Keep dirt, sand, and powder away from the inside of your splint or cast.

Don'ts Of Cast Care

1. Do not get your cast wet, unless you have a Gortex cast.

2. Do not insert any object objects such as coat hangers into the cast to relieve itching. Instead, use the cool setting on a hair dryer to blow air into the cast.

3. Do not apply powders or deodorants to itching skin. If itching persists, contact your doctor.

4. Do not pull out the cast padding. It is there to protect your skin.

5. Do not break or trim the cast edges.

Warning Signs Following Splint/Cast Application

After application of a splint or cast, it is very important to elevate your injured arm or leg for 24 to 72 hours. The injured area should be elevated well above the heart. Rest and elevation greatly reduce pain and speed the healing process by minimizing early swelling. If you experience any of the following warning signs, contact your doctor's office immediately for advice.

- Increased pain and swelling which is not controlled with ice, elevation, and/or pain medication

- A feeling that the splint or cast is too tight

- Numbness and tingling in your hand or foot

- Burning and stinging

- Excessive swelling below the cast

- Loss of active movement of toes or fingers, which requires an urgent evaluation by your doctor

- A feeling of a blister developing in your cast

- A feeling that your calf is becoming swollen, tight, and painful inside the cast

- You notice any unusual odor coming from inside the cast

- If the cast breaks or becomes too loose

- If the cast edges are causing skin problems

- If a fever develops

Proper Cast Removal

Never remove the cast yourself. You may cut your skin or prevent proper healing of your injury. Your doctor will use a cast saw to remove your cast. The saw vibrates, but does not rotate. If the blade of the saw touches the padding inside the hard shell of the cast, the padding will vibrate with the blade.

Chapter 20

Concussions

Jake banged his head hard when he was tackled, and he felt kind of weird afterward. He thought it was just another hit that he could shake off—and he wanted to stay on the field. After the game, though, he felt pretty sick. Should Jake have kept on playing?

Probably not. Jake may have had a concussion—and it was actually a bad idea for him to stay in the game.

What is a concussion and what causes it?

The brain is made of soft tissue and is cushioned by spinal fluid. It is encased in the hard, protective skull. When a person gets a head injury, the brain can slosh around inside the skull and even bang against it. This can lead to bruising of the brain, tearing of blood vessels, and injury to the nerves. When this happens, a person can get a concussion—a temporary loss of normal brain function. Most people with concussions recover just fine with appropriate treatment. But it's important to take proper steps if you suspect a concussion because it can be serious.

About This Chapter: "Concussions," May 2007, reprinted with permission from www.kidshealth.org. Copyright © 2007 The Nemours Foundation. This information was provided by KidsHealth, one of the largest resources online for medically reviewed health information written for parents, kids, and teens. For more articles like this one, visit www.KidsHealth.org, or www.TeensHealth.org.

Concussions and other brain injuries are fairly common. About every 21 seconds, someone in the United States has a serious brain injury. One of the most common reasons people get concussions is through a sports injury. High-contact sports such as football, boxing, and hockey pose a higher risk of head injury, even with the use of protective headgear.

People can also get concussions from falls, car accidents, bike and blading mishaps, and physical violence, such as fighting. Guys are more likely to get concussions than girls. However, in certain sports, like soccer, girls have a higher potential for concussion.

What are the signs and symptoms?

The signs of concussion are not always well recognized. And because of that, teens may put themselves at risk for another injury. For example, players may return to a game before they should, or a skateboarder may get back on the board and continue skating, thinking nothing's wrong. That's a problem, because if the brain hasn't healed properly from a concussion and someone gets another brain injury (even if it's with less force), it can be serious.

Repeated injury to the brain can lead to swelling, and sometimes people develop long-term disabilities, or even die, as a result of serious head injuries. So it's really important to recognize and understand the signals of a concussion.

Although we may think of a concussion as someone losing consciousness (passing out), a person can have a concussion and never lose consciousness.

Symptoms of a concussion may include:

- "seeing stars" and feeling dazed, dizzy, or lightheaded;
- memory loss, such as trouble remembering things that happened right before and after the injury;
- nausea or vomiting;
- headaches;

- blurred vision and sensitivity to light;

- slurred speech or saying things that don't make sense;

- difficulty concentrating, thinking, or making decisions;

- difficulty with coordination or balance (such as being unable to catch a ball or other easy tasks);

- feeling anxious or irritable for no apparent reason;

- feeling overly tired.

Different Grades Of Concussion: There are different grades of concussion:

- Someone with a grade 1 concussion can have some of the symptoms listed above, but with no loss of consciousness and with symptoms ending within 15 minutes.

- With a grade 2 concussion, there has been no loss of consciousness but the symptoms last longer than 15 minutes.

- In a grade 3 concussion, the person loses consciousness—even if it's just for a few seconds.

Knowing the different grades is important because how soon a player can safely return to a sports activity is tied to the grade of the concussion:

- With a grade 1 concussion, the player can resume play once symptoms have stopped. However, that player should stop play if he or she gets another head injury.

- A grade 2 concussion requires that a player stop playing and not return to any type of sport or physical activity that could cause a head injury for at least another week.

- Someone with a grade 3 concussion should see a doctor as quickly as possible.

What should you do if a friend or teammate has a concussion? Tell an adult or coach immediately. Even if the concussion seems mild, the player should sit out for the rest of the game. If the symptoms are severe (such as seizures or a very long period of unconsciousness) or they seem to be getting worse, that's an indication of a serious head injury. Get medical help right away.

What do doctors do?

If a doctor suspects that someone may have a concussion, he or she will ask about the head injury—such as how it happened and when—and the symptoms. The doctor may ask what seem like silly questions—things like "Who are you?" or "Where are you?" or "What day is it?" and "Who is the president?" Doctors ask these questions to check the person's level of consciousness and memory and concentration abilities.

The doctor will perform a thorough examination of the nervous system, including testing balance, coordination of movement, and reflexes. The doctor may ask the patient to do some activity such as running in place for a few minutes to see how well the brain functions after a physical workout.

Sometimes a doctor may order a CT scan (a special brain x-ray) or an MRI (a special non-x-ray brain image) to rule out bleeding or other serious injury involving the brain.

If the concussion isn't serious enough to require hospitalization, the doctor will give instructions on what to do at home, like having someone wake the person up at least once during the night. If a person with a concussion cannot be easily awakened, becomes increasingly confused, or has other symptoms such as vomiting, it may mean there is a more severe problem that requires contacting the doctor again.

The doctor will probably recommend that someone with a concussion take acetaminophen or other aspirin-free medications for headaches. The person also will have to take things easy at school or work.

Can concussions be prevented?

Some accidents can't be avoided. But you can do a lot to prevent a concussion by taking simple precautions:

- Always wear a seat belt in a car. If you drive, be attentive at all times, and obey speed limits, signs, and safe-driving laws to reduce the chances of having an accident. Driving rules and regulations were created to protect everyone. Never use alcohol or other drugs when you're behind the wheel. There's a reason it's illegal: Alcohol and drugs make your reaction time slower and impair your judgment, making you much more likely to have an accident.

• Wearing appropriate headgear and safety equipment when biking, blading, skateboarding, snowboarding or skiing, and playing contact sports can significantly reduce your chances of having a concussion. By wearing a bike helmet, for instance, you can reduce your risk of having a concussion by about 85%.

Taking good care of yourself after a concussion is essential. If you re-injure your brain during the time it is still healing, it will take even more time to completely heal. Each time a person has a concussion, it does additional damage. Having multiple concussions over a period of time has the same effect on a person as being knocked unconscious for several hours.

Preventing concussions is mostly common sense. The best thing you can do to protect your head is to use it!

♣ It's A Fact!!
After A Concussion

After a concussion, the brain needs time to heal. It's really important to wait until all symptoms of a concussion have cleared up before returning to normal activities. The amount of time someone needs to recover depends on how long the symptoms last. Healthy teens can usually resume their normal activities within a few weeks, but each situation is different. A doctor will monitor the person closely to make sure everything's OK.

Someone who has had a concussion and has not recovered within a few months is said to have postconcussion syndrome. The person may have the same problems described earlier—such as poor memory, headaches, dizziness, and irritability—but these will last for longer periods of time and may even be permanent.

If someone has continuing problems after a concussion, the doctor may refer him or her to a rehabilitation specialist for additional help.

Chapter 21

Facial Sports Injuries

Playing catch, shooting hoops, bicycling, on a scenic path or just kicking around a soccer ball have more in common than you may think. On the up side, these activities are good exercise and are enjoyed by thousands of Americans. On the down side, they can result in a variety of injuries to the face.

Many injuries are preventable by wearing the proper protective gear, and your attitude toward safety can make a big difference. However, even the most careful person can get hurt. When an accident happens, it's your response that can make the difference between a temporary inconvenience and permanent injury.

When Someone Gets Hurt

- Ask "Are you all right?" Determine whether the injured person is breathing and knows who and where they are.

- Be certain the person can see, hear, and maintain balance. Watch for subtle changes in behavior or speech, such as slurring or stuttering. Any abnormal response requires medical attention.

- Note weakness or loss of movement in the forehead, eyelids, cheeks, and mouth.

- Look at the eyes to make sure they move in the same direction and that both pupils are the same size.

- If any doubts exist, seek immediate medical attention.

When Medical Attention Is Required, What Can You Do?

- Call for medical assistance (911).

- Do not move the victim, or remove helmets or protective gear.

- Do not give food, drink, or medication until the extent of the injury has been determined.

- Remember HIV...be very careful around body fluids. In an emergency protect your hands with plastic bags.

> ♣ **It's A Fact!!**
> **What first aid supplies should you have on hand in case of an emergency?**
>
> - Sterile cloth or pads
> - Scissors
> - Ice pack
> - Tape
> - Sterile bandages
> - Cotton tipped swabs
> - Hydrogen peroxide
> - Nose drops
> - Antibiotic ointment
> - Eye pads
> - Cotton balls
> - Butterfly bandages

- Apply pressure to bleeding wounds with a clean cloth or pad, unless the eye or eyelid is affected or a loose bone can be felt in a head injury. In these cases, do not apply pressure but gently cover the wound with a clean cloth.

- Apply ice or a cold pack to areas that have suffered a blow (such as a bump on the head) to help control swelling and pain.

- Remember to advise your doctor if the patient has HIV or hepatitis.

Facial Fractures

Sports injuries can cause potentially serious broken bones or fractures of the face. Common symptoms of facial fractures include:

- swelling and bruising, such as a black eye;
- pain or numbness in the face, cheeks or lips;
- double or blurred vision;

- nosebleeds;
- changes in teeth structure or ability to close mouth properly.

It is important to pay attention to swelling because it may be masking a more serious injury. Applying ice packs and keeping the head elevated may reduce early swelling.

If any of these symptoms occur, be sure to visit the emergency room or the office of a facial plastic surgeon (such as an otolaryngologist-head and neck surgeon) where x-rays may be taken to determine if there is a fracture.

Upper Face

When you are hit in the upper face (by a ball for example) it can fracture the delicate bones around the sinuses, eye sockets, bridge of the nose, or cheek bones. A direct blow to the eye may cause a fracture, as well as blurred or double vision. All eye injuries should be examined by an eye specialist (ophthalmologist).

Lower Face

When your jaw or lower face is injured, it may change the way your teeth fit together. To restore a normal bite, surgeries often can be performed from inside the mouth to prevent visible scarring of the face; and broken jaws often can be repaired without being wired shut for long periods. Your doctor will explain your treatment options and the latest treatment techniques.

Soft Tissue Injuries

Bruises, cuts, and scrapes often result from high speed or contact sports, such as boxing, football, soccer, ice hockey, bicycling skiing, and snowmobiling. Most can be treated at home, but some require medical attention.

You should get immediate medical care when you have:

- deep skin cuts;
- obvious deformity or fracture;
- loss of facial movement;
- persistent bleeding;

- change in vision;
- problems breathing and/or swallowing;
- alterations in consciousness or facial movement.

Bruises

Also called contusions, bruises result from bleeding underneath the skin. Applying pressure, elevating the bruised area above the heart, and using an ice pack for the first 24 to 48 hours minimizes discoloration and swelling. After two days, a heat pack or hot water bottle may help more. Most of the swelling and bruising should disappear in one to two weeks.

Cuts And Scrapes

The external bleeding that results from cuts and scrapes can be stopped by immediately applying pressure with gauze or a clean cloth. When the bleeding is uncontrollable, you should go to the emergency room.

Scrapes should be washed with soap and water to remove any foreign material that could cause infection and discoloration of the skin. Scrapes or abrasions can be treated at home by cleaning with 3% hydrogen peroxide and covering with an antibiotic ointment or cream until the skin is healed. Cuts or lacerations, unless very small, should be examined by a physician. Stitches may be necessary, and deeper cuts may have serious effects. Following stitches, cuts should be kept clean and free of scabs with hydrogen peroxide and antibiotic ointment. Bandages may be needed to protect the area from pressure or irritation from clothes. You may experience numbness around the cut for several months. Healing will continue for six to 12 months. The application of sunscreen is important during the healing process to prevent pigment changes. Scars that look too obvious after this time should be seen by a facial plastic surgeon.

Nasal Injuries

The nose is one of the most injured areas on the face. Early treatment of a nose injury consists of applying a cold compress and keeping the head higher than the rest of the body. You should seek medical attention in the case of:

- breathing difficulties;

- deformity of the nose;

- persistent bleeding;

- cuts.

Bleeding

Nosebleeds are common and usually short-lived. Often they can be controlled by squeezing the nose with constant pressure for five to ten minutes. If bleeding persists, seek medical attention.

Bleeding also can occur underneath the surface of the nose. An otolaryngologist/facial plastic surgeon will examine the nose to determine if there is a clot or collection of blood beneath the mucus membrane of the septum (a septal hematoma) or any fracture. Hematomas should be drained so the pressure does not cause nose damage or infection.

Fractures

Some otolaryngologist-head and neck specialists set fractured bones right away before swelling develops, while others prefer to wait until the swelling is gone. These fractures can be repaired under local or general anesthesia, even weeks later.

Ultimately, treatment decisions will be made to restore proper function of the nasal air passages and normal appearance and structural support of the nose. Swelling and bruising of the nose may last for ten days or more.

Neck Injuries

Whether seemingly minor or severe, all neck injuries should be thoroughly evaluated by an otolaryngologist—head and neck surgeon. Injuries may involve specific structures within the neck, such as the larynx (voicebox), esophagus (food passage), or major blood vessels and nerves.

Throat Injuries

The larynx is a complex organ consisting of cartilage, nerves, and muscles with a mucous membrane lining all encased in a protective tissue (cartilage) framework.

The cartilages can be fractured or dislocated and may cause severe swelling, which can result in airway obstruction. Hoarseness or difficulty breathing after a blow to the neck are warning signs of a serious injury and the injured person should receive immediate medical attention.

✔ Quick Tip
Prevention Of Facial Sports Injuries

The best way to treat facial sports injuries is to prevent them. To insure a safe athletic environment, the following guidelines are suggested:

- Be sure the playing areas are large enough that players will not run into walls or other obstructions.

- Cover unremoveable goal posts and other structures with thick, protective padding.

- Carefully check equipment to be sure it is functioning properly.

- Require protective equipment—such as helmets and padding for football, bicycling, and in-line skating; face masks, head and mouth guards for baseball; ear protectors for wrestlers; and eyeglass guards or goggles for racquetball and snowmobiling are just a few.

- Prepare athletes with warm-up exercises before engaging in intense team activity.

- In the case of sports involving fast-moving vehicles, for example, snowmobiles or dirt bikes—check the path of travel, making sure there are no obstructing fences, wires, or other obstacles.

- Enlist adequate adult supervision for all children's competitive sports.

Chapter 22

Dental Injuries

There are a number of simple precautions you can take to avoid accident and injury to your teeth. One way to reduce the chances of damage to your teeth, lips, cheek, and tongue is to wear a mouthguard when participating in sports or recreational activities that may pose a risk. Avoid chewing ice, popcorn kernels, and hard candy, all of which can crack a tooth. Cut tape using scissors rather than your teeth.

Accidents do happen, and knowing what to do when one occurs can mean the difference between saving and losing a tooth.

Most dentists reserve time in their daily schedules for emergency patients. Call your dentist and provide as much detail as possible about your condition. Remember, pain is a signal that something is wrong—a problem that will not disappear even if the pain subsides. If you're concerned about visiting the dentist because you have limited or no dental insurance, ask your dentist if the practice offers a convenient outside monthly payment plan. If the answer is yes, you can submit an application online and get an immediate credit decision—and the emergency care you need.

About This Chapter: "Dental Emergencies and Injuries," © American Dental Association. Reprinted with permission.

Tips For Dealing With Dental Emergencies

Bitten Lip Or Tongue: Clean the area gently with a cloth and apply cold compresses to reduce any swelling. If the bleeding doesn't stop, go to a hospital emergency room immediately.

Broken Tooth: Rinse your mouth with warm water to clean the area. Use cold compresses on the area to keep any swelling down. Call your dentist immediately.

Jaw—Possibly Broken: Apply cold compresses to control swelling. Go to your dentist or a hospital emergency department immediately.

Knocked Out Tooth: Hold the tooth by the crown and rinse off the root of the tooth in water if it's dirty. Do not scrub it or remove any attached tissue fragments. If possible, gently insert and hold the tooth in its socket. If that isn't possible, put the tooth in a cup of milk and get to the dentist as quickly as possible. Remember to take the tooth with you!

Objects Caught Between Teeth: Try to gently remove the object with dental floss; avoid cutting the gums. Never use a sharp instrument to remove any object that is stuck between your teeth. If you can't dislodge the object using dental floss, contact your dentist.

Toothache: Rinse your mouth with warm water to clean it out. Gently use dental floss or an interdental cleaner to ensure that there is no food or other debris caught between the teeth. Never put aspirin or any other painkiller against the gums near the aching tooth because it may burn the gum tissue. If the pain persists, contact your dentist.

Chapter 23

Back And Neck Injuries

Spinal Injuries In Adolescent Athletes

Because of their age and involvement in vigorous activities and sports, adolescents risk injury to the spine (back bone). Certain types of sport activities increase the risk of injury, especially to the lower back. However, these athletes can take steps to prevent many types of spinal injuries.

Anatomy And Skeletal Development

The spine is made up of vertebrae (bones), intervertebral disks (shock absorbers between vertebrae), and the spinal cord and other nerves. The vertebrae and intervertebral disks protect the spinal cord, and they enable the torso to move in many directions.

Physes (growth plates) are areas on the ends of a child's bones where the bone grows. As the skeleton matures, the physes harden, and bones stop growing. Girls reach skeletal maturity at about 16½ years of age; boys, at about 17½ or 18.

About This Chapter: This chapter includes "Spinal Injuries in Adolescent Athletes," by Lawrence Parker, MD, *Hughston Health Alert*, Fall 1999; and "Cervical Spine Fractures," by Lawrence Parker, MD, *Hughston Health Alert*, Winter 1997. © Hughston Sports Medicine Foundation, Inc. Reprinted with permission. Both were reviewed in November 2007. Additional text under the heading "How Is Back Pain Treated" is excerpted from "Handout on Health: Back Pain," National Institute of Arthritis and Musculoskeletal and Skin Diseases (www.niams.nih.gov), September 2005.

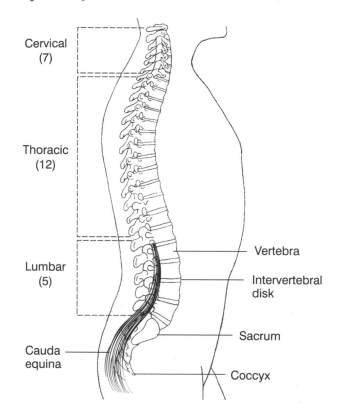

Figure 23.1. Side View Of Spine (Source: NIAMS, 2005).

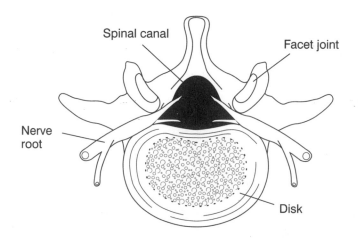

Figure 23.2. Normal Vertebra, Cross Section (Source: NIAMS, 2005).

Causes

Trauma and repetitive stress can cause back injury in adolescent athletes. Repetitive bending and twisting put athletes at risk for spinal injuries. During long training days, athletes are at increased risk of injury because their fatigued bodies cannot give full protection to the back. Using improper sport technique and having weak abdominal and tight leg muscles also can lead to injury.

The lumbar vertebrae (bones of the lower back) are more prone to injury in the growing adolescent, especially during sports participation. Ligaments and muscles that support the spine may not grow as fast as bone, and, therefore, they may become tight, putting increased stress on the spine.

Difficult maneuvers involving "flight" account for most spinal injuries. During these activities, the athlete is airborne and lands on a hard surface, such as the floor in gymnastics, or the water, such as in diving maneuvers. Other activities associated with spinal injuries include blocking in football, takedowns in wrestling, and use of heavy weights and attempts at complex free-weight lifts in weight training.

Specific Injuries

Spondylolysis And Spondylolisthesis: Putting repetitive stress on the vertebrae can cause a thin area of bone, called the pars interarticularis, to fracture (break). Spondylolysis refers to a fracture on one side of the pars interarticularis. In spondylolisthesis, the fracture has occurred on both sides of this area and the fractured vertebra has slipped forward against its neighboring vertebra. Repetitive hyperextension of the lower back, such as excessive back bends by gymnasts or by football linebackers, can lead to these conditions.

Disk Herniation: Intervertebral disks are made up of firm, gristle-like fibers that encompass a soft, fluid-like center. Disk material can bulge into the spinal canal and push on the spinal cord or another nerve.

In adolescents, disk herniation most commonly results from repetitive trauma to the back. In adolescents, a vertebral growth plate and its adjacent disk can become displaced into the spinal canal and push on the spinal cord. This condition is called slipped vertebral apophysis. It usually results from heavy lifting or from participation in sports that require very strenuous training, such as gymnastics.

♣ **It's A Fact!!**

Spine injuries such as sprains and fractures can cause either short-lived or chronic pain. Sprains are tears in the ligaments that support the spine, and they can occur from twisting or lifting improperly. Fractured vertebrae are often the result of osteoporosis, a condition that causes weak, porous bones. Less commonly, back pain may be caused by more severe injuries that result from accidents and falls.

Source: "Handout on Health: Back Pain," National Institute of Arthritis and Musculoskeletal and Skin Diseases (www.niams.nih.gov), September 2005.

Fractures: Blows to the back can cause fractures to certain parts of the vertebrae. Likewise, the physes and sacrum (tail bone) also can be fractured. Activities in which the athlete can get hit in the back or can fall from a great height can lead to spinal fractures.

Scheuermann Disease: This condition results in an exaggerated curve (hump) of the upper back involving at least two abnormally wedge-shaped vertebrae. The cause is not known.

Symptoms

Pain often accompanies back injuries. In many cases, activity makes the pain worse. To determine the seriousness of your back problem, pay attention to whether you have back pain at night, limited movement of the lower back, or pain that goes down the leg. If you have these symptoms, you need to seek treatment from a doctor.

Treatment

To treat a back injury, the adolescent athlete must stop playing the sport and participating in weight training, and he or she must see a doctor. The primary care doctor examines the athlete's back and, if necessary, refers the adolescent to an orthopaedic doctor. The doctor may prescribe a pain medication. Some adolescents need to wear a back brace as part of the treatment. A physical therapist instructs the athlete in appropriate conditioning, stretching, and strengthening exercises to rehabilitate the back and to enable him or her to return to sports participation.

After treatment, the doctor decides when the adolescent athlete can return to sports participation. Sometimes, the athlete has to decrease the intensity of practice or change the way he or she performs a particular activity.

You should be aware that the problem can reoccur. If it does, the adolescent will have to receive treatment again.

Prevention

Adults can help adolescent athletes prevent spinal injury. For example, coaches can institute shorter practices. Properly trained coaches, athletic trainers, parents, or other adults can supervise training sessions. They also can teach proper technique for weight training and various exercises.

Low back injury in adolescents is a serious problem. However, if diagnosed and treated properly, the athlete usually can return to vigorous activities.

Cervical Spine Fractures

The human spine comprises 24 vertebrae, or small bones containing the spinal cord. These vertebrae are grouped into three sections according to location: cervical spine (neck), thoracic spine (middle back), and lumbar spine (lower back). Soft tissues, such as ligaments (tissues that connect bones), muscles, and skin, surround and support the spine. Seven vertebrae form the

---

✔ Quick Tip
Which type of doctor should I see?

Many different types of doctors treat back pain, from family physicians to doctors who specialize in disorders of the nerves and musculoskeletal system. In most cases, it is best to see your primary care physician first. In many cases, he or she can treat the problem. In other cases, your doctor may refer you to an appropriate specialist.

Source: "Handout on Health: Back Pain," National Institute of Arthritis and Musculoskeletal and Skin Diseases (www.niams.nih.gov), September 2005.

cervical spine. This section of the spine connects the base of the head to the thorax (trunk and shoulders) and, with the help of soft tissues, supports the head. A fracture (break) of the cervical spine is commonly referred to as a broken neck.

Most injuries that involve the neck or cervical spine are the result of a violent collision that compresses the cervical spine against the shoulders. This force can be so great that a vertebra fractures or even bursts into small fragments. For example, striking your head against the bottom of a pool in shallow water or "spear" tackling using the crown of your helmet to stop an opposing football player can fracture the cervical spine.

Cervical spine injuries may also occur during motor vehicle accidents when the head is violently jerked either backwards or forwards. This type of accident may not cause a fracture but instead injure the muscles and ligaments of the neck. The resulting injury is a neck sprain, which is commonly called whiplash.

Regardless of the cause, cervical spine fractures are serious injuries; they may involve spinal cord damage that can result in partial or complete paralysis or even death.

If you suspect that someone has a neck injury, immediately contact emergency medical services. Do not move the person yourself—no matter how uncomfortable they look. Emergency medical technicians are trained in the proper treatment of people who have neck injuries. If you move a person who has a cervical spine fracture, you risk further injuring that person.

The surgeon will x-ray the injured person's spine to find out if the cervical spine is fractured. To treat the fractured spine, the surgeon first reduces it through traction. This process involves inserting tongs into the skull, attaching a pulley to the tongs, and attaching small weights to the other end of the pulley. The weights pull the head away from the shoulders just enough to enable the soft tissues around the spine to push the fractured bone back into place. After the fracture is reduced, the surgeon examines the spinal cord for damage. Because the spinal cord is soft tissue, it cannot be seen on an x-ray. Therefore, the surgeon injects a dye into the damaged area that coats the spinal cord and other soft tissues so they can be seen on an x-ray.

Most cervical spine fractures must be treated surgically. The surgeon chooses the treatment method based on the severity of the fracture. For example, the fractured vertebra may be fused to the healthy vertebra next to it, or it may be removed and replaced with a bone graft that is fused to the vertebrae on either side.

Cervical spine fractures and other neck injuries occur less frequently because people are more educated about how fractures occur and about how to prevent them. Protect yourself and your family by always wearing a seatbelt, supervising children and adolescents who are swimming and diving in lakes and pools, and using the proper equipment and training during athletic participation. If a significant neck injury does occur, be sure to contact your local emergency medical services for help.

How Is Back Pain Treated

Treatment for back pain generally depends on what kind of pain you experience: acute or chronic.

Acute Back Pain: Acute back pain usually gets better on its own and without treatment, although you may want to try acetaminophen, aspirin, or ibuprofen to help ease the pain. Perhaps the best advice is to go about your usual activities as much as you can with the assurance that the problem will clear up. Getting up and moving around can help ease stiffness, relieve pain, and have you back doing your regular activities sooner. Exercises are not usually advisable for acute back pain, nor is surgery.

Chronic Back Pain: Treatment for chronic back pain falls into two basic categories: the kind that requires an operation and the kind that does not. In the vast majority of cases, back pain does not require surgery. Doctors will almost always try nonsurgical treatments before recommending surgery. In a very small percentage of cases—when back pain is caused by a tumor, an infection, or a nerve root problem called cauda equina syndrome, for example—prompt surgery is necessary to ease the pain and prevent further problems.

Following are some of the more commonly used treatments for chronic back pain.

Nonoperative Treatments

Hot Or Cold: Hot or cold packs—or sometimes a combination of the two—can be soothing to chronically sore, stiff backs. Heat dilates the blood vessels, improving the supply of oxygen that the blood takes to the back and reducing muscle spasms. Heat also alters the sensation of pain. Cold may reduce inflammation by decreasing the size of blood vessels and the flow of blood to the area. Although cold may feel painful against the skin, it numbs deep pain. Applying heat or cold may relieve pain, but it does not cure the cause of chronic back pain.

Exercise: Although exercise is usually not advisable for acute back pain, proper exercise can help ease chronic pain and perhaps reduce its risk of returning. The following four types of exercise are important to general physical fitness and may be helpful for certain specific causes of back pain:

- **Flexion:** The purposes of flexion exercises, which are exercises in which you bend forward, are to 1) widen the spaces between the vertebrae, thereby reducing pressure on the nerves; 2) stretch muscles of the back and hips; and 3) strengthen abdominal and buttock muscles. Many doctors think that strengthening the muscles of the abdomen will reduce the load on the spine. One word of caution: If your back pain is caused by a herniated disc, check with your doctor before performing flexion exercises because they may increase pressure within the discs, making the problem worse.

- **Extension:** With extension exercises, you bend backward. They may minimize radiating pain, which is pain you can feel in other parts of the body besides where it originates. Examples of extension exercises are leg lifting while lying prone and raising the trunk while lying prone. The theory behind these exercises is that they open up the spinal canal in places and develop muscles that support the spine.

- **Stretching:** The goal of stretching exercises, as their name suggests, is to stretch and improve the extension of muscles and other soft tissues of the back. This can reduce back stiffness and improve range of motion.

- **Aerobic:** Aerobic exercise is the type that gets your heart pumping faster and keeps your heart rate elevated for a while. For fitness, it is important to get at least 30 minutes of aerobic (also called cardiovascular) exercise three times a week. Aerobic exercises work the large muscles of the body and include brisk walking, jogging, and swimming. For back problems, you should avoid exercise that requires twisting or vigorous forward flexion, such as aerobic dancing and rowing, because these actions may raise pressure in the discs and actually do more harm than good. In addition, avoid high-impact activities if you have disc disease. If back pain or your fitness level makes it impossible to exercise 30 minutes at a time, try three 10-minute sessions to start with and work up to your goal. But first, speak with your doctor or physical therapist about the safest aerobic exercise for you.

Medications: A wide range of medications are used to treat chronic back pain. Some you can try on your own. Others are available only with a doctor's prescription. The following are the main types of medications used for back pain.

- **Analgesics:** Analgesic medications are those designed specifically to relieve pain. They include over-the-counter acetaminophen (Tylenol) and aspirin, as well as prescription narcotics, such as oxycodone with acetaminophen (Percocet) or hydrocodone with acetaminophen (Vicodin). Aspirin and acetaminophen are the most commonly used analgesics; narcotics should only be used for a short time for severe pain or pain after surgery. People with muscular back pain or arthritis pain that is not relieved by medications may find topical analgesics helpful. These creams, ointments, and salves are rubbed directly onto the skin over the site of pain. They use one or more of a variety of ingredients to ease pain. Topical analgesics include such products as Zostrix, Icy Hot, and Ben Gay. (Brand names included in this chapter are provided as examples only, and their inclusion does not mean that these products are endorsed by the National Institutes of Health or any other government agency. Also, if a particular brand name is not mentioned, this does not mean or imply that the product is unsatisfactory.)

- **NSAIDs:** Nonsteroidal anti-inflammatory drugs (NSAIDs) are drugs that relieve both pain and inflammation, which may also play a role in some cases of back pain. NSAIDs include the nonprescription products ibuprofen (Motrin, Advil), ketoprofen (Actron, Orudis KT), and naproxen sodium (Aleve). More than a dozen others, including a subclass of NSAIDs called

COX-2 inhibitors, are available only with a prescription. All NSAIDs work similarly: by blocking substances called prostaglandins that contribute to inflammation and pain. However, each NSAID is a different chemical, and each has a slightly different effect on the body. Side effects of all NSAIDs can include stomach upset and stomach ulcers, heartburn, diarrhea, and fluid retention; however, COX-2 inhibitors are designed to cause fewer stomach ulcers. For unknown reasons, some people seem to respond better to one NSAID than another. It's important to work with your doctor to choose the one that's safest and most effective for you.

• **Other Medications:** Muscle relaxants and certain antidepressants have also been prescribed for chronic back pain, but their usefulness is questionable.

Traction: Traction involves using pulleys and weights to stretch the back. The rationale behind traction is to pull the vertebrae apart to allow a bulging disc to slip back into place. Some people experience pain relief while in traction, but that relief is usually temporary. Once traction is released, the stretch is not sustained and back pain is likely to return. There is no scientific evidence that traction provides any long-term benefits for people with back pain.

♣ **It's A Fact!!**
Warning: NSAIDs can cause stomach irritation or, less often, they can affect kidney function. The longer a person uses NSAIDs, the more likely he or she is to have side effects, ranging from mild to serious. Many other drugs cannot be taken when a patient is being treated with NSAIDs because NSAIDs alter the way the body uses or eliminates these other drugs. Check with your health-care provider or pharmacist before you take NSAIDs. Also, NSAIDs sometimes are associated with serious gastrointestinal problems, including ulcers, bleeding, and perforation of the stomach or intestine. People over age 65 and those with any history of ulcers or gastrointestinal bleeding should use NSAIDs with caution.

Source: "Handout on Health: Back Pain," National Institute of Arthritis and Musculoskeletal and Skin Diseases (www.niams.nih.gov/hi/topics/pain/backpain.htm), September, 2005.

Corsets And Braces: Corsets and braces include a number of devices, such as elastic bands and stiff supports with metal stays, that are designed to limit the motion of the lumbar spine, provide abdominal support, and correct posture. While these may be appropriate after certain kinds of surgery, there is little, if any, evidence that they help treat chronic low back pain. In fact, by keeping you from using your back muscles, they may actually cause more problems than they solve by causing lower back muscles to weaken from lack of use.

Behavioral Modification: Developing a healthy attitude and learning to move your body properly while you do daily activities—particularly those involving heavy lifting, pushing, or pulling—are sometimes part of the treatment plan for people with back pain. Other behavior changes that might help pain include adopting healthy habits, such as exercise, relaxation, and regular sleep, and dropping bad habits, such as smoking and eating poorly.

Injections: When medications and other nonsurgical treatments fail to relieve chronic back pain, doctors may recommend injections for pain relief. Following are some of the most commonly used injections, although some are of questionable value:

- **Nerve Root Blocks:** If a nerve is inflamed or compressed as it passes from the spinal column between the vertebrae, an injection called a nerve root block may be used to help ease the resulting back and leg pain. The injection contains a steroid medication and/or anesthetic and is administered to the affected part of the nerve. Whether the procedure helps or not depends on finding and injecting precisely the right nerve.

- **Facet Joint Injections:** The facet joints are those where the vertebrae connect to one another, keeping the spine aligned. Although arthritis in the facet joints themselves is rarely the source of back pain, the injection of anesthetics or steroid medications into facet joints is sometimes tried as a way to relieve pain. The effectiveness of these injections is questionable. One study suggests that this treatment is overused and ineffective.

- **Trigger Point Injections:** In this procedure, an anesthetic is injected into specific areas in the back that are painful when the doctor applies pressure to them. Some doctors add a steroid medication to the injection. Although the injections are commonly used, researchers have found that injecting anesthetics and/or steroids into trigger points provides no more relief than "dry needling," or inserting a needle and not injecting a medication.

- **Prolotherapy:** One of most talked-about procedures for back pain, prolotherapy is a treatment in which a practitioner injects a sugar solution or other irritating substance into trigger points along the periosteum (the tough, fibrous tissue covering the bones) to trigger an inflammatory response that promotes the growth of dense, fibrous tissue. The theory behind prolotherapy is that such tissue growth strengthens the attachment of tendons and ligaments whose loosening has contributed to back pain. As yet, studies have not verified the effectiveness of prolotherapy. The procedure is used primarily by chiropractors and osteopathic physicians.

Complementary And Alternative Treatments: When back pain becomes chronic or when medications and other conventional therapies do not relieve it, many people try complementary and alternative treatments. While such therapies won't cure diseases or repair the injuries that cause pain, some people find them useful for managing or relieving pain. Following are some of the most commonly used complementary therapies.

- **Manipulation:** Spinal manipulation refers to procedures in which professionals use their hands to mobilize, adjust, massage, or stimulate the spine or surrounding tissues. This type of therapy is often performed by osteopathic doctors and chiropractors. It tends to be most effective in people with uncomplicated pain and when used with other therapies. Spinal manipulation is not appropriate if you have a medical problem such as osteoporosis, spinal cord compression, or inflammatory arthritis (such as rheumatoid arthritis) or if you are taking blood-thinning medications such as warfarin (Coumadin) or heparin (Calciparine, Liquaemin).

- **Transcutaneous Electrical Nerve Stimulation (TENS):** TENS involves wearing a small box over the painful area that directs mild electrical impulses to nerves there. The theory is that stimulating the nervous system can modify the perception of pain. Early studies of TENS suggested it could elevate the levels of endorphins, the body's natural pain-numbing chemicals, in the spinal fluid. But subsequent studies of its effectiveness against pain have produced mixed results.

- **Acupuncture:** This ancient Chinese practice has been gaining increasing acceptance and popularity in the United States. It is based on the theory that a life force called Qi (pronounced chee) flows through the body along certain channels, which if blocked can cause illness. According to the theory, the insertion of thin needles at precise locations along these channels by practitioners can unblock the flow of Qi, relieving pain and restoring health. Although few Western-trained doctors would agree with the concept of blocked Qi, some believe that inserting and then stimulating needles (by twisting or passing a low-voltage electrical current through them) may foster the production of the body's natural pain-numbing chemicals, such as endorphins, serotonin, and acetylcholine. A consensus panel convened by the National Institutes of Health (NIH) in 1997 concluded that there is clear evidence this treatment is

✎ What's It Mean?

Cervical Spine: The upper portion of the spine closest to the skull. It is composed of seven vertebrae.

Disc: Circular pieces of cushioning tissue situated between each of the spine's vertebrae. Each disc has a strong outer cover and a soft jelly-like filling.

Herniated Disc: A potentially painful problem in which the hard outer coating of the disc is damaged, allowing the disc's jelly-like center to leak and cause irritation to adjacent nerves.

Kyphoplasty: A procedure for vertebral fractures in which a balloon-like device is inserted into the vertebra to help restore the height and shape of the spine and a cement-like substance is injected to repair and stabilize it.

Laminectomy: The surgical removal of the lamina (the back of the spinal canal) and spurs inside the canal that are pressing on nerves within the canal. The procedure is a major surgery requiring a large incision and a hospital stay.

Lumbar Spine: The lower portion of the spine. It is composed of five vertebrae.

Spondylolisthesis: A condition in which a vertebra of the lumbar (lower) spine slips out of place.

Vertebrae: The individual bones that make up the spinal column.

Source: "Handout on Health: Back Pain," National Institute of Arthritis and Musculoskeletal and Skin Diseases (www.niams.nih.gov), September 2005.

effective for some pain conditions, including postoperative dental pain. Although there is less convincing evidence to support using acupuncture for back pain and some other pain conditions, the panel concluded that acupuncture may be effective when used as part of a comprehensive treatment plan for low back pain, fibromyalgia, and several other conditions.

- **Acupressure:** As with acupuncture, the theory behind acupressure is that it unblocks the flow of Qi. The difference between acupuncture and acupressure is that no needles are used in acupressure. Instead, a therapist applies pressure to points along the channels with his or her hands, elbows, or even feet. (In some cases, patients are taught to do their own acupressure.) Acupressure has not been well studied for back pain.

- **Rolfing:** A type of massage, Rolfing involves using strong pressure on deep tissues in the back to relieve tightness of the fascia, a sheath of tissue that covers the muscles, that can cause or contribute to back pain. The theory behind Rolfing is that releasing muscles and tissues from the fascia enables the back to properly align itself. So far, the usefulness of Rolfing for back pain has not been scientifically proven.

Operative Treatments

Depending on the diagnosis, surgery may either be the first treatment of choice—although this is rare—or it is reserved for chronic back pain for which other treatments have failed. If you are in constant pain or if pain reoccurs frequently and interferes with your ability to sleep, to function at your job, or to perform daily activities, you may be a candidate for surgery.

In general, there are two groups of people who may require surgery to treat their spinal problems. People in the first group have chronic low back pain and sciatica, and they are often diagnosed with a herniated disc, spinal stenosis, spondylolisthesis, or vertebral fractures with nerve involvement. People in the second group are those with only predominant low back pain (without leg pain). These are people with discogenic low back pain (degenerative disc disease), in which discs wear with age. Usually, the outcome of spine surgery is much more predictable in people with sciatica than in those with predominant low back pain. Some of the diagnoses that may need surgery include herniated discs, spinal stenosis, spondylolisthesis, vertebral fractures, and discogenic low back pain (degenerative disc disease).

Chapter 24

Burners And Stingers

Burners and stingers are a common injury in contact or collision sports. The injury is named for the stinging or burning pain that spreads from the shoulder to the hand. This can feel like an electric shock or lightening bolt down the arm. This can be accompanied by a warm sensation.

Anatomy

Nerve roots exit the spinal canal of the neck and come together to form cords of nerves. These nerves ultimately provide sensation and motor innervation to the muscles of the arm.

The nerve roots are named for the level at which they exit the spinal canal. For example, the term C5 refers to cervical nerve root 5, which exits the spinal cord at the 5th cervical spinal body.

As the nerve roots move away from the spinal canal, they join to form larger bundles or cords. In the upper extremity this is called the brachial plexus. All of the nerve supply to the arms runs through this plexus. This is also a potential site of injury that can cause a burner or stinger.

About This Chapter: Reproduced with permission from Moseley C: *Your Orthopaedic Connection*. Rosemont, IL, American Academy of Orthopaedic Surgeons. © 2007 AAOS.

Cause

When a burner or stinger occurs, one potential area of injury is where the nerve root exits the spinal canal.

Burners and stingers are a common injury in contact sports. Athletes who engage in contact sports are more likely to suffer this injury. In fact, up to 70 percent of all college football players report having experienced a burner or stinger during their 4-year careers.

♣ **It's A Fact!!**
Nerves are stretched when the player takes a hit on the top of the shoulder, causing the neck to be driven one way and the arm to be driven the other way.

The two most common sports for burners and stingers are American football and wrestling.

Tackling or blocking in football is the most common athletic activity causing a burner or stinger. Football defensive players and lineman therefore frequently suffer this injury. Another possible mechanism is a fall onto the head, such as in a wrestling takedown or a football tackle.

In addition to the type of sport, another risk factor may be the size of the spinal canal. It has been suggested that athletes with recurrent stingers or burners may have a smaller spinal canal than players who do not suffer recurrent injury. This is a condition called cervical, or spinal, stenosis.

Symptoms

The injury is to the nerve supply of the upper limb, either at the neck or shoulder. In most cases, the injuries are temporary and symptoms resolve quickly.

- A burning or electric shock sensation is often felt.
- The arm may feel numb immediately following the injury, and weakness is common.
- The symptoms most commonly occur in one arm only.

- Symptoms usually last seconds to minutes, but in five percent to ten percent of cases, they can last hours, days, or even longer.

Diagnosis

An orthopedic surgeon makes the diagnosis based upon the history of injury and the symptoms. X-rays, magnetic resonance imaging (MRI), and other nerve studies are not usually needed.

More extensive examination is needed if there are any of the following symptoms:

- Weakness lasting more than several days

- Neck pain

- Symptoms in both arms

- History of recurrent stingers/burners

Nonsurgical Treatment

Treatment begins by removing the athlete from further injury. Athletes are not allowed to return to sports activity until their symptoms are completely gone. This can take a few minutes or several days. Athletes should never be allowed to return to sports if they have weakness or neck pain.

Although the injury gets better with time, the athlete may need to work with a trainer or therapist to regain strength and motion if the symptoms last for several days.

Chapter 25

Shoulder Injuries

What are the most common shoulder problems?

The most movable joint in the body, the shoulder is also one of the most potentially unstable joints. As a result, it is the site of many common problems. They include sprains, strains, dislocations, separations, tendinitis, bursitis, torn rotator cuffs, frozen shoulder, fractures, and arthritis. Specific shoulder problems will be discussed later in this chapter.

How common are shoulder problems?

According to the Centers for Disease Control and Prevention, about 13.7 million people in the United States sought medical care in 2003 for shoulder problems.

What are the structures of the shoulder and how does it function?

To better understand shoulder problems and how they occur, it helps to begin with an explanation of the shoulder's structure and how it functions.

About This Chapter: This chapter includes excerpts from "Questions and Answers about Shoulder Problems," National Institute of Arthritis and Musculoskeletal and Skin Diseases (NIAMS), March 2006. Additional text from Nicholas Institute for Sports Medicine and Athletic Trauma and Sports Injury Clinic is cited separately within the chapter.

The shoulder joint is composed of three bones: the clavicle (collarbone), the scapula (shoulder blade), and the humerus (upper arm bone) (see Figure 25.1). Two joints facilitate shoulder movement. The acromioclavicular (AC) joint is located between the acromion (part of the scapula that forms the highest point of the shoulder) and the clavicle. The glenohumeral joint, commonly called the shoulder joint, is a ball-and-socket-type joint that helps move the shoulder forward and backward and allows the arm to rotate in a circular fashion or hinge out and up away from the body. (The "ball," or humerus, is the top, rounded portion of the upper arm bone; the "socket," or glenoid, is a dish-shaped part of the outer edge of the scapula into which the ball fits.) The capsule is a soft tissue envelope that encircles the glenohumeral joint. It is lined by a thin, smooth synovial membrane.

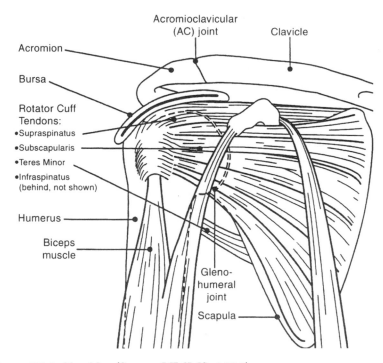

Figure 25.1. Shoulder (Source: NIAMS, 2006).

In contrast to the hip joint, which more closely approximates a true ball and socket joint, the shoulder joint can be compared to a golf ball and tee, in which the ball can easily slip off the flat tee. Because the bones provide little inherent stability to the shoulder joint, it is highly dependent on surrounding soft tissues such as capsule ligaments and the muscles surrounding the rotator cuff to hold the ball in place. Whereas the hip joint is inherently quite stable because of the encircling bony anatomy, it also is relatively immobile. The shoulder, on the other hand, is relatively unstable but highly mobile, allowing an individual to place the hand in numerous positions. It is in fact, one of the most mobile joints in the human body.

The bones of the shoulder are held in place by muscles, tendons, and ligaments. For example, the front of the joint capsule is anchored by three glenohumeral ligaments. The rotator cuff is a structure composed of tendons that work along with associated muscles to hold the ball at the top of the humerus in the glenoid socket and provide mobility and strength to the shoulder joint. Two filmy sac-like structures called bursae permit smooth gliding between bones, muscles, and tendons. They cushion and protect the rotator cuff from the bony arch of the acromion.

✎ What's It Mean?

Acromioclavicular (AC) Joint: The joint of the shoulder located between the acromion (part of the scapula that forms the highest point of the shoulder) and the clavicle (collarbone).

Capsule: A soft tissue envelope that encircles the glenohumeral joint and is lined by a thin, smooth, synovial membrane.

Humerus: The upper arm bone.

Tendons: Tough cords of tissue that attach the shoulder muscles to bone and assist the muscles in moving the shoulder.

Source: NIAMS, 2006.

What are the origins and causes of shoulder problems?

The shoulder is easily injured because the ball of the upper arm is larger than the shoulder socket that holds it. To remain stable, the shoulder must be anchored by its muscles, tendons, and ligaments.

Although the shoulder is easily injured during sporting activities and manual labor, the primary source of shoulder problems appears to be the natural age-related degeneration of the surrounding soft tissues such as those found in the rotator cuff. The incidence of rotator cuff problems rises dramatically as a function of age and is generally seen among individuals who are more than 60 years old. Often, the dominant and nondominant arm will be affected to a similar degree. Overuse of the shoulder can lead to more rapid age-related deterioration.

Shoulder pain may be localized or may be felt in areas around the shoulder or down the arm. Disease within the body (such as gallbladder, liver, or heart disease, or disease of the cervical spine of the neck) also may generate pain that travels along nerves to the shoulder. However, these other causes of shoulder pain are beyond the scope of this chapter, which will focus on problems within the shoulder itself.

How are shoulder problems diagnosed?

As with any medical issue, a shoulder problem is generally diagnosed using a three-part process:

- **Medical History:** The patient tells the doctor about any injury or other condition that might be causing the pain.

- **Physical Examination:** The doctor examines the patient to feel for injury and to discover the limits of movement, location of pain, and extent of joint instability.

- **Tests:** The doctor may order one or more of the tests listed below to make a specific diagnosis. These tests may include the following:

    - *Standard X-Ray:* A familiar procedure in which low-level radiation is passed through the body to produce a picture called a radiograph. An x-ray is useful for diagnosing fractures or other problems of the bones. Soft tissues, such as muscles and tendons, do not show up on x-rays.

    - *Arthrogram:* A diagnostic record that can be seen on an x-ray after injection of a contrast fluid into the shoulder joint to outline structures such as the rotator cuff. In disease or injury, this contrast fluid may either leak into an area where it does not belong, indicating a tear or opening, or be blocked from entering an area where there normally is an opening.

- *Ultrasound:* A noninvasive, patient-friendly procedure in which a small, hand-held scanner is placed on the skin of the shoulder. Just as ultrasound waves can be used to visualize the fetus during pregnancy, they can also be reflected off the rotator cuff and other structures to form a high-quality image of them. The accuracy of ultrasound for the rotator cuff is particularly high.

- *Magnetic Resonance Imaging (MRI):* A noninvasive procedure in which a machine with a strong magnet passes a force through the body to produce a series of cross-sectional images of the shoulder. Other diagnostic tests, such as one that involves injecting an anesthetic into and around the shoulder joint, are discussed in detail in other parts of this chapter.

What should I know about specific shoulder problems, including their symptoms and treatment?

The symptoms of shoulder problems, as well as their diagnosis and treatment, vary widely, depending on the specific problem. The following is important information to know about some of the most common shoulder problems.

Dislocation: The shoulder joint is the most frequently dislocated major joint of the body. In a typical case of a dislocated shoulder, either a strong force pulls the shoulder outward (abduction) or extreme rotation of the joint pops the ball of the humerus out of the shoulder socket. Dislocation commonly occurs when there is a backward pull on the arm that either catches the muscles unprepared to resist or overwhelms the muscles. When a shoulder dislocates frequently, the condition is referred to as shoulder instability. A partial dislocation in which the upper arm bone is partially in and partially out of the socket is called a subluxation.

Signs And Symptoms: The shoulder can dislocate either forward, backward, or downward. When the shoulder dislocates, the arm appears out of position. Other symptoms include pain, which may be worsened by muscle spasms; swelling; numbness; weakness; and bruising. Problems seen with a dislocated shoulder are tearing of the ligaments or tendons reinforcing the joint capsule and, less commonly, bone and/or nerve damage.

Diagnosis: Doctors usually diagnose a dislocation by a physical examination; x-rays may be taken to confirm the diagnosis and to rule out a related fracture.

Treatment: Doctors treat a dislocation by putting the ball of the humerus back into the joint socket, a procedure called a reduction. The arm is then stabilized for several weeks in a sling or a device called a shoulder immobilizer. Usually the doctor recommends resting the shoulder and applying ice three or four times a day. After pain and swelling have been controlled, the patient enters a rehabilitation program that includes exercises. The goal is to restore the range of motion of the shoulder, strengthen the muscles, and prevent future dislocations. These exercises may progress from simple motion to the use of weights.

After treatment and recovery, a previously dislocated shoulder may remain more susceptible to re-injury, especially in young, active individuals. Ligaments may have been stretched or torn, and the shoulder may tend to dislocate again. A shoulder that dislocates severely or often, injuring surrounding tissues or nerves, usually requires surgical repair to tighten stretched ligaments or reattach torn ones.

Sometimes the doctor performs surgery through a tiny incision into which a small scope (arthroscope) is inserted to observe the inside of the joint. After this procedure, called arthroscopic surgery, the shoulder is generally stabilized for about six weeks. Full recovery takes several months. Arthroscopic techniques involving the shoulder are relatively new, and some surgeons prefer to repair a recurrent dislocating shoulder by time-tested open surgery under direct vision. Usually following open surgery there are fewer repeat dislocations, and movement is improved, but there is often some loss of motion.

Separation: A shoulder separation occurs where the collarbone (clavicle) meets the shoulder blade (scapula). When ligaments that hold the joint together are partially or completely torn, the outer end of the clavicle may slip out of place, preventing it from properly meeting the scapula. Most often, the injury is caused by a blow to the shoulder or by falling on an outstretched hand.

Signs And Symptoms: Shoulder pain or tenderness and, occasionally, a bump in the middle of the top of the shoulder (over the acromioclavicular (AC) joint) are signs that a separation may have occurred.

Diagnosis: Doctors may diagnose a separation by performing a physical examination. They may confirm the diagnosis and determine the severity of the separation by taking an x-ray. While the x-ray is being taken, the patient makes the separation more pronounced by holding a light weight that pulls on the muscles.

Treatment: A shoulder separation is usually treated conservatively by rest and wearing a sling. Soon after injury, an ice bag may be applied to relieve pain and swelling. After a period of rest, a therapist helps the patient perform exercises that put the shoulder through its range of motion. Most shoulder separations heal within two or three months without further intervention. However, if ligaments are severely torn, surgical repair may be required to hold the clavicle in place. A doctor may wait to see if conservative treatment works before deciding whether surgery is required.

Rotator Cuff Disease—Tendinitis And Bursitis: These conditions are closely related and may occur alone or in combination.

Tendinitis is inflammation (redness, soreness, and swelling) of a tendon. In tendinitis of the shoulder, the rotator cuff and/or biceps tendon become inflamed, usually as a result of being pinched by surrounding structures. The injury may vary from mild inflammation to involvement of most of the rotator cuff. When the rotator cuff tendon becomes inflamed and thickened, it may get trapped under the acromion. Squeezing of the rotator cuff is called impingement syndrome.

Bursitis, or inflammation of the bursa sacs that protect the shoulder, may accompany tendinitis and impingement syndrome. Inflammation caused by a disease such as rheumatoid arthritis may cause rotator cuff tendinitis and bursitis. Sports involving overuse of the shoulder and occupations requiring frequent overhead reaching are other potential causes of irritation to the rotator cuff or bursa and may lead to inflammation and impingement.

If the rotator cuff and bursa are irritated, inflamed, and swollen, they may become squeezed between the head of the humerus and the acromion. Repeated motion involving the arms, or the effects of the aging process on shoulder movement over many years, may also irritate and wear down the tendons, muscles, and surrounding structures.

Signs And Symptoms: Signs of these conditions include the slow onset of discomfort and pain in the upper shoulder or upper third of the arm and/or difficulty sleeping on the shoulder. Tendinitis and bursitis also cause pain when the arm is lifted away from the body or overhead. If tendinitis involves the biceps tendon (the tendon located in front of the shoulder that helps bend the elbow and turn the forearm), pain will occur in the front or side of the shoulder and may travel down to the elbow and forearm. Pain may also occur when the arm is forcefully pushed upward overhead.

Diagnosis: Diagnosis of tendinitis and bursitis begins with a medical history and physical examination. X-rays do not show tendons or the bursae, but may be helpful in ruling out bony abnormalities or arthritis. The doctor may remove and test fluid from the inflamed area to rule out infection. Impingement syndrome may be confirmed when injection of a small amount of anesthetic (lidocaine hydrochloride) into the space under the acromion relieves pain.

Treatment: The first step in treating these conditions is to reduce pain and inflammation with rest, ice, and anti-inflammatory medicines such as aspirin and ibuprofen (Advil, Motrin). In some cases, the doctor or therapist will use ultrasound (gentle sound-wave vibrations) to warm deep tissues and improve blood flow. Gentle stretching and strengthening exercises are added gradually. These may be preceded or followed by use of an ice pack. If there is no improvement, the doctor may inject a corticosteroid medicine into the space under the acromion. While steroid injections are a common treatment, they must be used with caution because they may lead to tendon rupture. If there is still no improvement after six to 12 months, the doctor may recommend either arthroscopic or open surgery to repair damage and relieve pressure on the tendons and bursae.

Torn Rotator Cuff: Rotator cuff tendons often become inflamed from overuse, aging, or a fall on an outstretched hand or another traumatic cause. Sports or occupations requiring repetitive overhead motion or heavy lifting can also place a significant strain on rotator cuff muscles and tendons. Over time, as a function of aging, tendons become weaker and degenerate.

Eventually, this degeneration can lead to complete tears of both muscles and tendons. These tears are surprisingly common. In fact, a tear of the rotator cuff is not necessarily an abnormal situation in older individuals if there is no significant pain or disability. Fortunately, these tears do not lead to any pain or disability in most people. However, some individuals can develop very significant pain as a result of these tears and they may require treatment.

Signs And Symptoms: Typically, a person with a rotator cuff injury feels pain over the deltoid muscle at the top and outer side of the shoulder, especially when the arm is raised or extended out from the side of the body. Motions like those involved in getting dressed can be painful. The shoulder may feel weak, especially when trying to lift the arm into a horizontal position. A person may also feel or hear a click or pop when the shoulder is moved. Pain or weakness on outward or inward rotation of the arm may indicate a tear in a rotator cuff tendon. The patient also feels pain when lowering the arm to the side after the shoulder is moved backward and the arm is raised.

Diagnosis: A doctor may detect weakness but may not be able to determine from a physical examination where the tear is located. x-rays, if taken, may appear normal. An MRI or ultrasound can help detect a full tendon tear or a partial tendon tear.

Treatment: Doctors usually recommend that patients with a rotator cuff injury rest the shoulder, apply heat or cold to the sore area, and take medicine to relieve pain and inflammation. Other treatments might be added, such as electrical stimulation of muscles and nerves, ultrasound, or a cortisone injection near the inflamed area of the rotator cuff. If surgery is not an immediate consideration, exercises are added to the treatment program to build flexibility and strength and restore the shoulder's function. If there is no improvement with these conservative treatments and functional impairment persists, the doctor may perform arthroscopic or open surgical repair of the torn rotator cuff.

Treatment for rotator cuff disease usually depends on the severity of the injury, the age and health status of the patient, and the length of time a given patient may have had the condition. Patients with rotator cuff tendinitis or bursitis that does not include a complete tear of the tendon can usually be treated without surgery. Nonsurgical treatments include the use of anti-inflammatory medication and occasional steroid injections into the area of the inflamed rotator cuff, followed by rehabilitative rotator cuff strengthening exercises. These treatments are best undertaken with the guidance of a health-care professional such as a physical therapist, who works in conjunction with the treating physician.

Surgical repair of rotator cuff tears is best for:

- younger patients, especially those with small tears. Surgery leads to a high degree of successful healing and reduces concerns about the tear getting worse over time.

- individuals whose rotator cuff tears are caused by an acute, severe injury. These people should seek immediate treatment that includes surgical repair of the tendon.

Generally speaking, individuals who are older and have had shoulder pain for a longer period of time can be treated with nonoperative measures even in the presence of a complete rotator cuff tear. These people are often treated similarly to those who have pain, but do not have a rotator cuff tear. Again, anti-inflammatory medication, use of steroid injections, and rehabilitative exercises can be very effective. When treated surgically, rotator cuff tears can be repaired by either arthroscopic or traditional open surgical techniques.

Fracture: A fracture involves a partial or total crack through a bone. The break in a bone usually occurs as a result of an impact injury, such as a fall or blow to the shoulder. A fracture usually involves the clavicle or the neck (area below the ball) of the humerus.

Signs And Symptoms: A shoulder fracture that occurs after a major injury is usually accompanied by severe pain. Within a short time, there may be redness and bruising around the area. Sometimes a fracture is obvious because the bones appear out of position.

Diagnosis: X-rays can confirm the diagnosis of a shoulder fracture and the degree of its severity.

♣ It's A Fact!!

What is a fractured clavicle?

The collar bone (or clavicle) is the bone that runs along the front of the shoulder to the breast bone (sternum). This bone is usually fractured as a result of falling badly onto an outstretched arm or onto the shoulder or in a collision with an opponent in a contact sport such as rugby or American football. The likelihood of a clavicle fracture is increased if the playing surface is particularly hard.

The bone usually fractures in its middle third and is very painful. Symptoms of a fractured collar bone include the following:

• Pain on the collar bone

• Swelling

• A bony deformity may be seen or felt

What can the athlete do for a fractured collar bone?

• If you suspect you have a broken collar bone you should see a doctor immediately.

What can a doctor do?

• Immobilize the bone with a figure eight bandage.

• Provide pain relief.

• Advise on full rehabilitation and strengthening.

• Operate if necessary.

The injury is likely to take four to eight weeks to heal. You should not do any sports, or even running, until it has properly healed. However you may be able to cycle.

Source: Reprinted with permission from "Fractured Collar Bone," © 2007 Sports Injury Clinic. For more information, including video presentations, visit http://www.sportsinjuryclinic.net.

Treatment: When a fracture occurs, the doctor tries to bring the bones into a position that will promote healing and restore arm movement. If someone's clavicle is fractured, he or she must initially wear a strap and sling around the chest to keep the clavicle in place. After removing the strap and sling, the doctor will prescribe exercises to strengthen the shoulder and restore movement. Surgery is occasionally needed for certain clavicle fractures.

Fracture of the neck of the humerus is usually treated with a sling or shoulder stabilizer. If the bones are out of position, surgery may be necessary to reset them. Exercises are also part of restoring shoulder strength and motion.

Swimmer's Shoulder

"Swimmer's Shoulder," reprinted with permission from Nicholas Institute for Sports Medicine and Athletic Trauma (www.nismat.org), © 2007. All rights reserved.

What is swimmer's shoulder?

Swimmer's shoulder is an inflammatory condition caused by the mechanical impingement of soft tissue against the coracoacromial arch. This condition is most often caused by the repetitive overhead arm motion of the freestyle stroke. The pain associated with swimmer's shoulder may be caused by two different sources of impingement in the shoulder.

One type of impingement occurs during the pull-through phase of freestyle. The pull-through phase begins when the hand enters the water and terminates when the arm has completed pulling through the water and begins to exit the surface. At the beginning of pull-through, termed hand-entry, if a swimmer's hand enters the water across the mid-line of her body this will place the shoulder in a position of horizontal adduction which mechanically impinges the long head of the biceps against the anterior part of the coracoacromial arch.

A second type of impingement may occur during the recovery phase of freestyle. The recovery phase is the time of the stroke cycle when the arm is exiting the water and lasts until that hand enters the water again. As a swimmer fatigues it will become more difficult for her to lift her arm out of the water, and the muscles of the rotator cuff which work to externally rotate and depress the head of the humerus against the glenoid become less efficient. When these muscles are not working properly the supraspinatus muscle will be mechanically impinged between the greater tuberosity of the humerus and the middle and posterior portions of the coracoacromial arch.

These two repetitive use injuries can result in painful swimmer's shoulder.

Why do swimmers get swimmer's shoulder?

Swimmers may have shoulder pain for many reasons. Poor swimming technique is a major factor in shoulder pain. As mentioned previously, if a swimmer crosses mid-line upon hand-entry, this may cause impingement of the long head of the biceps tendon. As well, if a swimmer's hand enters the water with the thumb pointing down and the palm facing outwards, this can result in the same type of impingement.

Overtraining can lead to shoulder pain if the swimmer continues to swim with fatigued muscles. As the muscles fatigue they will work less efficiently which has two poor consequences. First, the muscles will have to work harder in a weakened condition. Second, the swimmer will have to perform more strokes to cover the same distance, which is overusing already fatigued muscles. Together these two factors can result in swimmer's shoulder.

Unilateral breathing may also cause swimmer's shoulder. Swimmers who consistently turn their heads to the same side to breathe are risking shoulder pain in the opposite shoulder as it has to work harder to support forward movement with the head turned to the side.

Overuse of certain training equipment may cause shoulder pain. The use of hand paddles that are much larger than the swimmer's hand, or those paddles that do not have drainage holes place great strain on the shoulder muscles during the pull-through phase of freestyle. Using a kickboard with arms fully extended in front of the swimmer can place the shoulder in a position of impingement. The longer the swimmers uses these items, or uses them incorrectly, the greater the risk of shoulder pain.

How can I prevent swimmer's shoulder?

Swimmer's shoulder can be prevented by using proper freestyle stroke. The hand should enter the water with the small finger first and the palm facing inward. When the hand enters the water it should not cross the middle of the body to avoid impingement. For further stroke instruction, seek the advice of a swimming coach.

Swimmers should avoid rapid increases in training distances or frequency of training as this is likely to wear out the shoulder muscles leaving them at risk for impingement and shoulder pain.

Stretching shoulder, chest, and neck muscles will help to prevent a swimming posture that is conducive to impingement. Generally, swimmers have tight neck, chest, and anterior shoulder muscles that cause them to assume a hunched over posture.

Tricep Stretch: Begin by raising your arm directly over your head with your palm facing front. Bend your elbow and try to reach the shoulder blade on the same side of you body. Use your opposite arm to push your elbow back.

Doorway Stretch To The Pectoralis Major: Begin by placing your elbow against the frame of a door. Keep the angle between your trunk and your arm at 90 degree. Rest your forearms against the door frame. Step forward with one foot to feel the stretch.

Infraspinatus Stretch: Extend your arm out directly in front of you and bend your elbow across your body. With your other hand gently pull your elbow across your body.

Levator Scapulae Stretch: Begin by placing one arm as in the first part of the triceps stretch. Look towards your opposite hip and use you free hand to gently pull your head towards your hip.

Upper Trapezius Stretch: Lean your head to the side trying to bring your ear towards your shoulder without lifting your shoulder.

Latissimus Dorsi Stretch: Raise both arms overhead and place palms together interlocking fingers. At shoulders lift arms upwards with fingers remaining intertwined.

Axial Extension: Pull your chin down and backwards as if trying to make a double chin.

Chapter 26

Elbow Injuries

Tennis Elbow (Lateral Epicondylitis)

What is tennis elbow/lateral epicondylitis?

Lateral epicondylitis, commonly known as tennis elbow, is a painful condition involving the tendons that attach to the bone on the outside (lateral) part of the elbow. Tendons anchor the muscle to bone. The muscle involved in this condition, the extensor carpi radialis brevis, helps to extend and stabilize the wrist. With lateral epicondylitis, there is degeneration of the tendon's attachment, weakening the anchor site and placing greater stress on the area. This can then lead to pain associated with activities in which this muscle is active, such as lifting, gripping, and/or grasping. Sports such as tennis are commonly associated with this, but the problem can occur with many different types of activities, athletic and otherwise.

What causes tennis elbow/lateral epicondylitis?

Overuse: The cause can be both non-work and work related. An activity that places stress on the tendon attachments, through stress on the extensor muscle-tendon unit, increases the strain on the tendon. These stresses can be from holding too large a racquet grip or from repetitive gripping and grasping activities, such as meat-cutting, plumbing, painting, weaving, etc.

Trauma: A direct blow to the elbow may result in swelling of the tendon that can lead to degeneration. A sudden extreme action, force, or activity could also injure the tendon.

Who gets tennis elbow/lateral epicondylitis?

The most common age group that this condition affects is between 30 to 50 years old, but it may occur in younger and older age groups, and in both men and women.

Signs And Symptoms Of Tennis Elbow/Lateral Epicondylitis

Pain is the primary reason for patients to seek medical evaluation. The pain is located over the outside aspect of the elbow, over the bone region known as the lateral epicondyle. This area becomes tender to touch. Pain is also produced by any activity which places stress on the tendon, such as gripping or lifting. With activity, the pain usually starts at the elbow and may travel down the forearm to the hand. Occasionally, any motion of the elbow can be painful.

What treatments are available for tennis elbow/lateral epicondylitis?

Conservative (Non-Surgical)

- *Activity Modification:* Initially, the activity causing the condition should be limited. Limiting the aggravating activity, not total rest, is recommended. Modifying grips or techniques, such as use of a different size racket and/ or use of 2-handed backhands in tennis, may relieve the problem.

- *Medication:* Anti-inflammatory medications may help alleviate the pain.

- *Brace:* A tennis elbow brace, a band worn over the muscle of the forearm, just below the elbow, can reduce the tension on the tendon and allow it to heal.

- *Physical Therapy:* May be helpful, providing stretching and/or strengthening exercises. Modalities such as ultrasound or heat treatments may be helpful.

- *Steroid Injections:* A steroid is a strong anti-inflammatory medication that can be injected into the area. No more than three injections should be given.

- *Shockwave Treatment:* A new type of treatment, available in the office setting, has shown some success in 50–60% of patients. This is a shock wave delivered to the affected area around the elbow, which can be used as a last resort prior to the consideration of surgery.

Surgery

Surgery is only considered when the pain is incapacitating and has not responded to conservative care, and symptoms have lasted more than six months. Surgery involves removing the diseased, degenerated tendon tissue. Two surgical approaches are available: traditional open surgery (incision) and arthroscopy—a procedure performed with instruments inserted into the joint through small incisions. Both options are performed in the outpatient setting.

Recovery

Recovery from surgery includes physical therapy to regain motion of the arm. A strengthening program will be necessary in order to return to prior activities. Recovery can be expected to take 4–6 months.

Little League Elbow

"Young Pitchers Can Strike Out Early from 'Little League Elbow'," June 29, 2004. © Baylor College of Medicine (www.bcm.edu).

Little leaguers who pitch too many innings when they are young may not be able to throw as many pitches later because of a serious injury called little league elbow.

✎ What's It Mean?

Ligament: A tough band of connective tissue that connects bones to bones.

Tendon: The flexible but tough connective tissue that attaches muscles to bones.

Source: Excerpted from "Questions and Answers about Knee Problems," National Institute of Arthritis and Musculoskeletal and Skin Diseases, May 2006.

"Young ball players who throw too much and try complicated pitches as early as age 10 can shorten their career by damaging the growth plate on the inside of the elbow," says Dr. David Lintner, an associate professor of orthopedic surgery at Baylor College of Medicine (BCM) in Houston. "Excessive pull to the area too many times can cause the growth plate in the elbow to separate and in extreme cases young players require surgery."

Little league elbow can be identified early by asking ball players about pain in their pitching arms, or more specifically about pain in the little bump on the inside of the elbow. If the pain is not ignored, the rest period is shorter and treatment does not require surgery to repair the damaged growth plate.

"The amount of throwing varies from player to player, but one thing that seems to be most helpful in preventing little league elbow is overseeing the kinds of pitches young kids throw, such as sidearm or breaking pitches and the curveball," says Lintner, also chief of sports medicine at BCM and an orthopedic surgeon at The Methodist Hospital. "All of these pitches are hazardous to the elbow and can lead to separation of the growth plate."

Pitchers under the age of 15 should not be throwing any of these pitches because they have less control of their arms, says Lintner. Ultimately, the rash of ligament injuries in teenage pitchers is related to overwork in younger years.

"A proper warm up is necessary, which includes jogging as well as light throwing before throwing full speed to loosen up the entire body and increase the blood flow all over their body to prevent injury, but parents and coaches still need to count the number of pitches thrown," says Lintner. "Kids shouldn't go from standing still to throwing the ball with full force."

> ### ✔ Quick Tip
> ### Elbow Fracture Recovery
>
> - Move your fingers.
>
> - Keep the cast dry and clean. Waterproof casts cannot be used for fractures with pins in place.
>
> - Your doctor will order pain medication for you to use at home. Follow the directions on the label carefully. If the pain medicine does not work, please call the orthopaedic nurse or doctor.
>
> Source: Cincinnati Children's Hospital Medical Center, 2007.

If the player's elbow begins to hurt, the player should stop throwing, ice it down, and see a sports medicine specialist for x-rays for any damage that may have already occurred. If the growth plate has not separated and surgery is not necessary, ice and rest will help the elbow to heal, Lintner says.

Elbow Fractures

"Elbow Fracture Care," © 2007 Cincinnati Children's Hospital Medical Center (www.cincinnatichildrens.com). Reprinted with permission.

How are elbow fractures treated?

Elbow fractures are broken bones, close to the elbow. Some children have fractures that may need only a cast for the bone to heal. Others may need to go to the operating room to have pins put in the bone to hold it in place while healing takes place.

If you need to have pins placed in the bone, a cast will be applied over the pins after the surgery is completed. The pins will be removed at the doctor's office after healing has taken place.

Care: There may be some swelling of the hand and/or fingers for 2–5 days after the fracture. Keep the elbow and hand elevated for the first 2–3 days by lying down on a couch or bed and propping the arm up with pillows, keep elbow and hand above the level of the heart.

Keeping an ice bag on the elbow will also help to reduce the swelling. Ice bags you can use include frozen vegetables such as peas or corn, commercial ice products such as "blue ice," or heavy plastic bags filled with ice. Cover the bags of ice with a dry thin towel to protect the cast from getting wet. If the swelling or pain increases or fingers become numb notify the orthopaedic nurse, or doctor.

Check your fingers often for movement, feeling and circulation during the first couple of days following surgery and/or cast placement. Notify your doctor of any decrease in circulation, decrease in the ability to move the fingers, or decreased feeling (numbness) in the fingers.

Pin Tract Infection: About 3% of patients can develop a pin tract infection. This usually starts about 1–4 weeks after pin placement. Signs of infection include:

- Increasing elbow pain or fussiness [in young children] after the first week;

- Fever;

- Drainage out of the cast.

If you develop any of these symptoms please call the orthopaedic nurse, or doctor.

Baths Only; No Showers (for fractures treated with pins and non-waterproof casts): You should place a plastic bag over the casted arm and tape it tight at the top (at the armpit). Never submerge the arm or allow water to run over it. Place the casted arm on the side of the tub and make to keep the cast out of the water. If it should get wet, immediately dry with a blow dryer using the cool setting only. If this does not dry the cast, call your doctor immediately for further instructions. A wet cast can cause skin sores if not taken care of right away.

Activities: You should avoid any activities that may increase the likelihood of tripping and falling. When you feel well enough and are no longer requiring (narcotic) pain medicine, you may return to school wearing a sling. Place a safety pin between the two sling layers, just in front of the elbow to help keep the sling from sliding off of the arm. You should wear the sling when out of bed until the cast is removed.

Cast Removal: After healing takes place you may have elbow stiffness that lasts for 3–4 weeks after the cast is removed. Children often hold their arm for the first few hours after their cast is removed due to elbow stiffness. The stiffness usually goes away spontaneously within a month after cast removal.

Pin Removal: Elbow pins are usually removed in the office in a matter of seconds. Although patients may be anxious or cry, it is not a painful procedure, so they need not be scared. Healthcare providers usually place an ace wrap over the pin sites which can be replaced with a Band-Aid the next day.

Physical Therapy: Physical therapy is usually not necessary. Patients are encouraged to swim once the skin pin holes have closed up (usually 1–2 days after cast removal), and you can play sports once you have near full motion (approximately 1–4 weeks after cast removal). Return of full range of motion may take up to three months.

Follow-Up: Your doctor will tell you when you need to return for follow-up care. Call the office as soon as you can to make the appointment. X-rays will be taken to determine how the healing is progressing.

Cincinnati Children's Hospital Medical Center

Contact Us: For additional information on this or any health topic, please call the Family Resource Center, 513-636-7606, or your pediatrician.

Chapter 27

Wrist And Hand Injuries

Wrist Sprains

What are sprains?

A sprain is an injury to a ligament. Ligaments are the connective tissues that connect bones to bones; they could be thought of as tape that holds the bones together at a joint (see Figure 27.1).

How do wrist sprains occur?

These types of injuries are common in falls and sports. The wrist is usually bent backwards when the hand hits the ground such as when someone slips or trips and falls. These injuries also frequently occur during sports such as football and snowboarding. After injury, the wrist will usually swell and may show bruising. It is usually very painful to move.

What are the most common types of wrist sprains?

The most common ligament to be injured in the wrist is the scapholunate ligament (see Figure 27.2). It is the ligament between two of the small bones in the wrist, the scaphoid bone and the lunate bone. There are many other

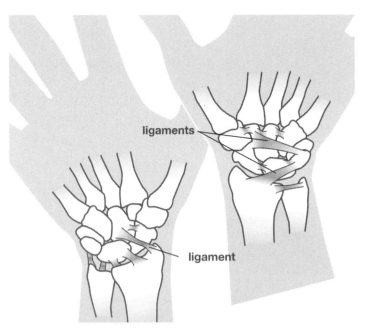

Figure 27.1. Ligaments of the wrist (© 2006 American Society for Surgery of the Hand).

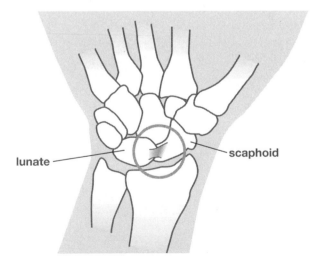

Figure 27.2. Diagram of the scapholunate ligament (circled) (© 2006 American Society for Surgery of the Hand).

ligaments in the wrist, but they are less frequently injured. Sprains can have a wide range of severity; minor sprains may have minimal stretch of the ligaments, and more severe sprains may have complete ruptures of the ligament(s).

How are these injuries treated?

Initially your doctor will examine your wrist, to check its flexibility and stability, and to see where it hurts. X-rays are taken to check the alignment of the wrist bones and to check for any fractures. Occasionally other studies such as magnetic resonance imaging (MRI) may be performed to help determine the diagnosis. Treatment may range from immobilization in a splint or cast to surgery. Surgery may consist of arthroscopic or open surgery. Arthroscopic surgery is performed through small (3–4 millimeter) holes in the skin where a camera and other special instruments are placed inside the wrist to confirm the diagnosis and potentially treat the ligament injury. Some injuries require open surgery in which an incision is made to repair and/or reconstruct the ligament. A variety of methods exist, which could include metal pins, screws, and other specialized devices. Patients are usually placed in a splint or cast after surgery which may need to remain on for 6–12 weeks after surgery. Your doctor will determine the best course of treatment.

Chronic Injuries

The term "chronic" refers to an old injury of greater than several months to years. If there is no or minimal cartilage damage, the ligament may be reconstructed as discussed above. If there is moderate to severe cartilage damage (arthritis), symptoms may be pain, stiffness, and swelling. These may be first treated with splinting and non-steroidal anti-inflammatory medicines, and later with cortisone injections. If these treatments fail, surgery may be an option. This may be a partial wrist fusion, removal of arthritic bones ("proximal row carpectomy"), wrist replacement, or complete wrist fusion. Your doctor will determine the best course of treatment.

Associated Injuries

Occasionally fractures occur along with wrist sprains. These may require additional surgery to repair the fracture with metal pins, screws, or plates. Cartilage damage may also be present which does not show up on the x-ray.

♣ It's A Fact!!

Wrist Fractures

Wrist fractures are common among children and the elderly. Children's bones are soft and tend to get buckle (torus) fractures, which are incomplete fractures on one side of the bone. Because bones become brittle with age, fractures are common among the elderly.

Wrist fractures most often occur when a person falls forward and then attempts to break the fall by throwing the hands forward. The impact of the hand on the ground and the sudden uptake of body weight by the wrist cause the ends of the radius and/or the ulna (the bones in the forearm) to buckle just above the wrist.

In older people, particularly those with osteoporosis, the radius may fracture just above the wrist, resulting in a backward angle. This is called a Colles' fracture.

The fracture may appear on an x-ray as a mild increase in density on the top side of the bone with a slight irregularity in the surface rather than a nice smooth line. Severe injuries will show evidence of a fracture through the entire bone.

Treatment may range from simple immobilization with a splint and sling to a lightweight fiberglass cast. If cast immobilization is insufficient to repair the fracture, surgery may be necessary and the break may need to be fixed with a plate and screws.

Causes: This injury is usually the result of trauma from a fall in which the person attempts to break the fall using the hands and arms. It is frequently associated with such sports as inline skating, skateboarding, running, or any other activity in which the hands may be called upon to prevent a foreword fall occurring at relatively high speed.

What you can expect from these injuries?

Despite optimal treatment, wrist sprains occasionally result in residual long term pain, stiffness, and swelling. The wrist is a complex group of bones, cartilage, and ligaments that are in a delicate balance for precise movements. Injury can upset this balance and damage previously well-tuned moving parts.

Symptoms

- History of a typical fall resulting in wrist injury

- Wrist pain

- Swelling just above the wrist

- Deformity of the arm just above the wrist (increased angulation)

- Unable to hold or lift object of any significant weight

First Aid

- Reassure the injured person.

- A fractured or dislocated hand, finger, or wrist should be placed and splinted in a normal resting position. Rest the fingers around a padded object such as a sock, wadded cloth, or rolled elastic bandage. If the hand or wrist is injured, place the object in the victim's palm, and use a circumferential wrap to maintain the position of the object. In order for the hand to maintain circulation, keep the fingertips uncovered. If the victim has a broken wrist, place a rigid splint on the underside of the wrist, hand, and forearm to restrict any motion. Broken fingers can be splinted independently or taped together with padding in between.

- Elevate the broken wrist, hand, or finger and place it in a sling.

- Use an ice pack over the wrist to help reduce swelling.

- Transport the victim to an emergency medical facility.

- DO NOT attempt to move the wrist or hand.

Source: Excerpted from "Colles' Wrist Fracture," © 2006 A.D.A.M., Inc. Reprinted with permission.

Future Treatments

There is much research underway searching for better methods to treat these serious injuries. They include stronger and more precise ligament reconstructions using either local tissues (tendons) or distant tissues (ligaments from the hand or foot).

Thumb Sprains

What are thumb sprains?

A sprain is an injury to a ligament. Ligaments are the connective tissues that connect bones to bones across a joint.

How do thumb sprains occur?

These types of injuries are common in sports and falls. The thumb is jammed into another player, the ground, or the ball. The thumb may be bent in an extreme position, causing a sprain. The thumb will usually swell and may show bruising. It is usually very painful to move.

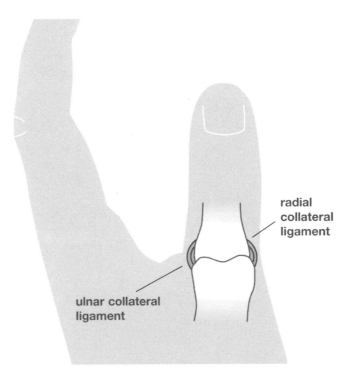

Figure 27.3. The ulnar collateral ligament (UCL) and the radial collateral ligament (RCL) help stabilize the thumb (© 2006 American Society for Surgery of the Hand).

What are the most common types of thumb sprains?

The most common ligament to be injured in the thumb is the ulnar collateral ligament (see Figure 27.3). Injury to this ligament is sometimes called "skier's thumb" because it is a common skiing injury. It occurs when the skier falls and the pole acts as a fulcrum in the hand to bend the thumb in an extreme position. This ligament may also be injured by jamming the thumb on the ground when falling or by jamming the thumb on a ball or other player. The radial collateral ligament (see Figure 27.3) may also be injured. It is much less commonly injured than the ulnar collateral ligament.

How are thumb sprains treated?

X-rays are usually taken to make sure the bones of the thumb and hand are not fractured. Your doctor will then examine the thumb to determine whether the ligament is torn. If the ligament is partially torn, it is usually treated in a cast or splint. Radial collateral ligament injuries are frequently treated this way as well. The end of a completely torn ulnar collateral ligament often gets trapped behind a tendon. Complete ulnar collateral ligament tears are most commonly treated with surgery to repair the ligament. Sometimes the remaining ligament tissue is of poor quality and the ligament must be reconstructed.

Chronic Injuries

The term "chronic" refers to an old injury of greater than several weeks duration. In this case, the joint may be unstable with symptoms of pain, especially with pinching. The joint may feel loose and strength may be decreased. These injuries may be treated by reconstruction of the ligament, or joint fusion if arthritis is present.

Associated Injuries

On occasion, fractures may occur along with thumb sprains. These may require additional surgery with repair using metal pins, screws, or plates. Cartilage damage may occur as well which does not show up on x-ray. This occasionally results in long-term pain and eventual arthritis. Some patients may benefit from cortisone injections or eventual surgery.

♣ **It's A Fact!!**
Boxer's Fracture

What is it?

Boxer's fracture is the common name for a break in the end of the small finger metacarpal bone. ·

What caused it?

It is usually caused by punching something harder than the hand, such as a wall or another person's head. The end of the metacarpal bone takes the brunt of the impact, which usually breaks through the narrowest area near the end (the "neck"), and bends down toward the palm.

What can you do to help?

Ice, elevation, and hangover help if needed.

What can a therapist do to help?

A therapist can make a splint to help protect the broken bone.

Hand Fractures

What is a fracture?

The hand is made up of many bones that form its supporting framework. This frame acts as a point of attachment for the muscles that make the wrist and fingers move. A fracture occurs when enough force is applied to a bone to break it. When this happens, there is pain, swelling, and decreased use of the injured part. Many people think that a fracture is different from a break, but they are the same (see Figure 27.4). Fractures may be simple with the bone pieces aligned and stable. Other fractures are unstable and the bone fragments tend to displace or shift. Some fractures occur in the shaft (main body) of the bone, others break the joint surface.

What can a doctor do to help?

A doctor can set the bone, but many times the bone falls back after being set. If the break is bad enough, it may be best to have the fracture set and then held in place with pins or other hardware.

How successful is treatment?

Casting or splinting the break is helpful to keep from injuring the area further, but without surgery, the break usually heals with a bend at the site of the break. The most reliable way to get the bones to heal straight is to use with pins or other orthopedic hardware. This works well in most people—but is not usually needed, as most people do just fine even if the bone heals with a bit of a bend.

What happens if you have no treatment?

Most of the time, the break heals without any real problem. However, if the bone heals with too much of a bend, it may mess up the action of the tendons which straighten the other finger joints, and result in a permanent bend in the middle knuckle of the finger.

Comminuted fractures (bone is shattered into many pieces) usually occur from a high energy force and are often unstable. An open (compound) fracture occurs when a bone fragment breaks through the skin. There is some risk of infection with compound fractures.

How does a fracture affect the hand?

Fractures often take place in the hand. A fracture may cause pain, stiffness, and loss of movement. Some fractures will cause an obvious deformity, such as a crooked finger, but many fractures do not. Because of the close relationship of bones to ligaments and tendons, the hand may be stiff and weak after the fracture heals. Fractures that involve joint surfaces may lead to early arthritis in those involved joints.

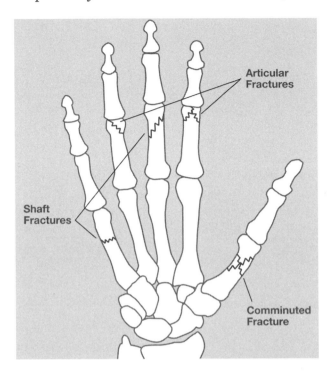

Figure 27.4. Examples of fractures in fingers (© 2006 American Society for Surgery of the Hand).

How are hand fractures treated?

Medical evaluation and x-rays are usually needed so that your doctor can tell if there is a fracture and to help determine the treatment. Depending upon the type of fracture, your hand surgeon may recommend one of several treatment methods.

A splint or cast may be used to treat a fracture that is not displaced, or to protect a fracture that has been set. Some displaced fractures may need to be set and then held in place with wires or pins without making an incision. This is called closed reduction and internal fixation.

Other fractures may need surgery to set the bone (open reduction). Once the bone fragments are set, they are held together with pins, plates, or screws (see Figure 27.5). Fractures that disrupt the joint surface (articular fractures)

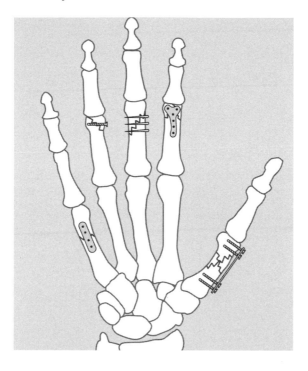

Figure 27.5. Examples of plates, pins, and screws used to join fractures while they heal (© 2006 American Society for Surgery of the Hand).

usually need to be set more precisely to restore the joint surface as smooth as possible. On occasion, bone may be missing or be so severely crushed that it cannot be repaired. In such cases, a bone graft may be necessary. In this procedure, bone is taken from another part of the body to help provide more stability.

Fractures that have been set may be held in place by an "external fixator," a set of metal bars outside the body attached to pins which are placed in the bone above and below the fracture site, in effect keeping it in traction until the bone heals.

Once the fracture has enough stability, motion exercises may be started to try to avoid stiffness. Your hand surgeon may determine when the fracture is sufficiently stable.

What types of results can I expect from surgery for hand fractures?

Perfect alignment of the bone on x-ray is not always necessary to get good function. A bony lump may appear at the fracture site as the bone heals and is known as a "fracture callus." This functions as a "spot weld." This is a normal healing process and the lump usually gets smaller over time. Problems with fracture healing include stiffness, shift in position, infection, slow healing, or complete failure to heal. Smoking has been shown to slow fracture healing. Fractures in children occasionally affect future growth of that bone. You can lessen the chances of complication by carefully following your hand surgeon's advice during the healing process and before returning to work or sports activities. A hand therapy program with splints and exercises may be recommended by your physician to speed and improve the recovery process.

Chapter 28

Growth Plate Injuries

What is the growth plate?

The growth plate, also known as the epiphyseal plate or physis, is the area of growing tissue near the ends of the long bones in children and adolescents. Each long bone has at least two growth plates: one at each end. The growth plate determines the future length and shape of the mature bone. When growth is complete—sometime during adolescence—the growth plates close and are replaced by solid bone.

Because the growth plates are the weakest areas of the growing skeleton—even weaker than the nearby ligaments and tendons that connect bones to other bones and muscles—they are vulnerable to injury. Injuries to the growth plate are called fractures.

Who gets growth plate injuries?

Growth plate injuries can occur in growing children and adolescents. In a child, a serious injury to a joint is more likely to damage a growth plate than the ligaments that stabilize the joint. Trauma that would cause a sprain in an adult might cause a growth plate fracture in a child.

About This Chapter: From "Questions and Answers about Growth Plate Injuries," National Institute of Arthritis and Musculoskeletal and Skin Disorders (NIAMS), August 2007.

Fractures can result from a single traumatic event, such as a fall or automobile accident, or from chronic stress and overuse. Most growth plate fractures occur in the long bones of the fingers (phalanges) and the outer bone of the forearm (radius). They are also common in the lower bones of the leg (the tibia and fibula).

What causes growth plate injuries?

Growth plate injuries can be caused by an event such as a fall or blow to the limb, or they can result from overuse. For example, a gymnast who practices for hours on the uneven bars, a long-distance runner, and a baseball pitcher perfecting his curve ball can all have growth plate injuries.

- Growth plate fractures occur twice as often in boys as in girls because girls' bodies mature at an earlier age than boys. As a result, their bones finish growing sooner, and their growth plates are replaced by stronger bone.

- One-third of all growth plate injuries occur in competitive sports such as football, basketball, or gymnastics, while about 20 percent of growth plate fractures occur as a result of recreational activities such as biking, sledding, skiing, or skateboarding.

Although many growth plate injuries are caused by accidents that occur during play or athletic activity, growth plates are also susceptible to other disorders, such as bone infection, that can alter their normal growth and development. Other possible causes of growth plate injuries include the following:

- **Child Abuse:** More than 1 million children each year are the victims of substantiated child abuse or neglect. The second most common injury among abused children is a fracture, and growth plate injuries are prevalent because the growth plate is the weakest part of the bone.

- **Injury From Extreme Cold (for example, frostbite):** Exposure to extreme cold can damage the growth plate in children and result in short, stubby fingers or premature degenerative arthritis (breakdown of the joint cartilage).

- **Radiation And Medications:** Research has suggested that chemotherapy given for childhood cancers may negatively affect bone growth.

Prolonged use of steroids for inflammatory conditions such as juvenile idiopathic arthritis can also harm bone growth.

- **Neurological Disorders:** Children with certain neurological disorders that result in sensory deficit or muscular imbalance are prone to growth plate fractures, especially at the ankle and knee. Children who are born with insensitivity to pain can have similar types of injuries.

- **Genetics:** The growth plates are where many inherited disorders that affect the musculoskeletal system appear. Scientists are just beginning to understand the genes and gene mutations involved in skeletal formation, growth, and development. This new information is raising hopes for improving treatment for children who are born with poorly formed or improperly functioning growth plates.

- **Metabolic Disease:** Disease states such as kidney failure and hormone disorders can affect the growth plates and their function. The bone growth of children with long-term conditions of this kind may be negatively affected.

How are growth plate fractures diagnosed?

A child who has persistent pain, or pain that affects athletic performance or the ability to move and put pressure on a limb, should never be allowed or expected to "work through the pain." Whether an injury is acute or due to overuse, it should be evaluated by a doctor, because some injuries, if left untreated, can cause permanent damage and interfere with proper growth of the involved limb.

The doctor will begin the diagnostic process by asking about the injury and how it occurred and by examining the child. The doctor will then use x-rays to determine if there is a fracture, and if so, the type of fracture. Often the doctor will x-ray not only the injured limb but the opposite limb as well. Because growth plates have not yet hardened into solid bone, neither the structures themselves nor injuries to them show up on x-rays. Instead, growth plates appear as gaps between the shaft of a long bone, called the metaphysis, and the end of the bone, called the epiphysis. By comparing x-rays of the injured limb to those of the non-injured limb, doctors can look for differences that indicate an injury.

Very often the x-ray is negative, because the growth plate line is already there, and the fracture is undisplaced (the two ends of the broken bone are not separated). The doctor can still diagnose a growth plate fracture on clinical grounds because of tenderness of the plate. Children do get ligament strains if their growth plates are open, and they often have undisplaced growth plate fractures.

Other tests doctors may use to diagnose a growth plate injury include magnetic resonance imaging (MRI), computed tomography (CT), and ultrasound.

Because these tests enable doctors to see the growth plate and areas of other soft tissue, they can be useful not only in detecting the presence of an injury, but also in determining the type and extent of the injury.

What kind of doctor treats growth plate injuries?

For all but the simplest injuries, your doctor will probably refer you to an orthopaedic surgeon (a doctor who specializes in bone and joint problems in children and adults) for treatment. Some problems may require the services of a pediatric orthopaedic surgeon, who specializes in injuries and musculoskeletal disorders in children.

How are growth plate injuries treated?

Treatment for growth plate injuries depends on the type of injury. In all cases, treatment should be started as soon as possible after injury and will generally involve a mix of the following:

✎ What's It Mean?

Epiphysis: The end of a long bone, which is initially separated by cartilage from the shaft of the bone and develops separately. It eventually fuses with the shaft (diaphysis) of the bone to form a complete bone.

Metaphysis: The growing portion of a long bone that lies between the ends of the bones (epiphyses) and the shaft (diaphysis).

Physis: The area of developing tissue near the end of the long bones in children and adolescents. The physis is also called the growth plate.

Immobilization: The affected limb is often put in a cast or splint, and the child is told to limit any activity that puts pressure on the injured area.

Manipulation Or Surgery: If the fracture is displaced (meaning the ends of the injured bones no longer meet as they should), the doctor will have to put the bones or joints back in their correct positions, either by using his or her hands (called manipulation) or by performing surgery. Sometimes the doctor needs to fix the break and hold the growth plate in place with screws or wire. After the procedure, the bone will be set in place (immobilized) so it can heal without moving. This is usually done with a cast that encloses the injured growth plate and the joints on both sides of it. The cast is left in place until the injury heals, which can take anywhere from a few weeks to two or more months for serious injuries. The need for manipulation or surgery depends on the location and extent of the injury, its effect on nearby nerves and blood vessels, and the child's age.

Strengthening And Range-Of-Motion Exercises: These are exercises designed to strengthen the muscles that support the injured area of the bone and to improve or maintain the joint's ability to move in the way that it should. Your doctor may recommend these after the fracture has healed. A physical therapist can work with you and your doctor to design an appropriate exercise plan.

Long-Term Follow-Up: Long-term follow-up is usually necessary to monitor the child's recuperation and growth. Evaluation includes x-rays of matching limbs at three- to six-month intervals for at least two years. Some fractures require periodic evaluations until the child's bones have finished growing. Sometimes a growth arrest line (a line on the x-ray where the bone stopped growing temporarily) may appear as a marker of the injury. Continued bone growth away from that line may mean there will not be a long-term problem, and the doctor may decide to stop following the patient.

Will the affected limb of a child with a growth plate injury still grow?

About 85 percent of growth plate fractures heal without any lasting effect. Whether an arrest of growth occurs depends on the treatment provided, and the following factors, in descending order of importance:

- **Severity Of The Injury:** If the injury causes the blood supply to the epiphysis to be cut off, growth can be stunted. If the growth plate is shifted, shattered, or crushed, the growth plate may close prematurely, forming a bony bridge or "bar." The risk of growth arrest is higher in this setting. An open injury in which the skin is broken carries the risk of infection, which could destroy the growth plate.

- **Age Of The Child:** In a younger child, the bones have a great deal of growing to do; therefore, growth arrest can be more serious, and closer surveillance is needed. It is also true, however, that younger bones have a greater ability to heal.

- **Which Growth Plate Is Injured:** Some growth plates, such as those in the region of the knee, are more involved in extensive bone growth than others.

- **Type Of Fracture:** The most serious fractures are: fractures that run through the epiphysis, across the growth plate, and into the metaphysis; fractures in which the end of the bone is crushed and the growth plate is compressed; and fractures in which a portion of the epiphysis, growth plate, and metaphysis is missing (this usually occurs with open wounds and compound fractures).

The most frequent complication of a growth plate fracture is premature arrest of bone growth. The affected bone grows less than it would have without the injury, and the resulting limb could be shorter than the opposite, uninjured limb. If only part of the growth plate is injured, growth may be lopsided and the limb may become crooked.

♣ **It's A Fact!!**

National Institute of Arthritis and Musculoskeletal and Skin Diseases (NIAMS) currently funds Core Centers for Musculoskeletal Disorders at major medical centers. These centers provide the resources for established, currently funded investigators who are often from different disciplines, to adopt a multidisciplinary approach to common research problems in musculoskeletal disorders.

The centers foster research to better understand the mechanisms of bone repair and regeneration, including fracture healing and development of techniques for growth plate repair.

Growth plate injuries at the knee have the greatest risk of complications. Nerve and blood vessel damage occurs most frequently there. Injuries to the knee have a much higher incidence of premature growth arrest and crooked growth.

What are researchers trying to learn about growth plate injuries?

Researchers continue to seek better ways to diagnose and treat growth plate injuries and to improve patient outcomes. Examples of such work include the following:

- Removal of a growth-blocking "bridge" or bar of bone that can form across a growth plate following a fracture: After the bridge is removed, fat, cartilage, or other materials are inserted in its place to prevent the bridge from forming again. Investigators are studying the use of cultured chondrocytes (cartilage cells grown in a dish) to replace the bridge.

- Use of gene therapy and/or other means to enhance the body's production of chondrocytes: These cells are essential to growth at the ends of the bones.

- Research on drugs that protect the growth plate during radiation treatment: One study of animals showed that the drug amifostine, in combination with pentoxifylline, selenium, or misoprostol, reduced the risk of limb-length discrepancies that can occur when radiation is used to treat cancer in a limb.

- A study of radiologic predictors for premature closure of the growth plate following fractures: By predicting the injuries most likely to result in arrested growth, doctors could opt to treat them differently and more aggressively.

- Research on cancer drugs to determine which ones are likely to affect the growth plates: One recent study, for example, showed that in rats the chemotherapy agent doxorubicin affected the growth plate of the tibia at the knee while two other agents, methotrexate and cisplatin, did not.

- Development of methods to regenerate musculoskeletal tissue by using principles of tissue engineering.

Chapter 29

Testicular Injuries

It hurts to even think about it. A baseball takes an unexpected bounce when you're crouched and waiting to field a grounder, an opponent misses a kick on the soccer field and his foot has only one place to go, or you're speeding along on your bike and you hit a big bump. All result in one really painful thing—a shot to the testicles, one of the most tender areas on a guy's body. Testicular injuries are relatively uncommon, but guys should be aware that they can happen. So how can you avoid injury?

Why Do Testicular Injuries Happen And What Can You Do?

If you're a guy who plays sports, likes to lift weights and exercise a lot, or leads an all-around active life, you've probably come to find out that the testicles are kind of vulnerable and can be injured in a variety of ways. Because they hang in a sac outside the body (the scrotum), the testicles are not protected by bones and muscles like other parts of your reproductive system and most of your other organs. Also, the location of the testicles makes them prime targets to be accidentally struck on the playing field or injured during strenuous exercise and activity.

About This Chapter: "Testicular Injuries," September 2007, reprinted with permission from www.kidshealth.org. Copyright © 2007 The Nemours Foundation. This information was provided by KidsHealth, one of the largest resources online for medically reviewed health information written for parents, kids, and teens. For more articles like this one, visit www.KidsHealth.org, or www.TeensHealth.org.

The good news is that because the testicles are loosely attached to the body and are made of a spongy material, they're able to absorb most collisions without permanent damage. Testicles, although sensitive, can bounce back pretty quickly and minor injuries rarely have long-term effects. Also, sexual function or sperm production will most likely not be affected if you have a testicular injury.

You'll definitely feel pain if your testicles are struck or kicked, and you might also feel nauseous for a short time. If it's a minor testicular injury, the pain should gradually subside in less than an hour and any other symptoms should go away. In the meantime, you can do a few things to help yourself feel better such as take pain relievers, lie down, gently support the testicles with supportive underwear, and apply ice packs to the area. At any rate, it's a good idea to avoid strenuous activity for a while and take it easy for a few days.

However, if the pain doesn't subside or you experience extreme pain that lasts longer than an hour; if you have swelling or bruising of the scrotum or a puncture of the scrotum or testicle; if you continue to have nausea and vomiting; or if you develop a fever, get to a doctor immediately. These are symptoms of a much more serious injury that needs to be addressed as soon as possible.

Serious Testicular Injuries

Examples of serious testicular injury are testicular torsion and testicular rupture. In the case of testicular torsion, the testicle twists around, cutting off its blood supply. This can happen due to a serious trauma to the testicles, strenuous activity, or even for no apparent reason.

Testicular torsion isn't common, but when it does happen, it most often occurs in guys ages 12 to 18. If it occurs, it is crucial to see a doctor as soon as possible—within 6 hours of the time the pain starts. Unfortunately, after 6 hours, there is a much greater possibility that complications could result, including reduced sperm production or the loss of the testicle. The problem may be fixed by a doctor manually untwisting the testicle. If that doesn't work, surgery will be necessary.

✔ Quick Tip
Seeing A Doctor

If you have to see a doctor, he or she will first need to know how long
you have been experiencing pain and how severe your discomfort is. To rule
out a hernia or other problem as the cause of the pain, the doctor will examine
your abdomen and groin. In addition, the doctor will look at your scrotum for
swelling, color, and damage to the skin and examine the testicle itself. Because
infections of the reproductive system or urinary tract can sometimes cause
similar pain, your doctor may do a urine test to rule out a urinary
tract infection or infection of the reproductive organs.

Testicular rupture can also happen, but it is a rare type of testicular trauma.
This can happen when the testicle receives a forceful direct blow or when the
testicle is crushed against the pubic bone (the bone that forms the front of the
pelvis), causing blood to leak into the scrotum. Testicular rupture, like testicular
torsion and other serious injuries to the testicles, causes extreme pain, swelling in
the scrotum, nausea, and vomiting. To fix the problem, surgery is necessary to
repair the ruptured testicle.

Preventing Testicular Injuries

It's a good idea to take precautions to avoid testicular injuries, especially
if you play sports, exercise a lot, or just live an all-around active life. Here are
some tips to keep your testicles safe and sound:

Protect Your Testicles: Always wear an athletic cup or athletic supporter
when playing sports or participating in strenuous activity. Athletic cups are
usually made of hard plastic, are worn over the groin area, and provide a
good degree of shielding and safety for the testicles. Cups are best used when
participating in sports where your testicles might get hit or kicked, like football, hockey, soccer, or karate. An athletic supporter, or jock strap, is basically
a cloth pouch that you wear to keep your testicles close to your body. Athletic supporters are best used when participating in strenuous exercise, cycling, or doing any heavy lifting.

Check Your Fit: Make sure the athletic cup and/or athletic supporter is the right size. Safety equipment that's too small or too big won't protect you as effectively.

Keep Your Doctor Informed: If you play sports, you probably have regular physical exams by a doctor. If you experience testicular pain even occasionally, talk to your doctor about it.

Be Aware Of The risks Of Your Sport Or Activity: If you play a sport or participate in an activity with a high risk of injury, talk to your coach or doctor about any additional protective gear you should use.

☞ **Remember!!**

Participating in sports and living an active life are great ways to stay fit and relieve stress. But it's important to make sure your testicles are protected. When you're exercising or playing sports, make sure that using protective gear is part of your routine and you'll be able to play hard without fear of testicular injury.

Chapter 30

Knee Injuries

If you've ever injured your knee, you're not alone. Knee injuries have actually become pretty common. One of the main reasons they're common is that with so many teens playing sports, knees can be overused, leading to several types of injuries, some of which can't be repaired. So what are some of these knee injuries and what can you do to prevent them?

What's In A Knee?

To understand knee injuries, first you have to understand the knee. The knee is a joint, which means it sits between the area where bones connect. It's actually the largest joint in the body. Your knees provide stability and flexibility for your body and allow your legs to bend, swivel, and straighten. The knee is made up of several body parts like bones, cartilage, muscles, ligaments, and tendons, all working as one. So when we talk about a knee injury, it could be stress or damage to any of these parts.

About This Chapter: "Knee Injuries," January 2006, reprinted with permission from www.kidshealth.org. Copyright © 2006 The Nemours Foundation. This information was provided by KidsHealth, one of the largest resources online for medically reviewed health information written for parents, kids, and teens. For more articles like this one, visit www.KidsHealth.org, or www.TeensHealth.org.

Bones And Cartilage

The knee sits in the middle of three bones: the tibia (your shin bone), the femur (your thigh bone), and the patella (the knee cap). The patella is a flat, triangular bone that protects the knee joint.

The ends of the femur and the patella are covered in articular cartilage. Articular cartilage acts like a cushion and to keep the femur, patella, and tibia from grinding against each other. On the top of the tibia, extra pads of cartilage called menisci help absorb the

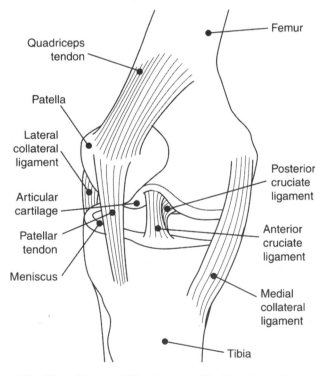

Figure 30.1. The Knee (Source: "Handout on Health: Sports Injuries," National Institute of Arthritis and Musculoskeletal and Skin Diseases, National Institutes of Health, NIH Publication No. 04-5278, April 2004.)

body's weight (if you're talking about one, it's called a meniscus). Each knee has two menisci—the inside (medial) meniscus and the outside (lateral) meniscus.

Muscles

The muscles in the knee include the quadriceps, a large muscle at the front of the thigh, and the hamstring, which is located at the back of the thigh. The quadriceps muscle helps you straighten and extend your leg, and the hamstring helps you bend your knee.

Tendons And Ligaments

Several tendons and ligaments work together to help the knee move naturally.

Tendons are like cables of strong tissue that connect muscles to bones. The tendons in the knee are the quadriceps tendon and the patellar tendon. The quadriceps tendon connects to the top of the patella (kneecap) and allows you to extend your leg. The patellar tendon connects to the bottom of your kneecap and attaches to the top of the tibia (shinbone).

Ligaments are like cables of strong tissue that connect bones to bones or cartilage to bones. There are four ligaments in the knee that help connect the femur to the tibia and keep your legs stable:

- **Medial Collateral Ligament (MCL):** The MCL connects your femur to your tibia along the inside of your knee. It keeps the inner part of your knee stable and helps control the sideways motion of your knee, like keeping it from bending inward.

- **Lateral Collateral Ligament (LCL):** The LCL connects your femur to your tibia along the outside of your knee. It keeps the outer part of your knee stable and helps control the sideways motion of your knee, like keeping it from bending outward.

- **Anterior Cruciate Ligament (ACL):** The ACL connects your femur to your tibia at the center of the knee. It helps control forward motion and rotation, like keeping your shinbone from sliding out in front of your thighbone.

- **Posterior Cruciate Ligament (PCL):** The PCL connects your femur to your tibia at the back of the knee. It helps control the knee's backward motion, like keeping the shinbone from sliding out under the thighbone.

Types Of Knee Injuries

Now that you know all about its working parts, you probably realize that there are a bunch of ways to injure a knee. Common causes for injuries are overuse (from repetitive motions, like in many sports), sudden stops or twists, or direct blows to the knee. Here are some of the more common injuries:

Sprains

A sprain means you've stretched or torn a ligament. Common knee sprains usually involve damage to the ACL or MCL. The most serious sprains involve complete tears of one or more of the knee ligaments. Symptoms of knee sprains include:

- a popping or snapping sound in the knee at the time of injury;
- pain that seems to come from within the knee, especially with movement;
- not being able to put any weight on that leg;
- swelling;
- fluid behind the kneecap;
- the knee feels loose or unstable.

Strains

A strain means you've partially or completely torn a muscle or tendon. With knee strains, you may feel symptoms similar to a sprain and may see bruises around the injured area.

Tendinitis

Tendinitis happens when a tendon gets irritated or inflamed. It is often caused by overuse. A person with tendinitis might have pain or tenderness when walking, or when bending, extending, or lifting a leg.

Meniscal Tears

Damage to the menisci is a really common sports injury, especially in sports where sudden changes in speed or side-to-side movements can cause them to tear. Meniscal injuries often occur together with severe sprains, especially those involving the ACL. Meniscal injuries can cause tenderness, tightness, and swelling around the front of the knee. Sometimes fluid collects around the knee (this is called effusion).

Fractures And Dislocations

A fracture is a cracked, broken, or shattered bone. You may have trouble moving that bone and it's likely there's a lot of pain. Patellar dislocation happens when the patella (the kneecap) is knocked off to the side of the knee joint, by twisting or some kind of impact. Sometimes it will go back to its normal position by itself, but usually it will need to be put back into place by a doctor. Symptoms include swelling and a lot of pain at the front of your knee. There will usually be an abnormal bulge on the side of your knee, and you may be unable to walk.

Cartilage Injuries

Sometimes a small piece of bone or cartilage softens or breaks off from the end of a bone, causing long-term knee pain. This is called osteochondritis desiccans (OCD). Symptoms of OCD include pain, swelling, an inability to extend the leg, and stiffness, catching, or popping sensations with knee movement. Treatment can include resting the knee, wearing a cast for a couple of months, and sometimes surgery in older teens. Chondromalacia happens when the cartilage in the knee joint softens because of injury, muscle weakness, or overuse, and the patella and the thighbone may rub together. This causes pain and aching, especially when a person walks up stairs or hills. Treatment may involve surgery.

Other Conditions Of The Knee

Bursitis

A bursa is a sac filled with fluid located near a joint. If a bursa in the knee becomes inflamed and swollen from overuse or constant friction, it can develop into a condition called bursitis. Symptoms of bursitis in the knee include warmth, tenderness, swelling, and pain on the front of the kneecap.

Osgood-Schlatter Disease

Osgood-Schlatter disease is a painful disorder caused by repetitive stress on the front end of the tibia where the patellar tendon connects to the bone. It happens most frequently in young athletes between the ages of 10 to 15 years. Symptoms include a bump below the knee joint that's painful to the touch and is also painful with activity. Pain is relieved with rest.

What Do Doctors Do?

There are different things a doctor may do to figure out whether you have a knee injury. Treatment for a knee injury usually depends on the type of injury you have.

First, your doctor will ask you questions about your symptoms, including what your usual activities are, especially any sports you play. The doctor will also want to know about other health conditions that lead to knee pain.

♣ It's A Fact!!

What Kinds Of Doctors Treat Knee Problems?

Injuries and diseases of the knees are usually treated by an orthopaedist (a doctor who treats problems with bones, joints, ligaments, tendons, and muscles).

Source: Excerpted from "Fast Fasts About Knee Problems," National Institute of Arthritis and Musculoskeletal and Skin Diseases (www.niams.nih.gov), March 2006.

The doctor will then examine the different parts of your knee, checking the bones, ligaments, and tendons for any signs of injury. The doctor will probably bend, twist, and turn your knee to look for any signs of an unstable knee joint. Don't be surprised if you're asked to get off the exam table and walk, bend over, or squat so your doctor can get a better look at your knee. Sometimes an x-ray of your knee is needed to get a good picture of your bones. A computerized axial tomography (CAT) scan or magnetic resonance imaging (MRI) may also be recommended so doctors can get a better three-dimensional picture.

For injuries like mild sprains, strains, and overuse, resting your knee may be one of the first treatments your doctor recommends. Remember RICE:

- Rest

- Ice

- Compression

- Elevation

If your doctor recommends RICE, you should rest your knee as much as possible, use ice packs for a couple of days to bring down swelling, use compression (ACE) bandages, and elevate the leg on pillows or other soft objects. For inflammation and pain, your doctor may prescribe anti-inflammatory medications like ibuprofen.

Other treatment for knee injuries may involve using a knee immobilizer (kind of like a brace or a sleeve that you wrap around your leg to keep it from moving too much), or having to wear a cast for a few weeks or months. You may also have to use crutches to get around for awhile.

For more serious knee injuries, your doctor might recommend you see an orthopedic surgeon, a doctor specially trained in the care of bone and joint diseases (also called an orthopedist). Orthopedists take care of many kinds of knee injuries, especially those involving sports and different types of accidents. He or she will know how to treat the injury and follow your progress as it heals.

Arthroscopy

If necessary, an orthopedist will perform arthroscopy, a type of surgery that takes a direct look at the inside of your knee joint.

During arthroscopy, the orthopedist first makes a small opening in the knee and inserts an arthroscope, a tiny tube-like tool, into the joint capsule. The arthroscope contains a lighted video camera on the end, and is wired to a television screen that the surgeon watches while moving the scope to pinpoint the exact knee problem. Most of the time, the doctor is able to fix the problem during the procedure, like repairing a torn ACL ligament.

Arthroscopy is often used to treat knee injuries such as ligament and meniscal tears, as well as other types of serious knee injuries. An orthopedist can also perform open surgery on the knee, which allows him or her to see the injury without the aid of a television screen.

Physical Therapy

Depending on the type of knee injury you have, your doctor may recommend rehabilitative physical therapy. Working with a physical therapist, you'll do specific exercises designed to take your knee joint through its range of motion to prevent stiffness and scarring as your knee heals. You may also need to do regular exercises to strengthen the muscles surrounding the knee. Physical therapy is commonly used to help a person recover after surgery.

You may be anxious for your knee to heal so you can get back to your sport and your normal life. But trying to rush your recovery after an injury or surgery can put you at risk for future injury and may further extend the healing process. Take your doctor or physical therapist's instructions seriously, and don't put your health in jeopardy by returning to your normal activities before you get the go-ahead from a health pro.

Preventing Knee Injuries

Preventing knee injuries from the start is a lot less painful and a lot less hassle than undergoing surgery. If you play sports, always wear appropriate protective equipment during practices and competitions. Kneepads and shin guards (as well as helmets and other protective gear) will help to protect you from injury. You'll also want to make sure you wear supportive shoes that are in good condition and are appropriate for your sport.

When it comes to your workouts, always warm up and cool down, and remember to work up to your training program slowly. Suddenly increasing the intensity or duration of your workouts can lead to overuse injuries. Try weightlifting to strengthen your muscles and stretching and yoga to improve your flexibility because strong, flexible muscles help support and protect joints. If you play only one sport, try conditioning and training year-round—even if it's at a lower intensity than during your competitive season—to maintain coordination and balance. That way you'll be less likely to injure yourself during your competitive season.

In growing kids and teens, imbalances in muscle flexibility and strength can lead to injuries and inflammation from overuse. Regular stretching can help. After an injury or surgery has healed, it is also important to continue a regular stretching or conditioning program to prevent another injury.

The way you move can also help you prevent knee injuries. If your sport involves a lot of jumping, make sure to bend your knees when you land, which takes pressure off of the ACL. Do you have to cut laterally or pivot frequently in your sport? Use your joints to crouch and bend at the knees and hips, reducing your chance of a ligament injury.

Remember, if you experience any symptoms of knee injuries or knee pain, don't hesitate to tell your coach, parent, or doctor. Limit your activities until you can get treatment or a diagnosis.

✔ Quick Tip
How Can People Prevent Knee Problems?

Some knee problems (such as those resulting from an accident) can't be prevented. But many knee problems can be prevented by doing the following:

- Warm up before playing sports. Walking and stretching are good warm-up exercises. Stretching the muscles in the front and the back of the thighs is a good way to warm up the knees.

- Make the leg muscles strong by doing certain exercises (for example, walking up stairs, riding a stationary bicycle, or working out with weights).

- Avoid sudden changes in the intensity of exercise.

- Increase the force or duration of activity slowly.

- Wear shoes that fit and are in good condition.

- Maintain a healthy weight. Extra weight puts pressure on the knees.

Source: Excerpted from "Fast Fasts About Knee Problems," National Institute of Arthritis and Musculoskeletal and Skin Diseases (www.niams.nih.gov), March 2006.

Chapter 31

Shin Splints

Shin splints are pains in the front of the lower legs caused by exercise. They usually appear after a period of relative inactivity.

Causes: Tibial shin splints are very common and affect both recreational and trained athletes. Runners are often affected. There are two types, tibial periostitis and posterior tibial shin splints. In tibial periostitis the bone itself is tender.

Anterior compartment syndrome affects the outer side of the front of the leg.

Stress fractures usually produce localized, sharp pain with tenderness one or two inches below the knee. A stress fracture is likely to occur two or weeks into a new training program or after beginning a harder training program.

Home Care: For posterior tibial and tibial periostitis shin splints, the healing process usually takes a week of rest with ice treatment for 20 minutes twice a day. Over-the-counter pain medications will also help. Do not resume running for another two to four weeks.

For anterior compartment syndrome, pain will usually subside as the muscles gradually accustom themselves to the intense exercise. Complete rest is probably not necessary.

For a stress fracture, a rest period of at least one month is required. Complete healing requires four to six weeks. Crutches can be used but typically are not necessary.

When To Contact A Medical Professional: Although shin splints are seldom serious, you may need to call your health care provider:

♣ **It's A Fact!!**
Shin splints can be caused by any of four types of problems, which are only occasionally serious. Most shin splints can be treated with rest.

- if the pain is prolonged and persistent, even with rest;

- if you are not sure your pain is caused by shin splints;

- if there is no progress with home treatment after several weeks.

What To Expect At Your Office Visit: The health care provider will perform a physical examination and will obtain your medical history. Medical history questions documenting your symptom in detail may include the following:

- *Time Pattern:* When did the pain develop? Is it present all of the time?

- *Quality:* Describe the pain. Is it a sharp pain?

- *Location:* Are both legs affected? Where exactly on the leg is the pain?

- *Aggravating Factors:* Have you recently begun exercising? Have you recently increased the amount that you exercise? Have you recently changed the type of exercise that you do?

- *Relieving Factors:* What have you done for the pain? How well did it work?

- *Other:* What other symptoms are also present?

The physical examination may include an examination of the legs.

Home treatment will be prescribed for any of the different types of shin splints. Surgical intervention might be indicated in the rare event that shin splints caused by an anterior compartment syndrome do not go away over time.

The pressure can be relieved by splitting the tough, fibrous tissue that surrounds the muscles. Surgery may also be necessary in the cases of non-healing stress fractures.

Chapter 32

Ankle Sprains

Sprained Ankle/Ankle Sprain

What is a sprained ankle?

A sprained ankle is a very common type of ankle injury. The most common is an inversion sprain where the ankle turns inwards damaging the ligaments on the outside of the ankle. A medial ligament sprain is rare but can occur particularly with a fracture. A sprain is stretching and or tearing of ligaments. (You sprain a ligament and strain a muscle).

The most common damage done in a sprained ankle is to the talofibular ligament. If the sprain is worse, there might also damage to the calcaneofibular ligament which is further back towards the back of the heel. In addition to the ligament damage there may also be damage to tendons, bone, and other joint tissues.

How are ankle sprains treated?

Treatment of a sprained ankle can be separated into immediate first aid and longer term rehabilitation and strengthening.

About This Chapter: This chapter includes text reprinted with permission from "Sprained Ankle/Ankle Sprain," "Assessment and Diagnosis of the Ankle Sprain," and "Rehabilitation (Sprained Ankle)," © 2007 Sports Injury Clinic. For more information, including video presentations, visit http://www.sportsinjuryclinic.net.

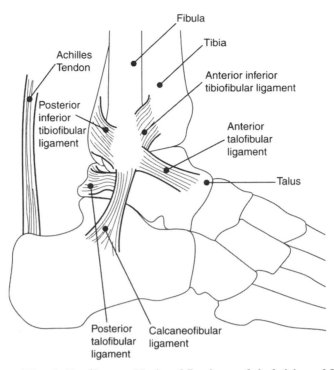

Figure 32.1. The Ankle. (Source: National Institute of Arthritis and Musculoskeletal and Skin Diseases, National Institutes of Health, NIH Publication No. 04-5278, April 2004.)

Immediate first aid for ankle sprains: Aim to reduce the swelling by DR. ICE (diagnosis, rest, ice, compression, elevation) as soon as possible. Getting the diagnosis right from the start is important.

- **D** is for diagnosis. It is important to get the correct diagnosis from the start. If other factors such as an avulsion sprain (where a bone fragment is pulled away from the bone) are suspected then treatment may be different.

- **R** is for rest. It is important to rest the injury to reduce pain and prevent further damage. If you need crutches then use them. People with crutches get more sympathy. Many therapists advocate partial weight bearing as soon as pain will allow. This is thought to accelerate rehabilitation.

- **I** is for ice or cold therapy. Applying ice and compression can ease the pain, reduce swelling, reduce bleeding (initially), and encourage blood flow (when used later).

- **C** is for compression. This reduces bleeding and helps reduce swelling. A Louisiana wrap bandaging technique is excellent for providing support and compression to a recently injured ankle. [A Louisiana ankle wrap guide with streaming video clips is available online; visit http://www.sportsinjuryclinic.net.]

- **E** is for elevation. Elevation uses gravity to reduce bleeding and reduces swelling by allowing fluids to flow away from the site of injury.

♣ It's A Fact!!

A sprained ankle is classified into three categories depending on severity:

First Degree Ankle Sprain

- Some stretching or perhaps tearing of the lateral ankle ligaments
- Little or no joint instability
- Mild pain
- Little or no swelling
- Some joint stiffness or difficulty walking or running

Second Degree Ankle Sprain

- Some tearing of the ligament fibres
- Moderate instability of the joint
- Moderate to severe pain and difficulty walking
- Swelling and stiffness in the ankle joint

Third Degree Ankle Sprain

- Total rupture of a ligament
- Gross instability of the joint
- Severe pain initially followed by no pain
- Severe swelling

So put your feet up and get someone else to wait on you.

In addition to immediate first aid the athlete can do the following:

• Protect the injured ankle by taping or an ankle support. Tape can also be used during the rehabilitation phase to protect the joint and give proprioceptive feedback to the ankle without risking further injury. When partial weight bearing, an ankle support or taping method can protect the lateral ligaments (allowing them to rest) while ensuring forwards and backwards motion is allowed—keeping the rest of the joint healthy.

What can a sports injury specialist do about it?

• A sports injury specialist will undertake a thorough assessment of the injury so time is not wasted treating the wrong condition.

• A doctor may prescribe anti-inflammatory medication to help with pain and swelling.

• Reduce swelling by compression devices or taping techniques.

• Use ultrasound and laser treatment.

• Use cross friction massage.

• Prescribe a full ankle rehabilitation program.

Assessment And Diagnosis Of Ankle Sprains

The following information is for information purposes only. We recommend seeking professional advice before attempting any rehabilitation.

What are the aims of assessment?

• To assess the degree of instability.

• Grade of ligament damage.

• Identify any reduction in range of motion or reduced strength.

• Identify any other additional or associated injuries such as an avulsion sprain where a piece of bone at the end of a ligament has come away from the main bone itself.

It is important to understand that no single test can give a conclusive answer or diagnosis but can help to build an overall picture of the problem in the therapist's head from where they use professional judgment and experience to make a diagnosis.

How is the assessment done?

As with any sports injury the therapist will usually follow a set procedure to diagnose an injury. The following is one example:

- Read medical records if available or x-rays. Previous treatment should be taken into account when diagnosing an injury, even one as simple as an ankle sprain.

- Listening—asking a number of questions to build up a picture of what might have happened. For example:

  - How did it happen?

  - Was there any pain at the time?

  - Was the pain sudden onset or gradual?

  - Was there any swelling and was it sudden onset or gradual? A sudden swelling often indicates a bleeding into the joint rather than a gradual increase in synovial fluid within the joint.

  - Did you hear any noises? This could indicate ligaments tearing or bones breaking.

  - Did you apply any emergency procedures such as RICE?

  - Is there anything you do which makes it worse/better?

  - Is this the first time you have injured the ankle in this way or is it recurrent?

- The therapist will observe the patient as they stand and when lying or sitting on a couch with the legs out in front. They will look for any abnormal position, deformity, and, of course, swelling.

Active Movements

- The patient moves the foot from plantar flexion to dorsi flexion.

- Looking for reduction in normal range of movement and any pain in performing these movements.

- Then repeat moving from eversion (turning outward) to inversion (turning inward).

Passive Movements

- The therapist moves the ankle and foot from plantarflexion (downward movement) to dorsiflexion (upward movement) and then inversion to eversion looking again at range of movement, comparing one foot with the other and noting painful movements.

- The athlete remains relaxed and does not resist or actively move the foot or ankle. Any pain at the extreme range of inversion may indicate ligament damage as it is the ligament that is being stressed.

- The anterior drawer test is a special test which assesses the integrity of the ankle ligaments, particularly the anterior talofibular ligament and the calcaneofibular ligament.

Resisted Movements

- The therapist gently resists the athlete as they try to move the ankle from inversion to eversion.

- Pain when performing this test may be an indication of tendon damage or inflammation (possibly peroneal tendons) as it is the tendons connecting muscle to bone that are stressed when performing this test.

Functional Tests

- These can only be performed if pain allows. A badly injured ankle will not be capable of performing these tests.

- The lunge test involves the athlete leaning forwards over one knee keeping the heel of the front foot in contact with the ground. It measures dorsiflexion in comparison to the uninjured ankle.

- Other tests include one leg standing balance (eyes closed) test and hopping tests. Hopping on a recently injured ankle is definitely to be avoided, but this test may be of benefit much later in the rehabilitation process.

Palpation (Touching And Feeling)

- Finally the therapist will touch or feel certain points of the ankle to identify any specific painful areas.

- The following are usual points to palpate: distal fibula (bottom of the fibula bone), lateral malleolus (bony bit on the outside of the ankle— peroneal tendon dislocation/inflammation), lateral ligaments (most likely to be painful), talus (bone at the top of the ankle which the tibia or shin bone sits on), peroneal tendon, base of 5th metatarsal (where the peroneus brevis attaches to) and medial ankle ligaments.

Does it need an x-ray?

If the sprain is severe and the athlete has trouble weight bearing an x-ray may be beneficial in identifying possible fractures. However, an experienced sports medicine professional should be capable of palpating to identify if the pain is worse on the bone (lateral or medial malleolus) or on the ligament itself.

The therapist should then record any significant signs or symptoms and test results for future reference and as a record of what was found.

Rehabilitation (Sprained Ankle)

The following guide is intended for information purposes only. We recommend seeking professional advice before attempting any rehabilitation.

♣ **It's A Fact!!**

What are the aims of rehabilitation?

The aims of rehabilitation of an ankle sprain can be broken down into separate phases:

- Decrease initial pain and swelling.
- Improve mobility and flexibility.
- Improve the strength of the joint.
- Re-establish neural control and coordination.
- Return to full fitness.

What happens during Phase 1, the early phase?

Decreasing pain and swelling: This should start as soon as possible after you have injured the ankle. This phase can last from two days to two weeks (or more) depending on how bad the injury is.

- Protection of the ankle from further injury by taping, splints, or a cast or brace. Research has suggested that limited stress on the ankle can promote faster and stronger healing. By allowing the ankle to move forwards and backwards (in the sagittal plane) and not laterally, the ankle can keep moving but strain on the injured ligaments is significantly reduced.

- A useful support at this stage is the Aircast gel type ankle support which prevents most sideways movement but still allows limited use of the ankle. The cold gel can also be beneficial by compressing and reducing swelling. This support is useful in the early stages but will not prevent sprains and re-injury during later stages and functional rehabilitation.

- The Louisiana wrap strapping technique using a cohesive bandage can also be beneficial in applying compression and support and is quick and easy to apply.

- The Open Basketweave taping technique also accomplishes early medial and lateral protection while allowing plantarflexion and dorsiflexion.

- Rest: This is essential. Use crutches with partial weight bearing to get about if necessary. A healing ligament needs a certain amount of stress to heal properly but overdoing it early on in the rehabilitation process can prevent healing.

- Isometric exercises can be performed early on so long as they are not too painful. Avoid inversion and eversion though as this will stress the injured ligaments.

- Ice: Use cold therapy throughout the rehabilitation process. Apply ice for 20 minutes every hour initially for the first day then reduce this to four to five times a day from then on. In the acute stage ice will constrict blood vessels and further bleeding. Longer term benefits include reduction of pain and muscle spasm.

- Ice should not be used for longer than 30 minutes at a time as nerve palsy may occur. Ice should be used for as long as it is beneficial. As soon as the rehabilitation process plateaus the therapist may decide to change to heat to progress further. However this may not be for weeks or even months sometimes.

- Compression: Use a tube grip bandage or taping. Even better are products that specifically apply compression at the same time as cooling. The Open Basketweave taping technique also contributes to compression and helps to control swelling (edema).

- Elevation: Put your feet up and read all about your injury. Elevating the leg will help swelling run away from the site of the injury. Elevate the leg while icing and for 10 minutes after.

What happens during Phase 2, the rehabilitation phase?

The rehabilitation phase begins when swelling stops increasing and pain lessens. This means the ligaments have reached the point in the healing process where they are not in danger of being re-injured from mild stress.

Improve Mobility And Flexibility

- Manual joint mobilization in the anterior/posterior direction (forwards and backwards).

- Seated wobble board exercises may be beneficial for an ankle that has reduced mobility. Initially plantarflexion/dorsiflexion and then progress to inversion/eversion as pain allows.

- For the first two to seven days after injury you can start to move the ankle straight up and down but do not turn it in or out. This will help increase mobility and start to strengthen it up. Do as much as pain will allow. Try two sets of 40 reps while the ankle is iced and elevated and build up on that.

- As swelling and pain lessen you can start to invert and evert the ankle (move the soles of you feet inwards and upwards and the outwards and upwards). This will start to put more stress on the damaged structures so be careful not to do too much.

• Stretching the Achilles tendon regularly is important. Having available a specific Achilles stretching board throughout the day can help to ensure a few minutes stretching a day.

Strengthening The Ankle Joint

• Again as the ankle improves you can start to do strengthening exercises where you pull the foot and toes up and hold for 10 seconds and then push down and hold for 10 seconds. This can also be done for inversion and eversion as pain allows. Try three sets of 10 reps twice a day and build on that.

• Continue to apply cold therapy to the joint regularly, at least three times a day for 20 minutes.

• If you see no further improvement with ice then start to apply heat in the form of a hot bath/bucket or via a specialist with ultrasound.

• Strapping and taping may still be beneficial.

• You should be able to maintain fitness by swimming or cycling if pain allows.

Re-Establish Coordination And Proprioception

Proprioception exercises are thought to be important in avoiding recurrent ankle sprains. Early weight bearing is thought to help reduce proprioception loss. Try balancing on one leg with your eyes closed. This will improve proprioception (the neuromuscular control you have over your muscles). This will have been damaged when you injured the ankle. Aim to be able to balance for one minute without wobbling.

A wobble board is a useful tool to have. It is a flat board that you stand on with a semi-spherical bottom. By balancing on this you strengthen the ankle and improve proprioception. A series of progressive wobble board exercises can be seen on the website http://www.sportsinjuryclinic.net.

What happens during the return to full fitness/functional training phase?

In order to start the functional rehabilitation phase (activity and sports specific training) it is important the athlete has full range of motion and 80 to 90% of pre-injury strength. When you can comfortably do all of the above then you are ready to start Phase 3 and begin your return to activity.

Cardiovascular (CV) exercise is important and should begin the first day after injury depending on what pain will allow. It is important that the athlete maintain some kind of CV exercise not just for the physical benefits but for psychological well being as well. Stationary cycling, hand cycle ergometer, running in water, and swimming are all possibilities depending on severity of injury and what pain will allow.

Running may begin as soon as walking is pain free. It is a good idea to tape the ankle before starting running training particularly during early sessions

✔ Quick Tip
How can ankle sprains be prevented?

It is estimated that 30 to 40% of all ankle inversion sprains end in re-injury. To avoid being one of the 30 to 40% it is important not to stop the rehabilitation process but continue with it until full fitness is regained. It is a common complaint that once an athlete goes over on the ankle they become prone to doing the same thing again. If the original sprain is a bad one and joint laxity has resulted then it may be, for certain sports where fast changes of direction are required, that strapping of the ankle or wearing a brace is necessary to prevent re-injury.

If the sprain does not result in joint laxity then a recurrence may be avoided by the following:

Re-establish proprioception: This involves lots of balancing exercises on one leg—essential to avoid re-injury. If you start to turn the ankle over then you will find you automatically right it without even thinking about it. If the proprioception is damaged then you lose this ability.

Strengthening the ankle: This will provide a far more stable joint. Also, if the ankle does start to turn and the proprioceptors work properly, the ankle starts to right itself, the muscles need to be strong enough to pull the ankle back in a split second.

until confidence, proprioception, and strength has returned. A laced ankle brace can also provide support and is less expensive in the long run, particularly if laxity in the ligaments means a support needs to be worn permanently.

Running should begin on a clear flat surface such as a running track. Grass or bumpy surfaces will increase the risk of re-injury. Jog the straights and walk the curves. Speed should be gradually increased over time to a sprint.

Sports specific drills using cones can be introduced: changing direction, running in a figure 8 pattern, and zigzagging between cones.

Chapter 33

Achilles Tendon Problems

Achilles Tendonitis

What is Achilles tendonitis?

It is estimated that Achilles tendonitis (sometimes spelled "tendinitis") accounts for around 11% of all running injuries. The Achilles tendon is the large tendon at the back of the ankle. It connects the large calf muscles (gastrocnemius and soleus) to the heal bone (calcaneus) and provides the power in the push-off phase of the gait cycle. The Achilles tendon can become inflamed through overuse as well as a number of contributory factors. The Achilles tendon has a poor blood supply which is why it is slow to heal.

Achilles tendonitis can be acute or chronic. Acute Achilles tendonitis may happen as a result of overuse or training too much, too soon especially on hard surfaces or up hills.

About This Chapter: This chapter includes text reprinted with permission from "Achilles Tendonitis," "Achilles Tendon Rupture (Partial)," "Treatment and Rehabilitation of Achilles Tendon Partial Rupture," and "Total Achilles Tendon Rupture," © 2007 Sports Injury Clinic. For more information, including video presentations, visit http://www.sportsinjuryclinic.net.

What are the symptoms of Achilles tendonitis?

Symptoms for acute inflammation of the Achilles tendon include the following:

- Pain on the tendon during exercise. Achilles pain will gradually come on with prolonged exercise but will go away with rest.

- Swelling over the Achilles tendon.

- Redness over the skin.

- You can sometimes feel a creaking when you press your fingers into the tendon and move the foot.

Chronic Achilles tendonitis may often follow on from acute Achilles tendonitis if the acute tendon injury is not treated properly or allowed to heal. Chronic Achilles tendonitis is a difficult condition to treat, particularly in older athletes who appear to suffer more often. The pains experienced during the acute phase of the injury tend to disappear after a warm up but return when training has stopped. Eventually the injury gets worse and worse until it is impossible to run.

♣ It's A Fact!!
What causes Achilles tendonitis?

- Overuse. Too much too soon is the basic cause of overuse injuries, however other factors can make an overuse injury more likely.

- Running up hills will mean the Achilles tendon has to stretch more than normal on every stride. This is fine for a while but will mean the tendon will fatigue sooner than normal.

- Overpronation (feet which roll in) can place an increased strain on the Achilles tendon. As the foot rolls in (flattens) the lower leg rotates inwards also; this twists the Achilles tendon, placing twisting stresses as well as stresses along its length.

- Wearing high heels consistently and then expecting to run five miles in flat running shoes puts abnormal strain on the Achilles tendon making it stretch further than it is comfortable.

Symptoms for chronic Achilles tendonitis are similar to those of acute tendonitis as well as the following:

- Pain and stiffness in the Achilles tendon especially in the morning. This pain may be described as diffuse along the tendon rather than specific.

- There may nodules or lumps in the Achilles tendon, particularly 2 cm above the heel.

- Pain in the tendon when walking especially up hill or up stairs.

- Chronic tendonitis differs from acute tendonitis in that it is more of a long term persistent problem.

How is Achilles tendonitis treated?

What The Athlete Can Do

- Rest and apply cold therapy or ice (not directly onto the skin).

- Wear a heel pad to raise the heel and take some of the strain off the Achilles tendon. This should be a temporary measure while the Achilles tendon is healing.

- See a sports injury professional who can advise on treatment and rehabilitation.

What A Sports Injury Therapist Or Doctor Can Do

- Prescribe anti-inflammatory medication.

- Identify the causes and prescribe orthotics or a change in training methods.

- Tape the back of the leg to support the tendon.

- Apply a plaster cast if it is really bad.

- Use ultrasound treatment.

- Apply sports massage techniques.

- Prescribe a rehabilitation program.

- Some might give a steroid injection, however an injection directly into the tendon is not recommended. Some specialists believe this can increase the risk of a total rupture.

• Scan with an MRI (magnetic resonance imagine) or ultrasound

If you look after this injury early enough you should make a good recovery. It is important you rehabilitate the tendon properly after it has recovered or the injury will return. If you ignore the early warning signs and do not look after this injury then it may become chronic which is very difficult to treat.

✔ Quick Tip
What products may help treat Achilles tendonitis?

Please consult your therapist before using any products to ensure they are compatible with your treatment program:

• **Cold Therapy Wraps:** Can be wrapped around to apply cold and compression reducing pain and inflammation.

• **Arch Support Insoles:** Orthotic type insoles which give firm support for the arch of the foot can help prevent over pronation and improve foot biomechanics. Overpronation of the foot causes the Achilles tendon to twist, increasing the stress on it.

• **Slant Board:** This is excellent for applying an accurate and gradual stretch to the calf muscles. It is easy to identify difference in calf muscle flexibility when stretching both legs at once. Stretching can be progressively increased and a much greater degree of stretching is possible over Achilles stretches on the floor.

• **Achilles Tendon Strap:** This wraps around the ankle and applies gentle pressure onto the Achilles tendon. It works by reducing the shock and tension in the Achilles tendon in the same was as a tennis elbow support works.

• **Heel Pads:** Can slightly raise the heels which temporarily shortens the calf muscles reducing stress on the Achilles tendons. Also reduces shock which may also reduce stresses on the tendon.

• **Night Splint:** Is worn overnight to apply a very gentle stretch and prevent tightening of the Achilles tendon and plantar fascia. Mainly advertised as plantar fasciitis night splints, they are also excellent for Achilles/calf muscle flexibility.

Achilles Tendon Rupture

What is a partial Achilles tendon rupture?

A partial Achilles tendon rupture can occur in athletes from all sports but particularly running, jumping, throwing, and racket sports. The tendon tears but not completely. Scar tissue will form which is likely to lead to inflammation of the tendon. Often the athlete will not feel the Achilles tendon rupture at the time but will become aware of it later when the tendon has cooled down.

Symptoms of a partial Achilles tendon rupture include the following:

- A sudden sharp pain in the Achilles tendon. (Sometimes the athlete will not feel a sharp pain at the time of the tear but pain will come on when cooled down).

- When returning to exercise after a short period of rest, there may be a sharp pain which disappears when warmed up only to return when stopped.

- Stiffness in Achilles tendon first thing in the morning.

- A small swelling in the tendon.

How is partial Achilles rupture treated?

What The Athlete Can Do

- R.I.C.E. (rest, ice, compress, elevate) for the first two to three days.

- See a sports injury specialist or doctor who can advise on treatment and rehabilitation.

- A proper diagnosis is essential. If the rupture is a complete Achilles tendon rupture then immediate surgery is usually indicated. A Thompson test is one way of determining if a total rupture may be present.

What A Sports Injury Specialist Or Doctor Can Do

- Correctly diagnose the injury; a Thompson test is one way of assessing the Achilles tendon.

- Tape the Achilles tendon to support it.

- Use ultrasound.

- Prescribe a rehabilitation program.

- They might put you in a plaster cast for four to six weeks.

- Operate (surgery)

Treatment And Rehabilitation Of Achilles Tendon Partial Rupture

What are the aims of rehabilitation for a partial rupture of the Achilles tendon?

The following guidelines are for information purposes only. We recommend seeking professional advice before starting any rehabilitation.

Aims Of Rehabilitation

- Control initial pain and swelling.

- Improve mobility and flexibility.

- Improve the strength of the tendon.

- Return to full fitness.

It may be a month before swelling is reduced and the injury has healed enough to progress into stretching and strengthening exercises.

Controlling Pain And Swelling.

- Apply cold therapy. This can be in the form of ice. Do not apply directly to the skin: place a wet tea towel around the ice or use a specialist product. Apply compression after or during the cold therapy to help reduce swelling.

- NSAIDs (nonsteroidal anti-inflammatory drugs, for example, ibuprofen) may help reduce the inflammation in the early stages. It is important to always check with your doctor before taking any medication. You should not take ibuprofen if you have asthma. Avoid taking medication for more than a week. The effectiveness may be reduced later in rehabilitation and may even hinder healing.

- Rest the injury from aggravating activities. If the athlete cannot walk without pain then they may need to use crutches. When the athlete can tolerate walking, place a 2 cm heal raise into shoes to raise the heal, shorten the Achilles tendon, and reduce the load on the tendon. Continue to rest the tendon until able to tolerate a strengthening program. With an injury of this kind, it may be a month or more before the athlete can attempt strengthening of the tendon.

- Taping the Achilles tendon may help to reduce the load on it as the athlete returns to walking, especially if they have no choice and have to get about, for example at work.

Increasing Mobility And Flexibility

When the swelling has gone down and pain is reduced the athlete may be able to begin to stretch the tendon. It may be as soon as a week after injury but it may be up to a month depending on severity. Begin with mobility exercises as soon as pain will allow. This may be within a few days but could be over a week depending on how bad the injury is.

Strengthening

- When pain and swelling have gone then strengthening exercises can begin.

- Start very slowly and progress slowly (double leg heel drop taking most of the weight on the uninjured leg).

- It is important that the tendon is strengthened in the stretched position by allowing the heels to drop below the toes.

- If you feel pain during, after, or the next day then you may need to rest and take a step back.

- Continue stretching throughout the rehabilitation process. Stretch well before and after strengthening sessions.

- Stretching exercises can be done on a daily basis, especially if the loads are light in the early stages.

- Strengthening should be continued for many weeks after you have returned to full fitness.

- Apply ice to the tendon at the end of a strengthening session to help prevent inflammation.

Return To Fitness

When the ankle has regained full flexibility, there is no pain or swelling, and strengthening exercises can be tolerated without adverse reaction then a gentle running program can begin. This may be up to three months after the initial injury depending on severity.

Start gentle jogging on a firm surface. Gradually build up until you can comfortably jog for 45 minutes. It is unlikely that you will be able to return to competition within four to six months. Below is an example of a gradual return to running program.

- Day 1: Walk 4 minutes jog 2 minutes repeat four times

- Day 2: Rest

- Day 3: Walk 4 minutes jog 3 minutes repeat three times

- Day 4: Rest

- Day 5: Walk 3 minutes jog 4 minutes repeat four times

- Day 6: Rest

- Day 7: Walk 2 minutes jog 6 minutes repeat four times

Continue this gradual progression until you can confidently run and resume normal training.

Gradually increase the duration of your runs. No more than 10% per week is usually recommended. If your sport demands sprinting then gradually increase the speed.

Continue with the stretching and strengthening program. It is important to do these even if you do not gain pain at this stage. Continue for at least three months. Continue to ice the tendon after training. You should now be ready to start back in full training but never neglect stretching and strengthening of the Achilles tendon or the injury might return.

Total Achilles Tendon Rupture

The Achilles tendon is the tendon that runs from your calf muscle at the back of your lower leg and inserts in at the back of the heel. It is more commonly injured in older men who are recreational athletes. Injury sometimes occurs following a history of inflammation or degeneration of the tendon but nearly always results from a sudden event such as pushing off hard on the toes or suddenly bending the foot upwards.

Symptoms of a total Achilles tendon rupture include the following:

- A sudden sharp pain as if someone has whacked you in the back of the leg with something.

- This will often be accompanied by a load crack or bang.

- You will be unable to walk properly and unable to stand on tiptoe.

- There may be a gap felt in the tendon.

- There will be a lot of swelling.

- A positive result for a Thompson test (for more information about a Thompson test, visit http://www.sportsinjuryclinic.net).

♣ It's A Fact!!

A total Achilles tendon rupture nearly always results from a sudden event such as pushing off hard on the toes or suddenly bending the foot upwards.

How is a total Achilles tendon rupture treated and rehabilitated?

What The Athlete Can Do

- Seek professional help immediately. The sooner you get this injury operated on the more chance you have of making a full recovery. Any longer than two days and you are in trouble.

- Apply ice.

What A Sports Injury Specialist Or Doctor Can Do

- Confirm the diagnosis.

- Operate on the tendon.

- Sometimes the leg is put in a plaster cast and allowed to heal without surgery. This is generally not the preferred method. It takes longer to heal and longer to start on rehabilitation.

How long might you be out of training for?

You can expect to be out of competition for six to nine months after surgery. This is increased to 12 months if you just have the Achilles immobilized in plaster instead of surgery. There is also a greater risk of re-injury if you do not have the surgery.

Chapter 34

Plantar Fasciitis

Anatomy

The plantar fascia is a thick, broad, inelastic band of fibrous tissue that courses along the bottom (plantar surface) of the foot. It is attached to the heel bone (calcaneus) and fans out to attach to the bottom of the metatarsal bones in the region of the ball of the foot. Because the normal foot has an arch, this tight band of tissue (plantar fascia) is at the base of the arch. In this position, the plantar fascia acts like a bowstring to maintain the arch of the foot.

Plantar fasciitis refers to an inflammation of the plantar fascia. The inflammation in the tissue is the result of some type of injury to the plantar fascia. Typically, plantar fasciitis results from repeated trauma to the tissue where it attaches to the calcaneus.

This repeated trauma often results in microscopic tearing of the plantar fascia at or near the point of attachment of the tissue to the calcaneus. The result of the damage and inflammation is pain.

If there is significant injury to the plantar fascia, the inflammatory reaction of the heel bone may produce spike-like projections of new bone called heel spurs. The spurs are not the cause of the initial pain of plantar fasciitis; they are the result of the problem. Most heel spurs are painless. Occasionally, they are associated with pain and discomfort and require medical treatment or even surgical removal.

Plantar fasciitis (heel-spur syndrome) is a common problem among people active in sports, especially runners. It typically starts as a dull, intermittent pain in the heel and may progress to sharp, constant pain. Often, it is usually worse in the morning or after sitting, and then decreases as the patient begins to walk around. In addition, the pain usually increases after standing or walking for long periods of time and at the beginning of a sporting activity.

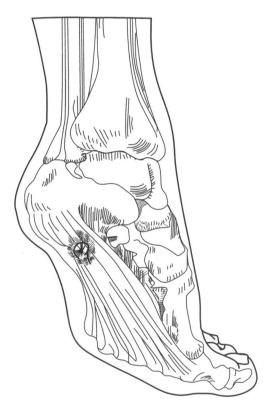

Figure 34.1. Plantar (Bottom) View Of Foot (original image provided by the Center for Orthopaedics and Sports Medicine; redrawn for Omnigraphics by Stephen G. Wesley).

Often people who develop plantar fasciitis have several risk factors for doing so. They include:

- flat feet;

- high arched, rigid feet;

- increasing age and family tendency;

- running on toes, hills, or very soft surfaces (sand);

- poor arch support in shoes;

- rapid change in activity level.

Treatment

Fortunately, the majority of cases of plantar fasciitis respond favorably to non-operative treatment. However, the recovery time varies tremendously from patient to patient. While some patients may be healed after six weeks of treatment, others may require six months or longer for recovery. In addition, the methods of treatment that may work for one patient, may not be successful in another patient. Typically, the methods of treatment that are attempted include anti-inflammatory mediation, icing, stretching, activity modification, and heel inserts.

In addition, it is necessary to avoid the activities that are known to aggravate the fasciitis. This includes any activity that involves repeated impact of the heel on a hard surface, such as running. Sometimes, cortisone injections are necessary to achieve satisfactory healing.

If the pain persists, it may be necessary to run additional diagnostic studies to rule other, less common, causes of heel pain such as stress fractures, nerve compression injuries, or collagen disorders of the skin.

Rarely, surgical treatment is necessary. However, when the non-surgical treatments have been tried and they have failed, surgery may be indicated for the relief of heel pain. Most of these surgical procedures can be completed on an outpatient basis in less than one hour. The surgery can be accomplished under local anesthesia or minimal sedation administrated by a trained anesthesiologist.

Surgical treatment options include:

• Surgical removal/release of the fascia. A small incision is made on the inside of the heel and the inflamed tissue is removed or released.

• Removal of bone spurs. During the same operation that is used to separate the connective tissue from the heel bone, the offending heel spur can be removed.

♣ **It's A Fact!!**
Postoperative Care

Immediately after either operation, a cast may or may not be used to support and immobilize the foot for two or three weeks. Crutches may be helpful for greater comfort and mobility while the foot heals.

When the cast has been removed, three to four weeks of physical therapy will speed healing and reduce swelling.

Chapter 35

Foot Injuries

The foot is a complex structure of 26 bones and 33 joints, layered with an intertwining web of over 120 muscles, ligaments, and nerves. It serves the following functions:

- Supports weight

- Acts as a shock absorber

- Serves as a lever to propel the leg forward

- Helps to maintain balance by adjusting the body to uneven surfaces

About Foot Pain

Given what the foot must endure, it is not surprising that about 75% of Americans experience foot pain at some point in their lives. Foot pain is generally defined by one of three sites of origin: the toes, the forefoot, and the hindfoot.

- **The Toes:** Toe problems most often occur because of the pressure imposed by ill-fitting shoes.

- **The Forefoot:** The forefoot is the front of the foot. Pain originating here usually involves one of the following bone groups: The metatarsal

About This Chapter: Excerpted from "Foot Pain: In-Depth Report," © 2007 A.D.A.M., Inc. Reprinted with permission.

bones (five long bones that extend from the front of the arch to the bones in the toe); the sesamoid bones (two small bones embedded at the top of the first metatarsal bone, which connects to the big toe).

- **The Hindfoot:** The hindfoot is the back of the foot. Pain originating here can extend from the heel, across the sole (known as the plantar surface), to the ball of the foot (the metatarsophalangeal joint).

> **♣ It's A Fact!!**
>
> Foot injuries are very common and often result from athletic activities. It is important to wear the right shoe for the specific sport. For example, a running shoe that is cushioned may not offer the support necessary for playing tennis.
>
> Many foot injuries can be treated by the individual without a doctor's care. Injuries such as sprains and strains can benefit from the "RICE" treatment: Rest, Ice, Compression, and Elevation.

Correct Walking And Foot Exercises

Correct Walking: In addition to wearing proper shoes and socks, walk often and correctly to prevent foot injury and pain. The head should be erect, the back straight, and the arms relaxed and swinging freely at the side. Step out on the heel, move forward with the weight on the outside of the foot, and complete the step by pushing off the big toe.

Foot Exercises: Exercises specifically for the toe and feet are easy to perform and help strengthen them and keep them flexible. Helpful exercises include the following:

- Raise and curl the toes 10 times, holding each position for a count of five.

- Put a rubber band around both big toes and pull the feet away from each other. Count to five. Repeat 10 times.

- Pick up a towel with the toes. Repeat five times.

- Pump the foot up and down to stretch the calf and shin muscles. Perform for two or three minutes.

Shoes

In general, the best shoes are well cushioned and have a leather upper, stiff heel counter, and flexible area at the ball of the foot. The heel area should be strong and supportive, but not too stiff, and the front of the shoe should be flexible. New shoes should feel comfortable right away, without a breaking in period.

Getting The Correct Fit: Well-fitted shoes with a firm sole and soft upper are the best way to prevent nearly all problems with the feet. They should be purchased in the afternoon or after a long walk, when the feet have swelled. There should be a ½ inch of space between the longest toe and the tip of the shoe (remember, the longest toe is not always the big toe), and the toes should be able to wiggle upward. A person should stand when being measured, and both feet should be sized, with shoes bought for the larger-sized foot. It is important to wear the same socks as you would regularly wear with the new shoes. Women who are accustomed to wearing pointed-toe shoes may prefer the feel of tight-fitting shoes, but with wear their tastes will adjust to shoes that are less confining and properly fitted.

The Sole: Ideally, the shoe should have a removable insole. Thin, hard soles may be the best choice for older people. Some research suggests that thick soles may even be responsible for foot injury in younger adults who engage in high-impact exercise.

The Heel: High heels are the major cause of foot problems in women. Although people believe that foot binding is a problem limited to Chinese women of the past, many fashionable high heels are designed to constrict the foot by up to an inch. Women who insist on wearing high-heeled shoes should at least look for shoes with wide toe room, reinforced heels that are relatively wide, and cushioned insoles. They should also keep the amount of time they spend wearing high heels to a minimum.

> ♣ **It's A Fact!!**
> Foot pain is fairly common even in children. Heel pain is common in very active children ages 8–13, when high-impact exercise can irritate growth centers of the heel.

Laces: The way shoes are laced can be important for preventing specific problems. Laces should always be loosened before putting shoes on. People with narrow feet should buy shoes with eyelets farther away from the tongue than people with wider feet. This makes for a tighter fit for narrower feet and looser for wider. If, after tying the shoe, less than an inch of tongue shows, then the shoes are probably too wide. Tightness should be adjusted both at the top of the shoe and at the bottom. Where high arches cause pain, eyelets should be skipped to relieve pressure.

Special-Purpose Footwear

People should avoid extreme variations between their exercise, street, and dress shoes.

Exercise And Sports: Shoes purchased for exercise should be specifically designed for a person's preferred sport. For instance, a running shoe should especially cushion the forefoot, while tennis shoes should emphasize ankle support. Athletic socks are almost as important as shoes. Experts often recommend padded acrylic socks.

Shoes for Sports

- *Aerobic Dancing:* Sufficient cushioning to absorb shock and pressure, which should be many times greater than shock from walking. Arches that maintain side-to-side stability. Thick upper leather support. Box-toe. Orthotics may be required for people with ankles that over-turn inward or outward. Soles should allow for twisting and turning.

- *Cycling:* Rigid support across the arch to prevent collapse during pedaling. Heel lift. Cross-training or combo hiking/cycling shoes may be sufficient for the casual biker. Toe clips or specially designed shoe cleats for serious cyclers. In some cases, orthotics may be needed to control arch and heel and balance forefoot.

- *Running:* Sufficient cushioning to absorb shock and pressure. Fully bendable at the ball of the foot. Sufficient traction on sole to prevent slipping. Consider insole or orthotic with arch support for problem feet.

- *Tennis:* Allows side-to-side sliding. Low-traction sole. Snug fitting heel with cushioning. Padded toe box with adequate depth. Soft-support arch.

> ## ♣ It's A Fact!!
> ## Sports And Aerobic Dancing
>
> People who engage in regular high-impact aerobic exercise are at risk for plantar fasciitis, heel spurs, sesamoiditis, shin splints, Achilles tendon, and stress fractures. In one study of aerobic dance instructors, for example, nearly one-third reported injuries in the feet and ankles. Even young athletes are at risk for stress fracture, particularly if they exercise six or seven days a week. Women are at higher risk for stress fractures than men are.

- *Walking:* Lightweight. Breathable upper material (leather or mesh). Wide enough to accommodate ball of the foot. Firm padded heel counter that does not bite into heel or touch anklebone. Low heel close to ground for stability. Good arch support. Front provides support and flexibility.

Foot Injury Treatment

If you suspect that bones in a toe or foot have been broken or fractured, you should call a doctor, who will probably order x-rays. It should be noted that a person is often able to walk even if a foot bone has been fractured, particularly if it is a chipped bone or a toe fracture.

Over-The-Counter Pain Relievers

Over-the-counter nonsteroidal anti-inflammatory drugs (NSAIDs) are commonly used to treat mild pain caused by muscle inflammation. Aspirin is the most common NSAID. Others include ibuprofen (Motrin, Advil, Nuprin, Rufen), ketoprofen (Actron, Orudis KT), naproxen (Aleve, Naprelan), and tolmetin (Tolectin). A gel containing ibuprofen can be applied to sore joints. Acetaminophen (Tylenol) is not an NSAID, and although it is a mild pain reliever, it will not reduce inflammation. It is important to note that high doses or long-term use of any NSAID can cause gastrointestinal disturbances, with sometimes serious consequences, including dangerous bleeding. No one should take NSAIDs for prolonged periods without consulting a doctor.

RICE (Rest, Ice, Compression, And Elevation)

The acronym RICE stands for rest, ice, compression, and elevation, the four basic elements of immediate treatment for an injured foot.

- Rest. Patients should get off injured feet as soon as possible.

- Ice. Ice is particularly important to reduce swelling and promote recovery during the first 48 hours. A bag or towel containing ice should be wrapped around the injured area on a repetitive cycle of 20 minutes on, 40 minutes off.

- Compression. An Ace bandage should be lightly wrapped around the area.

- Elevation. The foot should be elevated on several pillows.

Toe Pain

Corns: A corn is a type of callus, a protective layer of dead skin cells that form due to repeated friction. It is cone-shaped and has a knobby core that points inward. This core can put pressure on a nerve and cause sharp pain. Corns can develop on the top or between toes. If a corn develops between the toes, it is may be called a soft corn if it is kept pliable by the moisture from perspiration.

To prevent corns and calluses and relieve discomfort if they develop:

- Do not wear shoes that are too tight or too loose. Wear well-padded shoes with open toes or a deep toe box (the part of the shoe that surrounds the toes). If necessary, have a cobbler stretch the shoes in the area where the corn or callus is located.

- Wear thick socks to absorb pressure, but do not wear tight socks or stockings.

- Apply petroleum jelly or lanolin hand cream to corns or calluses to soften them.

- Use doughnut-shaped pads that fit over a corn and decrease pressure and friction. They are available at most drug stores.

- Place cotton, lamb's wool, or mole skin between the toes to cushion any corns in these areas.

Bursitis: Bursitis is an inflammation of the fluid filled sacs that protect the toe joints.

Ingrown Toenails: Ingrown toenails can occur on any toe but are most common on the big toes. They usually develop when tight-fitting or narrow shoes put too much pressure on the toenail and force the nail to grow into the flesh of the toe. Incorrect toenail trimming can also contribute to the risk of developing an ingrown toenail. Fungal infections, injuries, abnormalities in the structure of the foot, and repeated impact on the toenail from high-impact aerobic exercise can also produce ingrown toenails.

Toenails should be trimmed straight across and long enough so that the nail corner is not visible. If the nail is cut too short, it may grow inward. If the nail does grow inward, do not cut the nail corner at an angle. This only trains the nail to continue growing inward. When filing the nails, file straight across the nail in a single movement, lifting the file before the next stroke. Do not saw back and forth. A cuticle stick can be used to clean under the nail.

Bunions: A bunion is a deformity that usually occurs at the head of one of the five long bones (the metatarsal bones) that extend from the arch and connect to the toes. Bunions can be caused by several conditions:

- Narrow high-heeled shoes with pointed toes can put enormous pressure on the front of the foot.

- Injury in the joint may cause a bunion to develop over time.

- Genetics play a role in 10–15% of all bunions.

- Flat feet, gout, arthritis, and occupations (such as ballet) that place undue stress on the feet can also increase the risk for bunions.

Pressure and pain from bunions and bunionettes can be relieved by wearing appropriate shoes, such as soft, wide, low-heeled leather shoes that lace up; athletic shoes with soft toe boxes; and open shoes or sandals with straps that don't touch the irritated area.

A thick doughnut-shaped, moleskin pad can protect the protrusion. In some cases, an orthotic can help redistribute weight and take pressure off the bunion. Nonsteroidal anti-inflammatory drugs (NSAIDs) or corticosteroid injections may offer some pain relief. If discomfort persists, surgery may be necessary particularly for more serious conditions, such as hallux valgus. There are over 100 surgical variations ranging from removing the bump to realigning the toes.

Forefoot Pain

The incidence of forefoot pain and deformity increases with age. With early diagnosis, conservative therapy is often successful in treating common disorders of the forefoot. When a cause cannot be determined, any pain on the ball of the foot is generally referred to as metatarsalgia. It is most likely caused by improper footwear, particularly high heels, or by high-impact activities.

Calluses: Calluses are composed of the same material as corns, hardened patches of dead skin cells. Calluses, however, develop on the ball or heel of the foot. The skin on the sole of the foot is ordinarily about 40 times thicker than skin anywhere else on the body, but a callus can even be twice as thick. A protective callus layer naturally develops to guard against excessive pressure and chafing as people get older and the padding of fat on the bottom of the foot thins out. If calluses get too big or too hard, they may pull and tear the underlying skin.

Neuromas: A neuroma usually means a benign tumor of a nerve. However, Morton neuroma, also called interdigital neuroma, is not actually a tumor. It is a thickening of the tissue surrounding the nerves leading to the toes. Morton neuroma usually develops when the bones in the third and fourth toes pinch together, compressing a nerve. It can also occur in other locations. The nerve becomes enlarged and inflamed. The inflammation causes a burning or tingling sensation and cramping in the front of the foot. Tight, poorly-fitting shoes, injury, arthritis, or abnormal bone structure may also cause this condition.

Pain from Morton neuroma can be reduced by massaging the affected area. Roomier shoes (box-toe shoes), pads of various sorts, and cortisone injections in the painful area are also helpful. A combination of cortisone injections and shoe modifications provides better immediate relief than changes in footwear alone.

Stress Fracture: A stress fracture in the foot, also called fatigue or march fracture, usually results from a break or rupture in any of the five metatarsal bones (mostly the second or third). These fractures are caused by overuse during strenuous exercise, particularly jogging and high-impact aerobics. Women are at higher risk than men are. A fracture in the first metatarsal bone, which leads to the big toe, is uncommon because of the thickness of this bone. If it occurs, however, it is more serious than a fracture in any of the other metatarsal bones because it dramatically changes the pattern of normal walking and weight bearing.

Patients should seek treatment if pain persists for three weeks. In a study of young athletes, treatment after that time was associated with a lower chance for returning to their sport. Surgery may be needed if conservative measures fail. In most cases, however, stress fractures heal by themselves if rigorous activities are avoided. It is best to wear low-heeled shoes with stiff soles. Some physicians recommend moderate exercise, particularly swimming and walking. Occasionally, a physician may recommend wearing a special wooden shoe and a compressive wrap to make walking more comfortable.

Sesamoiditis: Sesamoiditis is an inflammation of the tendons around the small, round bones that are embedded in the head of the first metatarsal bone, which leads to the big toe. Sesamoid bones bear much stress under ordinary circumstances; excessive stress can strain the surrounding tendons. Often there is no clear-cut cause, but sesamoid injuries are common among people who participate in jarring, high-impact activities, such as ballet, jogging, and aerobic exercise.

Rest and reducing stress on the ball of the foot are the first lines of treatment for sesamoiditis. A low-heeled shoe with a stiff sole and soft padding inside is all that is usually required. In severe cases, surgery may be necessary.

Heel Pain

The heel is the largest bone in the foot. Heel pain is the most common foot problem and affects two million Americans every year. It can occur in the front, back, or bottom of the heel.

Plantar Fasciitis And Heel Spurs: Plantar fasciitis is a common foot problem that accounts for one million office visits per year. Plantar fasciitis occurs from small tears and inflammation in the wide band of tendons and ligaments that stretches from the heel to the ball of the foot. This band, much like the tensed string in a bow, forms the arch of the foot and helps to serve as a shock absorber for the body. The term plantar means the sole of the foot, and fascia refers to any fibrous connective tissue in the body. Most people with plantar fasciitis experience pain in the heel with their first steps in the morning. The pain also often spreads to the arch. The condition can be temporary or may become chronic if the problem is ignored. In such cases, resting provides relief, but only temporarily.

Heel spurs are calcium deposits that can develop under the heel bone as result of the inflammation that occurs with plantar fasciitis. Heel spurs and plantar fasciitis are sometimes blamed interchangeably for pain, but plantar fasciitis can occur without heel spurs, and spurs commonly develop without causing any symptoms at all.

The cause of plantar fasciitis is often unknown. It is usually associated with overuse during high-impact exercise and sports and accounts for up to 9% of all running injuries. Because the condition often occurs in only one foot, however, factors other than overuse are likely to responsible in many cases. Other causes of this injury include poorly fitting shoes, lack of calf flexibility, or an uneven stride that causes an abnormal and stressful impact on the foot.

Embarking on an exercise program as soon as possible and using NSAIDs, splints, or heel pads as needed reduces the risk for future surgery. Pain that is not relieved by NSAIDs may require more intensive treatments, including leg supports and even surgery.

Bursitis Of The Heel: Bursitis of the heel is an inflammation of the bursa, a small sack of fluid, beneath the heel bone. Nonsteroidal anti-inflammatory drugs (NSAIDs) such as aspirin or ibuprofen (Advil) and steroid injections will help relieve pain from bursitis. Applying ice and massaging the heel are also beneficial. A heel cup or soft padding in the heel of the shoe reduces direct impact when walking.

Haglund Deformity: Haglund deformity, known medically as posterior calcaneal exostosis, is a bony growth surrounded by tender tissue on the back of the heel bone. It develops when the back of the shoe repeatedly rubs against the back of the heel, aggravating the tissue and the underlying bone. It is commonly called pump bump because it frequently occurs with high heels. (It can also develop in runners, however.)

Applying ice followed by moist heat will help ease discomfort from a pump bump. Nonsteroidal anti-inflammatory drugs (NSAIDs) such as aspirin or ibuprofen (Advil) will also reduce pain. Your doctor may recommend an orthotic device to control heel motion. Corticosteroid injections are not recommended because they can weaken the Achilles tendon.

Achilles Tendonitis: Achilles tendonitis is an inflammation of the tendon that connects the calf muscles to the heel bone. It is caused by small tears in the tendon from overuse or injury and is most common in people who engage in high-impact exercise, particularly jogging, racquetball, and tennis.

An inflamed or torn Achilles tendon causes intense pain and affects mobility.

People at highest risk for this disorder from these activities are those with a shortened Achilles tendon. Such people tend to roll their feet too far inward when walking, and may bounce when they walk. A shortened tendon can be due to an inborn structural abnormality, or it can develop from regularly wearing high heels.

Evidence is uncertain about the best way to treat either acute or chronic Achilles tendonitis. Some approaches include treatments to relieve pain and reduce inflammation, gentle stretching, and laser therapy. If pain continues, the ruptured tendon will require a cast and perhaps surgery. Although some experts believe a cast is sufficient in many cases, without an operation, the tendon has a 38% chance of rupturing again. Some experts suggest surgery for active persons and nonsurgical treatment for older people.

Excessive Pronation: Pronation is the normal motion that allows the foot to adapt to uneven walking surfaces and to absorb shock. Excessive pronation occurs when the foot has a tendency to turn inward and stretch and pull the fascia. It can cause not only heel pain, but also hip, knee, and lower back problems.

Arch Pain

Tarsal Tunnel Syndrome: Tarsal tunnel syndrome results from compression of a nerve that runs through a narrow passage behind the inner ankle bone down to the heel. It can cause pain anywhere along the bottom of the foot. It is often associated with diabetes, back pain, or arthritis. It may also be caused by injury to the ankle or by a growth, abnormal blood vessels, or scar tissue that press against the nerve. Magnetic resonance (MR) imaging and the dorsiflexion-eversion test are being used to diagnose this syndrome.

Pain from tarsal tunnel syndrome may be relieved by treatment with orthotics, specially designed shoe inserts, to help redistribute weight and take pressure off the nerve. Corticosteroid injections may also help. Surgery is sometimes performed, particularly if symptoms persist for more than a year, although its benefits are under some debate.

Flat Foot: Flat foot, or pes planus, is a defect of the foot that eliminates the arch. The condition is most often inherited. Arches, however, can also fall in adulthood, in which case the condition is sometimes referred to as posterior tibial tendon dysfunction (PTTD). This occurs most often in women over 50, but it can occur in anyone.

♣ It's A Fact!!
The force exerted on the foot with each step is about 50% greater than the person's body weight. In a typical day, the feet support several hundred tons.

Children with flat feet often outgrow them, particularly tall, slender children with flexible joints. One expert suggests that if an arch forms when the child stands on tip-toes, then the child will probably outgrow the condition. For certain children, minimally invasive surgery to implant temporary corrective screws into the arch may be an option.

Abnormally High Arches: An overly-high arch (hollow foot) can cause problems. Army studies have found that recruits with the highest arches have the most lower-limb injuries and that flat-footed recruits have the least. Contrary to the general impression, the hollow foot is much more common than the flat foot.

Chapter 36

Guidelines For Returning To Play

Return To Play

Injuries are a common occurrence for those who exercise. Whether it be an overuse problem (tendinitis) or an acute traumatic injury (fracture or sprain), many injuries require restriction of and/or change in your exercise program.

The amount of time away from exercise varies according to the type of injury, severity of injury, body part involved, and other situational factors. Although there are steps to promote healing, it still takes time.

Injuries involve dysfunction or disruption of some component of the musculoskeletal system. Depending on the type and severity of the injury, these may cause pain, swelling, stiffness, weakness, or decreased range of motion. Improvement in these symptoms occurs with the healing process, but this does not necessarily mean the injury is completely healed.

Actions You Can Take To Decrease
Or Control The Initial Symptoms

- **Protect:** Protect the affected area from further injury.

About This Chapter: "Return to Play," reprinted with permission of the American College of Sports Medicine. Copyright © 2005 American College of Sports Medicine. This brochure is a product of ACSM's Consumer Products Committee.

- **Rest:** Initially resting and protecting the injured part will result in less swelling and a more rapid recovery.

- **Ice:** Ice packs on the affected area decrease swelling and help control pain. This is especially helpful in the first 48 to 72 hours after injury, but can continue to be used to minimize discomfort.

- **Compression:** Wrapping or bracing of the injured part allows for control of initial swelling and decreases motion.

- **Elevation:** Elevation of the injured part, especially if it is kept above the heart, helps decrease swelling and pain.

Healing Time

As stated before, healing time depends on site, severity, and type of injury. For example, a mild ankle sprain may heal in two to four weeks, while a fracture of the leg may take eight to 12 weeks. However, healing usually proceeds in certain stages.

- Swelling and pain decreases or disappears in the first 24 to 72 hours.

- Discoloration (bruising) usually subsides within ten to 14 days.

- Range of motion increases over seven to 14 days, although stiffness and weakness may persist.

♣ It's A Fact!!

When an injury occurs, it may result in weakness due to tissue damage and disuse, in addition to decreased control over the damaged body part. Regaining strength and coordination of the injured body part should be considered part of the rehabilitation and healing process, and an injury should not be considered healed until this process is accomplished. Attempting to return to an activity before proper healing of the injury puts you at risk for reinjury or an additional injury. Consultation with a sports medicine professional may aid in the initial treatment and rehabilitation, and the determination of when to return to play.

Guidelines For Return To Play

- **Pain-Free Full Range Of Motion:** The injured body part should have full movement and flexibility with little or no discomfort.

- **Return Of Strength:** The injured body part should be approximately equal (90–95 percent) to the opposite side before returning to full activity.

- **Minimal Pain Or Swelling:** Some mild discomfort, stiffness and/or swelling during or after exercise is to be expected during the initial return to activity. This responds well to ice therapy.

- **Functional Retraining:** You should be able to perform the specific motions and actions required for your sport effectively before returning to activity. For example, retraining a lower-extremity injury in basketball should involve the ability to run, stop, change directions, and jump.

- **Progressive Return To Activity:** Consider starting at 50 percent of normal activity and progress up as tolerated. An informal guideline you can use is to progress activity 10–15 percent increase per week if the previous level of activity does not result in increased symptoms during exercise or the day after exercise.

- **Continue General Conditioning With Cross-Training:** Using an alternative exercise allows maintenance of general cardiovascular fitness while not interfering with the healing of an injury. For example, ankle or knee injuries may do well with bicycling or swimming.

- **Mental Confidence In Ability To Do Exercise:** You must feel that you and your injury are ready to perform at the level required for your particular activity.

If you have any questions about how the above guidelines apply to your particular injury, consultation with a sports medicine professional would be advisable.

Part Three

Preventing Sports Injuries

Chapter 37

Getting Hurt Doesn't Have To Happen

Lots of teens are injured while playing sports—but getting hurt doesn't have to happen. A few sports injury prevention steps can help to keep everyone in the game. Read on to learn the basics of sports and exercise safety.

Essential Equipment

Did you know that playing tennis with a badly strung (too loose or too tight) racquet while wearing worn-out shoes can be just as dangerous as playing football without shoulder pads? Using the wrong—or improperly fitted—equipment is a major reason why teens get injured.

The equipment you wear while participating in sports and other activities is key to preventing injuries. Start with helmets: They are important for sports such as football, hockey, baseball, softball, biking, skateboarding, in-line skating, skiing, and snowboarding—to name just a few.

- Always wear a helmet made for the sport you're playing.

- When choosing a bike helmet, look for a sticker that says the helmet meets the safety standard set by the Consumer Product Safety Commission

(CPSC), a part of the United States government that creates safety standards for bike helmets and other safety equipment.

• If you use a multisport helmet for in-line skating and skateboarding, it is not considered safe for bicycle riding unless it has the CPSC sticker.

• Any helmet should fit snugly but comfortably on your head and shouldn't tilt backward or forward.

Eye protection also is a must for many sports:

• The most protective eye gear is made from a plastic called polycarbonate and has been tested especially for sports use.

• Face masks or polycarbonate guards or shields that attach to a helmet are worn in sports such as football, ice hockey, and softball and baseball when batting.

> **✔ Quick Tip**
> If you wear glasses, you'll probably need prescription polycarbonate goggles—don't just wear your regular glasses when you're on the court or field.

• Goggles are often worn for soccer, basketball, racquet sports, snowboarding, street hockey, and baseball and softball when fielding.

• All eye protection should fit securely and have cushions above your eyebrows and over your nose.

Mouth guards can protect your mouth, teeth, and tongue:

• You should wear a mouth guard if you play a contact sport or other sport where head injury is a risk, such as football, basketball, hockey, volleyball, martial arts, boxing, or wrestling.

• Mouth guards can be fitted for your mouth by a dentist or purchased at sports stores.

• If you wear a retainer, always take it out before you start to exercise, practice, or play.

Wrist, knee, and elbow guards are important gear, too:

• If you in-line skate, skateboard, or ride a scooter, you should wear guards.

• Elbow and wrist guards can prevent arm and wrist fractures, and knee guards can shield your knees from cuts and breaks.

If you play certain sports, especially contact sports, pads are essential:

- All kinds of sports, from hockey to in-line skating, use pads. There are shin, knee, elbow, wrist, chest, shoulder, hip, and thigh pads.

- Check with your coach or doctor to find out what kinds of pads you might need for your sport.

Some guys may also need to wear a protective cup:

- Guys who play hockey, football, basketball, baseball, soccer, and other contact sports should use a cup.

- For noncontact sports that involve running, guys should wear an athletic supporter.

- If you're unsure, ask your coach, athletic trainer, or parent if you need a cup for your sport.

And last but not least, the right footwear can keep you from tripping and falling:

- You know that sports like football, baseball, softball, and soccer require cleats. But you may not realize that sports like skateboarding and biking need special types of shoes, too. Ask your coach or doctor what shoes are best for your sport.

- Replace shoes and cleats that have worn out or are no longer supportive.

Not only is the right kind of equipment important, so is the right fit. If you don't know if your equipment fits properly, check with a coach, gym teacher, athletic trainer, or parent to make sure you have the right size and that you're wearing it correctly. Many sporting goods stores can also help you find the right fit. The bottom line: Wearing the right equipment with the right fit dramatically decreases your chances of getting hurt.

Warm Up To Keep Your Game Up

Don't rush into any sport or exercise without warming up first—muscles that haven't been properly prepared tend to be injured more easily. Start out with some light cardiovascular activities, such as easy jogging, jumping jacks, or brisk walking, just to get your muscles going. Follow your brief warm-up with some stretches. (Stretching works best after a warm-up because your tissues are more elastic [flexible] due to the increase in heat and blood flow to the muscles).

In addition to warm-ups and stretches, practice sessions are also an excellent preparation for most sports or activities. If you belong to a team, attend as many team practices and games as possible. This will put you in top physical condition and help you and your teammates work together—and knowing how your teammates play will help prevent injuries.

Even if you don't belong to a team, you can use regular workouts and practices to enhance your performance and lessen the chance of injuries. Remember, if a tool isn't used, it gets rusty, so keep yourself in top shape with regular practice. For instance, try doing tennis drills or practicing your serve before starting a set. Shoot some baskets or play a quick game of one-on-one with a friend. Practice gets your brain and body to work together while improving your performance.

Although you should practice regularly, don't overdo it. Sudden increases in training frequency, duration, or intensity might produce better performance at first but can lead to injuries later. Your doctor or coach can help you develop a training and conditioning program that's appropriate for your age and level of development.

Staying Off The Court When You're Hurt

If you've been injured and you try to come back too soon, you run the great risk of reinjuring yourself—maybe even more seriously than before. Don't let anyone—including yourself, your parents, your friends, or even your coach—pressure you into playing before your body is fully healed. Your doctor, coach, or trainer will give you specific advice on when you should return to your sport or activity.

Taking time to heal is particularly important if you've had a concussion. Lots of athletes try to come back too quickly after getting a concussion—because they can't see an injury, they think they're OK to play. But jumping back into the game too soon puts a player at greater risk for another concussion—and that can lead to a dangerous brain injury. So always get clearance from your doctor to play again if you've had a concussion.

Many athletes use pain relievers to avoid pain. If you feel persistent pain, don't use pain relievers to mask it, though. Taking large amounts of pain relievers—or, worse yet, taking pain relievers for a long time in order to play— can be dangerous. Pain is the body's way of signaling it's not happy with what you're doing. If you have a lot of pain, seek treatment so you can resolve what's causing it.

Be sure to seek medical treatment whenever you experience:

- moderate to severe pain;
- pain that interferes with daily activity or sleep;
- swelling of the injured area;
- an inability to perform normal activities.

The same advice goes for a cold or flu virus—don't play if you're sick. You won't be able to concentrate if your head is stuffed up and your nose is running faster than you are, and your lack of concentration can put you at risk for injury. It's better to wait until you feel better, so you can have a safe season.

The Rules Of The Game

Rules and regulations usually exist for a good reason—to keep you and your teammates in the game and to avoid injuries. Do yourself a favor and learn the rules thoroughly—and then follow them. Rules aren't restrictions. They're designed to promote safety so that everyone can enjoy the game. For example, a late hit in football after the referee's whistle has blown leads to a pretty big penalty. This rule is important because a player could be seriously injured if he or she is not expecting a tackle after play has stopped.

♣ It's A Fact!!
Sometimes rules may not be directly related to a sport or activity but need to be followed anyway. For instance, if you're in-line skating, skateboarding, or riding a bike, pay strict attention to all traffic laws, especially when riding on busy public streets.

Proper techniques also promote safety. This goes for any sport, from motor racing to baseball. Baseball players know not to spike the opposing player who's covering the bag, even when sliding hard into second base. And when two tennis players rush the net, an expertly angled volley is the correct shot— not a hard smash socked directly at an opponent's face.

Another example of a safe technique occurs in weight lifting. Weightlifters should take a breath between each repetition. Exhale on the pushing phase of a lift. So if you're doing a bench press, let the bar come down to your chest, and if you're pushing up, breathe out. Holding your breath can raise your blood pressure, and if you're pressing a lot of weight this can lead to a black-out or fainting spell.

So whether you're following rules, regulations, or proper techniques, re-member that they aren't there to restrict you—they're there to keep you safe and injury free.

Chapter 38

Understanding Bones, Muscles, And Joints

Every time you sprint through the halls because you're late for class, score against your opponents during a game, or shoot pool with friends, you're using your bones, muscles, and joints. Without these important body parts, you'd be seriously sidelined—you'd be unable to sit, stand, walk, or do any of the activities you do every day.

From our head to our toes, our bones provide support for our bodies and help form our shape. The skull protects the brain and forms the shape of our face. The spinal cord, a pathway for messages between the brain and the body, is protected by the backbone, or spinal column. The ribs form a cage that shelters the heart, lungs, liver, and spleen, and the pelvis helps protect the bladder, intestines, and in girls, the reproductive organs. Although they're very light, bones are strong enough to support our entire weight.

Joints occur where two bones meet. They make the skeleton flexible—without them, movement would be impossible.

Muscles are also necessary for movement: They're the masses of tough, elastic tissue that pull our bones when we move.

About This Chapter: "Bones, Muscles, and Joints: The Musculoskeletal System," March 2007, reprinted with permission from www.kidshealth.org. Copyright © 2007 The Nemours Foundation. This information was provided by KidsHealth, one of the largest resources online for medically reviewed health information written for parents, kids, and teens. For more articles like this one, visit www.KidsHealth.org, or www.TeensHealth.org.

What Are The Bones And What Do They Do?

The human skeleton has 206 bones. Our bones begin to develop before birth. When the skeleton first forms, it is made of flexible cartilage, but within a few weeks it begins the process of ossification (pronounced: ah-suh-fuh-**kay**-shun). Ossification is when the cartilage is replaced by hard deposits of calcium phosphate and stretchy collagen, the two main components of bone. It takes about 20 years for this process to be completed.

♣ It's A Fact!!
Together, our bones, muscles, and joints—along with tendons, ligaments, and cartilage—form our musculoskeletal systems and enable us to do everyday physical activities.

The bones of kids and young teens are smaller than those of adults and contain "growing zones" called growth plates. These plates consist of columns of multiplying cartilage cells that grow in length, and then change into hard, mineralized bone. These growth plates are easy to spot on an x-ray. Because girls mature at an earlier age than boys, their growth plates change into hard bone at an earlier age.

Bone building continues throughout your life, as your body constantly renews and reshapes the bones' living tissue. Bone contains three types of cells: osteoblasts (pronounced: **ahs**-tee-uh-blastz), which make new bone and help repair damage; osteocytes (pronounced: **ahs**-tee-o-sites), which carry nutrients and waste products to and from blood vessels in the bone; and osteoclasts (pronounced: **ahs**-tee-o-klasts), which break down bone and help to sculpt and shape it. Osteoclasts are very active in kids and teens, working on bone as it is remodeled during growth. They also play an important role in the repair of fractures.

Bones are made up of calcium, phosphorus, sodium, and other minerals, as well as the protein collagen. Calcium is needed to make bones hard, which allows them to support your weight. Bones also store calcium and release some into the bloodstream when it's needed by other parts of the body. The amounts of certain vitamins and minerals that you eat, especially vitamin D and calcium, directly affect how much calcium is stored in the bones.

The soft bone marrow inside many of our bones is where most of the blood cells flowing through our bodies are made. The bone marrow contains special cells called stem cells, which produce the body's red blood cells and platelets. Red blood cells carry oxygen to the body's tissues, and platelets help with blood clotting when a person has a cut or wound.

Bones are made up of two types of material—compact bone and cancellous bone. Compact bone is the solid, hard outside part of the bone. It looks like ivory and is extremely strong. Holes and channels run through it, carrying blood vessels and nerves from the periosteum, the bone's membrane covering, to its inner parts. Cancellous (pronounced: **kan**-suh-lus) bone, which looks like a sponge, is inside the compact bone. It is made up of a mesh-like network of tiny pieces of bone called trabeculae (pronounced: truh-**beh**-kyoo-lee). The spaces in this network are filled with red marrow, found mainly at the ends of bones, and yellow marrow, which is mostly fat.

Bones are fastened to other bones by long, fibrous straps called ligaments (pronounced: **lih**-guh-mentz). Cartilage (pronounced: **kar**-tul-ij), a flexible, rubbery substance in our joints, supports bones and protects them where they rub against each other.

What Are The Muscles And What Do They Do?

Bones don't work alone—they need help from the muscles and joints. Muscles pull on the joints, allowing us to move. They also help the body perform other functions so we can grow and remain strong, such as chewing food and then moving it through the digestive system.

The human body has more than 650 muscles, which make up half of a person's body weight. They are connected to bones by tough, cord-like tissues called tendons, which allow the muscles to pull on bones. If you wiggle your fingers, you can see the tendons on the back of your hand move as they do their work.

Humans have three different kinds of muscle:

- Skeletal muscle is attached to bone, mostly in the legs, arms, abdomen, chest, neck, and face. Skeletal muscles are called striated (pronounced: **stry**-ay-ted) because they are made up of fibers that have horizontal stripes when viewed under a microscope. These muscles hold the skeleton together, give the body shape, and help it with everyday movements (they are known as voluntary muscles because you can control their movement). They can contract (shorten or tighten) quickly and powerfully, but they tire easily and have to rest between workouts.

- Smooth, or involuntary, muscle is also made of fibers, but this type of muscle looks smooth, not striated. Generally, we can't consciously control our smooth muscles; rather, they're controlled by the nervous system automatically (which is why they are also called involuntary). Examples of smooth muscles are the walls of the stomach and intestines, which help break up food and move it through the digestive system. Smooth muscle is also found in the walls of blood vessels, where it squeezes the stream of blood flowing through the vessels to help maintain blood pressure. Smooth muscles take longer to contract than skeletal muscles do, but they can stay contracted for a long time because they don't tire easily.

- Cardiac (pronounced: **kar**-dee-ak) muscle is found in the heart. The walls of the heart's chambers are composed almost entirely of muscle fibers. Cardiac muscle is also an involuntary type of muscle. Its rhythmic, powerful contractions force blood out of the heart as it beats.

Even when you sit perfectly still, there are muscles throughout your body that are constantly moving. Muscles enable your heart to beat, your chest to rise and fall as you breathe, and your blood vessels to help regulate the pressure and flow of blood through your body. When we smile and talk, muscles are helping us communicate, and when we exercise, they help us stay physically fit and healthy.

The movements your muscles make are coordinated and controlled by the brain and nervous system. The involuntary muscles are controlled by structures deep within the brain and the upper part of the spinal cord called the brain stem. The voluntary muscles are regulated by the parts of the brain known as the cerebral motor cortex and the cerebellum.

When you decide to move, the motor cortex sends an electrical signal through the spinal cord and peripheral nerves to the muscles, causing them to contract. The motor cortex on the right side of the brain controls the muscles on the left side of the body and vice versa.

The cerebellum (pronounced: ser-uh-**beh**-lum) coordinates the muscle movements ordered by the motor cortex. Sensors in the muscles and joints send messages back through peripheral nerves to tell the cerebellum and other parts of the brain where and how the arm or leg is moving and what position it's in. This feedback results in smooth, coordinated motion. If you want to lift your arm, your brain sends a message to the muscles in your arm and you move it. When you run, the messages to the brain are more involved, because many muscles have to work in rhythm.

Muscles move body parts by contracting and then relaxing. Your muscles can pull bones, but they can't push them back to their original position. So they work in pairs of flexors and extensors. The flexor contracts to bend a limb at a joint. Then, when you've completed the movement, the flexor relaxes and the extensor contracts to extend or straighten the limb at the same joint. For example, the biceps muscle, in the front of the upper arm, is a flexor, and the triceps, at the back of the upper arm, is an extensor. When you bend at your elbow, the biceps contracts. Then the biceps relaxes and the triceps contracts to straighten the elbow.

What Are The Joints And What Do They Do?

Joints allow our bodies to move in many ways. Some joints open and close like a hinge (such as knees and elbows), whereas others allow for more complicated movement—a shoulder or hip joint, for example, allows for backward, forward, sideways, and rotating movement.

Joints are classified by their range of movement. Immovable, or fibrous, joints don't move. The dome of the skull, for example, is made of bony plates, which must be immovable to protect the brain. Between the edges of these plates are links, or joints, of fibrous tissue. Fibrous joints also hold the teeth in the jawbone.

Partially movable, or cartilaginous (pronounced: kar-tuh-**lah**-juh-nus), joints move a little. They are linked by cartilage, as in the spine. Each of the vertebrae in the spine moves in relation to the one above and below it, and together these movements give the spine its flexibility.

Freely movable, or synovial (pronounced: sih-**no**-vee-ul), joints move in many directions. The main joints of the body—found at the hip, shoulders, elbows, knees, wrists, and ankles—are freely movable. They are filled with synovial fluid, which acts as a lubricant to help the joints move easily. There are three kinds of freely movable joints that play a big part in voluntary movement:

- Hinge joints allow movement in one direction, as seen in the knees and elbows.

- Pivot joints allow a rotating or twisting motion, like that of the head moving from side to side.

- Ball-and-socket joints allow the greatest freedom of movement. The hips and shoulders have this type of joint, in which the round end of a long bone fits into the hollow of another bone.

Things That Can Go Wrong With The Bones, Muscles, And Joints

As strong as bones are, they can break. Muscles can weaken, and joints (as well as tendons, ligaments, and cartilage) can be damaged by injury or disease. The following are problems that can affect the bones, muscles, and joints in teens:

Arthritis: Arthritis (pronounced: ar-**threye**-tus) is the inflammation of a joint, and people who have it experience swelling, warmth, pain, and often have trouble moving. Although we often think of arthritis as a condition that affects only older people, arthritis can also occur in children and teens. Health problems that involve arthritis in kids and teens include juvenile rheumatoid arthritis (JRA), lupus, Lyme disease, and septic arthritis (a bacterial infection of a joint).

> ♣ **It's A Fact!!**
> *Does cracking knuckles give you arthritis?*
> Though people sometimes say you'll get arthritis (a painful joint condition) if you crack your knuckles a lot, knuckle cracking has not been scientifically proven to cause arthritis. It is a fact, though, that cracking your knuckles is annoying!

Fracture: A fracture occurs when a bone breaks; it may crack, snap, or shatter. After a bone fracture, new bone cells fill the gap and repair the break. Applying a strong plaster cast, which keeps the bone in the correct position until it heals, is the usual treatment. If the fracture is complicated, metal pins and plates can be placed to better stabilize the fracture while the bone heals.

Muscular Dystrophy: Muscular dystrophy (pronounced: **mus**-kyoo-lur **dis**-truh-fee) is an inherited group of diseases that affect the muscles, causing them to weaken and break down over time. The most common form in childhood is called Duchenne muscular dystrophy, and it most often affects boys.

Osgood-Schlatter Disease (OSD): Osgood-Schlatter disease is an inflammation (pain and swelling) of the bone, cartilage, and/or tendon at the top of the shinbone, where the tendon from the kneecap attaches. OSD usually strikes active teens around the beginning of their growth spurts, the approximately two-year period during which they grow most rapidly.

Osteomyelitis: Osteomyelitis (pronounced: os-tee-oh-my-uh-**lie**-tus) is a bone infection that is often caused by Staphylococcus aureus (pronounced: sta-fuh-low-**kah**-kus **are**-ee-us) bacteria, though other types of bacteria can cause it, too. In kids and teens, osteomyelitis usually affects the long bones of the arms and legs. Osteomyelitis often develops after an injury or trauma.

Osteoporosis: In osteoporosis (pronounced: ahs-tee-o-puh-**row**-sus), bone tissue becomes brittle, thin, and spongy. Bones break easily, and the spine sometimes begins to crumble and collapse. Although the condition usually affects older people, girls with female athlete triad and teens with eating disorders can get the condition. Exercising regularly and getting plenty of calcium when you're a kid and teen can prevent or delay you from getting osteoporosis later in life.

Repetitive Stress Injuries: Repetitive stress injuries (RSIs) are a group of injuries that happen when too much stress is placed on a part of the body, resulting in inflammation (pain and swelling), muscle strain, or tissue damage. This stress generally occurs from repeating the same movements over and over again. RSIs are becoming more common in kids and teens because they spend more time than ever using computers. Playing sports like tennis that involve repetitive motions can also lead to RSIs. Kids and teens who spend a lot of time playing musical instruments or video games are also at risk for RSIs.

Scoliosis: Every person's spine curves a little bit; a certain amount of curvature is necessary for people to move and walk properly. But three to five people out of 1,000 have a condition called scoliosis (pronounced: sko-lee-o-sus), which causes the spine to curve too much. The condition can be hereditary, so a person who has scoliosis often has family members who have it.

Strains And Sprains: Strains occur when a muscle or tendon is overstretched. Sprains are an overstretching or a partial tear of the ligaments. Strains usually happen when a person takes part in a strenuous activity when the muscles haven't properly warmed up or the muscle is not used to the activity (such as a new sport or playing a familiar sport after a long break). Sprains, on the other hand, are usually the result of an injury, such as twisting an ankle or knee. Both strains and sprains are common in teens because they're active and still growing.

Tendinitis: Tendinitis (pronounced: ten-duh-ny-tus) is a common sports injury that usually happens after overexercising a muscle. The tendon and tendon sheath become inflamed, which can be painful. Resting the muscles and taking anti-inflammatory medication can help to relieve this condition.

Chapter 39

Warming Up, Stretching, And Cooling Down

Ben wants to start exercising regularly, but feels dumb asking how. He knows that in order to run or ride a bike he can't just start sprinting or pedaling like a maniac. He needs to prepare his body for these activities, but has heard mixed things about stretching before working out.

Here are the cold, hard facts on warming up, stretching, and cooling down.

The Basics Of Warming Up

It's important to warm up your body before any physical activity. Warming up goes a long way toward preparing the body for exercising, both physically and mentally. It also helps prevent injuries.

The term "warm-up" describes many light-aerobic and cardiovascular activities, which are separate from stretching. (Stretching works best when performed after warming up.) When you warm up, you are literally warming up the temperature of both your body and your muscles.

About This Chapter: "Stretching," September 2006, reprinted with permission from www.kidshealth.org. Copyright © 2006 The Nemours Foundation. This information was provided by KidsHealth, one of the largest resources online for medically reviewed health information written for parents, kids, and teens. For more articles like this one, visit www.KidsHealth.org, or www.TeensHealth.org.

Warming up also:

- increases your heart and respiratory rate;
- boosts the amount of nutrients and oxygen delivered to your muscles;
- prepares the body for a demanding workout;
- makes it easier to burn calories;
- extends your workout;

Types Of Warm-Ups

You can use many types of warm-up activities to prepare your body for intense physical exercise. Often a warm-up activity is simply the activity you are about to do but at a slower pace. For example, if you're about to go for a brisk run, warm up with a light jog, and if you're going to go for a swim, do a couple of slow freestyle warm-up laps.

Only after this light warm-up, which should last about five to ten minutes, should you attempt to stretch.

Stretching

Stretching used to be considered the main activity before a workout. That has all changed now. Stretching is still a beneficial activity prior to working out, but only after you have sufficiently warmed up. The reason for this is that stretching cold muscles can directly contribute to pulled and torn muscles. It's also now known that stretching is important after a workout as well.

Stretching properly may reduce muscle injuries and provides these benefits:

- An increase in flexibility and joint range of motion
- Correct exercise posture

> ✔ Quick Tip
> **Muscle Groups**
>
> To increase flexibility, include these muscle groups in your stretching routine:
>
> - Shoulders (deltoid and rotator cuff)
> - Back (muscles of the lower, middle, and upper back)
> - Thighs (hamstring and quad)
> - Calves (gastrocnemius and soleus)
> - Arms (biceps, triceps, and forearm muscles)

- Relaxed muscles

- Better sports coordination

Stretching has to be done right to have benefits, though. Here are some tips on stretching properly:

- **Stop if it hurts.** Stretching should never hurt. If you have reached a point in your stretch where it hurts, relax to where it feels comfortable and hold the stretch.

- **Maintain each stretch for 10–30 seconds.** Holding a stretch for any less won't sufficiently lengthen the muscle. Stretch the muscles gradually and don't force it. Avoid bobbing. Bobbing or bouncing while stretching may damage the muscle you are stretching. This damage may even cause scar tissue to form. Scar tissue tightens muscles and can get in the way of flexibility.

- **Remember to breath.** Breathing is a necessary part of any workout, including stretching.

- **Practice equality.** Even if you are a righty, it doesn't mean that you should neglect the left side of your body. Make sure you stretch both sides equally, so all of your muscles are evenly ready for action.

If you play a sport, you should do warm-ups that go with that sport. The same is true for stretching. These types of stretches are known as sports-specific stretches, and they focus on the muscles that are used for your particular sport. For instance, if you play baseball you might focus on your shoulder for throwing or your forearm for batting.

Cooling Down After Your Workout

The most efficient way of slowing down a car or bike isn't by riding straight into a brick wall. The same way you have to gradually slow down either your bike or your car, you need to slow down your body after a workout or exercise: five to ten minutes of slowed-down, easy activities will go a long way in helping your body recover from a workout.

Your cool-down routine can vary from workout to workout. It should include light aerobic activity and stretching. If you're running at a quick pace, you can slow down to a steady walk to cool down. Cooling down and stretching at the end of a workout help to:

- slow your heart rate to a normal speed;

- return your breathing to its regular pace;

- avoid stiffness and soreness of the muscles;

- reduce any risk of dizziness and lightheadedness;

- relax the muscles.

Whether you are new to working out or have been playing a sport your entire life, adding a good before-and-after routine to your workout will give you the best chance of avoiding injuries and may even help improve your performance.

Chapter 40

Hard Facts About Helmets

Protect Yourself... Wear A Helmet!

What do bicycling, horseback riding, baseball, and in-line skating all have in common? Helmets! The trick is that different sports require a different type of helmet to help protect participants from the different types of head injuries common to that particular sport.

All helmets are not created equal; beyond picking the right helmet for the sport, buyers should look inside the helmet for information on standards the helmet complies with. Bike helmets for example should carry a Consumer Product Safety Commission (CPSC), Snell, American Society for Testing and Materials (ASTM), or American National Standards Institute (ANSI) sticker or label.

Fit Is Key

A loose helmet cannot protect the head as well as one that is properly fit. The Bicycle Helmet Safety Institute suggests buying a brand and size that fits well prior to adjustments and then using the adjustable straps and/or sizing pads to ensure a snug fit. Select a helmet that fits you now, not a helmet to "grow into."

About This Chapter: This chapter includes "Protect Yourself... Wear a Helmet," © 2004 National Safety Council (www.nsc.org). Reprinted with permission; and "How to Fit a Bicycle Helmet," © 2007 Bicycle Helmet Safety Institute (www.helmets.org). Reprinted with permission.

♣ **It's A Fact!!**

Helmets...Fact Or Fiction?

Fiction: Helmets aren't cool.

Fact: Who says helmets can't be cool? If you're shopping for a helmet, there are lots of options, so you can pick out your favorite color. Or decorate your helmet with stickers and reflectors to show your personal style. Helmets are designed to help prevent injuries to your head because a serious fall or crash can cause permanent brain damage or death. And that's definitely not cool.

Fiction: Helmets just aren't comfortable.

Fact: Today's helmets are lightweight, well ventilated, and have lots of padding. Try on your helmet to make sure it fits properly and comfortably on your head before you buy it.

Fiction: Really good riders don't need to wear helmets.

Fact: Bike crashes or collisions can happen at any time. Even professional bike racers get in serious wrecks. In three out of four bike crashes, bikers usually get some sort of injury to their head.

Source: From "Hard Facts about Helmets," BAM! (Body and Mind), Centers for Disease Control and Prevention, 2002.

Helmets Save Lives

- According to the Bicycle Helmet Safety Institute, a bicycle helmet reduces the risk of serious head and brain injury by 85%.

- More than 70,000 persons need hospital emergency room treatment each year for injuries related to skateboarding according to the CPSC.

- Head injuries cause three-quarters of about 900 bicycle deaths each year, according to the Bicycle Helmet Safety Institute, a helmet advocacy program of the Washington, D.C.–area Bicyclist Association.

- Another 82,000 people suffer brain injuries each year while playing sports such as baseball and football, etc., according to the Brain Injury Association in Alexandria, Virginia.

- Brain surgeons and doctors across the U.S. agree that wearing helmets can save lives.

Both children and adults should wear the appropriate helmet when participating in the following sports or any recreational activity where head injuries are a risk:

- All-terrain vehicle (ATV) riding

- Baseball

- Bicycling

- Football

- Horse-back riding

- In-line skating

- Rock climbing

- Skateboarding

- Softball

For handling sports-related injuries and other emergencies, everyone should be trained in first aid.

How To Fit A Bicycle Helmet

Your Objective: Snug, Level, Stable

You want the helmet to be comfortably touching the head all the way around, level and stable enough to resist even violent shakes or hard blows, and stay in place. It should be as low on the head as possible to maximize side coverage and held level on the head with the strap comfortably snug.

Be Prepared For The Worst

Heads come in many sizes and shapes. You should be prepared for the possibility that the helmet you are trying to fit may not be compatible with

♣ **It's A Fact!!**

Your helmet should sit flat on your head—make sure it is level and is not tilted back or forward. The front of the helmet should sit low—about two finger widths above your eyebrows to protect your forehead. The straps on each side of your head should form a "Y" over your ears, with one part of the strap in front of your ear and one behind—just below your earlobes. If the helmet leans forward, adjust the rear straps. If it tilts backward, tighten the front straps. Buckle the chinstrap securely at your throat so that the helmet feels snug on your head and does not move up and down or from side to side.

Source: From "Hard Facts about Helmets," BAM! (Body and Mind), Centers for Disease Control and Prevention (CDC), 2002.

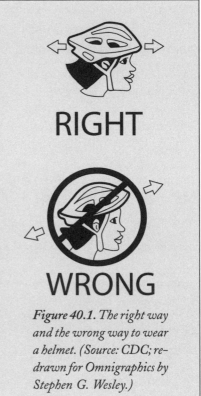

Figure 40.1. The right way and the wrong way to wear a helmet. (Source: CDC; redrawn for Omnigraphics by Stephen G. Wesley.)

this particular head. And unfortunately, you should expect to spend ten to fifteen minutes to get your helmet properly fitted.

1. Adjust The Fit Pads Or Ring

Helmets that fit with pads come with at least one set of foam fitting pads, and if you got a second set of thicker pads it can be used to customize the shape. For starters, you can often remove the top pad entirely or use the thinnest ones. This lowers the helmet on the head, bringing its protection down further on the sides. It may reduce the flow of cooling air slightly, but probably not enough to notice.

Adjust the side fit pads by using thicker pads if your head is narrow and there is a space, or add thicker pads in the back for shorter heads. You may also move pads around, particularly on the "corners" in the front and rear.

Leaving some gaps will improve air flow. The pads should touch your head evenly all the way around, without making the fit too tight. The pads may compress slightly over time, but not much, so do not count on that to loosen the fit. The helmet should sit level on the head, with the front just above the eyebrows, or if the rider uses glasses, just above the frame of the glasses. If you walk into a wall, the helmet should hit before your nose does!

There are also helmets on the market that use a fitting ring rather than side pads for adjustment. With these one-size-fits-all models you begin by adjusting the size of the ring. Some of them may require the ring so tight for real stability on your head that they feel binding, but loosening the ring can produce a sloppy fit, indicating that the helmet is not for you.

2. Adjust The Straps

Now put the helmet on and fasten the buckle. Be sure the front is in front! You want to adjust it to the "eye-ear-mouth" test developed by the Bicycle Coalition of Maine:

- When you look upward the front rim should be barely visible to your eye.
- The Y of the side straps should meet just below your ear.
- The chin strap should be snug against the chin so that when you open your mouth very wide you feel the helmet pull down a little bit.

With the helmet in position on your head, adjust the length of the rear straps, then the length of the front straps, to locate the Y fitting where the straps come together just under your ear. That may involve sliding the straps across the top of the helmet to get the length even on both sides. Then adjust the length of the chin strap so it is comfortably snug. If it cuts into the chin and is not comfortable, it is too tight. Now pay attention to the rear stabilizer if the helmet has one. It can keep the helmet from jiggling in normal use and make it feel more stable, but only a well-adjusted strap can keep it on in a crash.

When you think the straps are about right, shake your head around violently. Then put your palm under the front edge and push up and back. Can you move the helmet more than an inch or so from level, exposing your bare forehead? Then you need to tighten the strap in front of your ear, and perhaps loosen the rear strap behind your ear. Again, the two straps should meet just below your ear. Now reach back and grab the back edge. Pull up. Can you move the helmet more than an inch? If so, tighten the rear strap.

For a final check, look in a mirror or look at the wearer whose helmet you are fitting. Move the helmet side to side and front to back, watching the skin around the eyebrows. It should move slightly with the helmet. If it does not, the fit pads are probably too thin in front or back.

When you are done, your helmet should be level, feel solid on your head, and be comfortable. It should not bump on your glasses (if it does, tighten the nape strap). It should pass the eye-ear-mouth test. You should forget you are wearing it most of the time, just like a seat belt or a good pair of shoes. If it still does not fit that way, keep working with the straps and pads, or try another helmet.

Note: With a helmet that fits this well on a child, you must be sure the child removes the helmet before climbing trees and playing on playground equipment. Otherwise there is a risk of catching the helmet and being strangled! That doesn't happen in normal bike riding, even in crashes, but it can happen while climbing trees or monkey bars.

Finally, you want the straps to stay adjusted. Some helmets—even expensive ones—do not have locking pieces on the side where the straps come together under your ear. If you can move the side buckle with your hand, it will migrate in use. We call that "strap creep," and it is a major problem. If your helmet has non-locking side pieces, that means you have to either put on a rubber band and snug it up under the side buckle, or you will need to sew the straps when you have the fit just right. If you use heavy thread you only need five or six stitches to hold it. It's an extra chore, but worth it.

Chapter 41

Sports Eye Safety

More than 40,000 people a year suffer eye injuries while playing sports. For all age groups, sports-related eye injuries occur most frequently in baseball, basketball and racquet sports. Almost all sports-related eye injuries can be prevented. Whatever your game, whatever your age, you need to protect your eyes.

Recommended Sports Eye Protectors

Baseball

Recommended Protection

- Faceguard (attached to helmet) made of polycarbonate material
- Sports eyeguards

Injuries Prevented

- Scratches on the cornea

About This Chapter: This chapter begins with "Sports Eye Safety" and continues with "Recommended Sports Eye Protectors," and "Tips for Buying Sports Eye Protectors," reprinted with permission from Prevent Blindness America. Copyright 2007. All rights reserved. For additional information, call the Prevent Blindness America toll-free information line at 1-800-331-2020, or visit www.preventblindness.org.

- Inflamed iris
- Blood spilling into the eye's anterior chamber
- Traumatic cataract
- Swollen retina

Basketball

Recommended Protection

- Sports eyeguards

Injuries Prevented

- Fracture of the eye socket
- Scratches on the cornea
- Inflamed iris
- Blood spilling into the eye's anterior chamber
- Swollen retina

Soccer

Recommended Protection

- Sports eyeguards

Injuries Prevented

- Inflamed iris
- Blood spilling into the eye's anterior chamber
- Swollen retina

Football

Recommended Protection

- Polycarbonate shield attached to a faceguard
- Sports eyeguards

✔ **Quick Tip**

Take the following steps to avoid sports eye injuries:

- Wear proper safety goggles (lensed polycarbonate protectors) for racquet sports or basketball.
- Use batting helmets with polycarbonate face shields for youth baseball.
- Use helmets and face shields approved by the U.S. Amateur Hockey Association when playing hockey.
- Know that regular glasses don't provide enough protection.

Source: From "Sports Eye Safety," © 2007 Prevent Blindness America.

Injuries Prevented

- Scratches on the cornea

- Inflamed iris

- Blood spilling into the eye's anterior chamber

- Swollen retina

Hockey

Recommended Protection

- Wire or polycarbonate mask

- Sports eyeguards

Injuries Prevented

- Scratches on the cornea

- Inflamed iris

- Blood spilling into the eye's anterior chamber

- Traumatic cataract

- Swollen retina

Tips For Buying Sports Eye Protectors

The following guidelines can help you find a pair of eyeguards right for you:

- If you wear prescription glasses, ask your eye doctor to fit you for prescription eyeguards. If you're a monocular athlete (a person with only one eye that sees well), ask your eye doctor what sports you can safely participate in. Monocular athletes should always wear sports eyeguards.

- Buy eyeguards at sports specialty stores or optical stores. At the sports store, ask for a sales representative who's familiar with eye protectors to help you.

- Don't buy sports eyeguards without lenses. Only "lensed" protectors are recommended for sports use. Make sure the lenses either stay in place or pop outward in the event of an accident. Lenses that pop in against your eyes can be very dangerous.

- Fogging of the lenses can be a problem when you're active. Some eyeguards are available with anti-fog coating. Others have side vents for additional ventilation. Try on different types to determine which is most comfortable for you.

- Check the packaging to see if the eye protector you select has been tested for sports use. Also check to see that the eye protector is made of polycarbonate material. Polycarbonate eyeguards are the most impact resistant.

- Sports eyeguards should be padded or cushioned along the brow and bridge of the nose. Padding will prevent the eyeguards from cutting your skin.

- Try on the eye protector to determine if it's the right size. Adjust the strap and make sure it's not too tight or too loose. If you purchased your eyeguards at an optical store, an optical representative can help you adjust the eye protector for a comfortable fit.

Until you get used to wearing a pair of eyeguards, it may feel strange, but bear with it! It's a lot more comfortable than an eye injury.

♣ **It's A Fact!!**
Prevent Blindness America recommends that athletes wear sports eyeguards when participating in sports. Prescription glasses, sunglasses, and even occupational safety glasses do not provide adequate protection. Sports eyeguards come in a variety of shapes and sizes. Eyeguards designed for use in racquet sports are now commonly used for basketball and soccer and in combination with helmets in football, hockey, and baseball. The eyeguards you choose should fit securely and comfortably and allow the use of a helmet if necessary. Expect to spend between $20 and $40 for a pair of regular eyeguards and $60 or more for eyeguards with prescription lenses.

Source: From "Tips for Buying Sports Eye Protectors,"
© 2007 Prevent Blindness America.

Chapter 42

Protect Your Teeth With A Mouthguard

Do I need a mouth protector?

Anyone who participates in a sport that carries a significant risk of injury should wear a mouth protector. This includes a wide range of sports like football, hockey, basketball, baseball, gymnastics, and volleyball.

Mouth protectors, which typically cover the upper teeth, can cushion a blow to the face, minimizing the risk of broken teeth and injuries to the soft tissues of the mouth. If you wear braces or another fixed dental appliance on your lower jaw, your dentist may suggest a mouth protector for these teeth as well.

What are the advantages of using a mouth protector?

Accidents can happen during any physical activity. A mouth protector can help cushion a blow to the face that otherwise might result in an injury to the mouth. A misdirected elbow in a one-on-one basketball game or a spill off a bicycle can leave you with chipped or broken teeth, nerve damage to a tooth, or even tooth loss. A mouth protector can limit the risk of such injuries as well as protect the soft tissues of your tongue, lips, and cheek lining.

About This Chapter: "Mouthguards: Frequently Asked Questions (FAQ)," an undated document, © American Dental Association. Reprinted with permission.

A properly fitted mouth protector will stay in place while you are wearing it, making it easy for you to talk and breathe.

Are there different types of mouth protectors?

There are three types of mouth protectors:

1. **Stock:** Stock mouth protectors are inexpensive and come pre-formed, ready to wear. Unfortunately, they often don't fit very well. They can be bulky and can make breathing and talking difficult.

2. **Boil And Bite:** Boil and bite mouth protectors also can be bought at many sporting goods stores and may offer a better fit than stock mouth protectors. They should be softened in water, then inserted and allowed to adapt to the shape of your mouth. If you don't follow the directions carefully you can wind up with a poor-fitting mouth protector.

3. **Custom-Fitted:** Custom-fitted mouth protectors are made by your dentist for you personally. They are more expensive than the other versions, but because they are customized they can offer a better fit than anything you can buy off the shelf.

I wear braces. Can I use a mouth protector?

A properly fitted mouth protector may be especially important for people who wear braces or have fixed bridge work. A blow to the face could damage

> ✔ **Quick Tip**
> **Take Care Of The Mouthguard**
>
> Patients need to take care of their mouthguards by doing the following:
>
> • Rinse before and after each use or brush with toothbrush and toothpaste
>
> • Occasionally clean the mouthguard in cool, soapy water and rinse thoroughly
>
> • Transport the mouthguard in a sturdy container that has vents
>
> • Make sure not to leave the mouthguard in the sun or in hot water
>
> • Check for wear and replace the mouthguard when necessary
>
> Source: Excerpted from "Protecting Teeth with Mouthguards," © 2006 American Dental Association. Reprinted with permission.

the brackets or other fixed orthodontic appliances. A mouth protector also provides a barrier between the braces and your cheek or lips, limiting the risk of soft tissue injuries.

Talk to your dentist or orthodontist about selecting a mouth protector that will provide the best protection. Although mouth protectors typically only cover the upper teeth, your dentist or orthodontist may suggest that you use a mouth protector on the lower teeth if you have braces on these teeth too.

If you have a retainer or other removable appliance, do not wear it during any contact sports.

Chapter 43

Skin Protection Tips For Athletes

Without Proper Treatment, Skin Infections Can Sideline Your Season

When most people think about sports, they think about competition, teamwork, dedication, and team spirit. Rarely do athletes consider that they could be exposed to infections ranging from athlete's foot to serious skin conditions that could bench them, disrupt team dynamics, and jeopardize their health. With proper diagnosis and treatment, skin infections do not have to sideline athletes or hinder their performance.

Speaking in March, 2006, at the 64th Annual Meeting of the American Academy of Dermatology, dermatologist Brian B. Adams, M.D., M.P.H., associate professor in the department of dermatology at the University of Cincinnati in Ohio, discussed the importance of early recognition, diagnosis, and treatment of skin infections to minimize downtime and prevent team epidemics.

"Athletes are particularly susceptible to skin infections because of several factors including skin-to-skin contact with other athletes and athletic equipment, increased sweating which can impair the main barrier of the skin, and susceptibility of skin trauma," said Dr. Adams. "It is important to recognize the signs of infection or other skin problems so they can be treated quickly and efficiently to minimize loss of training time for athletes and, sometimes, entire teams."

Skin Infections

Skin problems can differ from sport to sport and athletes at all levels, from Olympians to weekend warriors, can experience skin infections related to their sport. One of the most common infections found in many sports is impetigo. A superficial infection of the skin, impetigo particularly affects athletes with skin-to-skin contact like wrestlers and rugby and football players. Impetigo, which is characterized by yellow, crusted, well-defined lesions, responds well to topical or oral antibiotics. Infected areas and lesions should be bandaged or infected athletes should not practice or compete until treatment has been determined effective. "Impetigo is highly contagious and can spread rapidly through teams or competitors," said Dr. Adams. "In many states, a physician's note is required before wrestlers diagnosed with impetigo will be allowed to compete again."

Another common skin infection is herpes simplex, which also is transmitted by skin-to-skin contact. Studies show that wrestling and rugby athletes are particularly susceptible, having a 33 percent chance of transmission. Herpes simplex causes blisters and sores anywhere on the skin. The highly contagious infection needs to be quickly detected and treated to prevent transmission to other team members or competitors. Treatment consists of warm compresses and antiviral agents.

A major challenge with herpes simplex is that many athletes are infected with the virus before skin lesions are visible. Athletes can take oral antiviral agents daily during the season to prevent contracting herpes simplex. Dr. Adams warns that if the virus is left untreated, there can be unnecessary complications. "Athletes who have contracted the virus should refrain from skin-to-skin activity for approximately four to seven days following the beginning of treatment," said Dr. Adams.

Another contagious infection is furunculosis, an infection characterized by the presence of furuncles or deep sores of the skin, which are also called boils. Furunculosis has caused epidemics among high school, college, and even professional teams. It is commonly seen in football players at the site of turf burns and is more common in certain positions; for example, a lineman is ten times more likely to be affected than a quarterback because they tend to have more contact with the turf. Treatment is typically a warm, moist compress applied three to four times daily for 10 minutes at a time and oral or topical antibiotics, though a physician may need to drain larger boils. Without treatment, the boil will likely heal in 10 to 20 days.

A fourth infection, tinea corporis gladiatorum, also known as ringworm, is one of the most common infections in wrestling and has caused epidemics, infecting between 24 to 77 percent of a team. This infection appears on the head, neck, and extremities as a well-defined, red, scaly patch. Treatment options include the use of both topical and oral antifungal agents, and athletes can take an oral antifungal agent weekly to prevent contracting the infection during their sports season. "Athletes, wrestlers in particular, are advised to refrain from their sport for five days after beginning treatment to ensure the infection is not transmitted to other athletes," said Dr. Adams.

Foot Infections

Athletes depend on their feet for most of their movement and need to pay special attention to keeping their feet healthy. One type of infection of the foot is pitted keratolysis, also known as "sweaty sock syndrome." This infection can be caused by wearing tight or restricting footwear and excessive sweating during exercise. The infection is characterized by crater-like pits on the surface of the feet and toes, particularly weight-bearing areas. Treatment consists of the application of topical antibiotics. "The best prevention is to wear breathable shoes and socks and to remove sweaty footwear immediately after exercise," recommended Dr. Adams.

Another foot infection is plantar verruca, or foot warts, which occurs most often in swimmers, rowers, and cross-country runners. This infection can be transmitted via the shower or locker room floor and can sometimes take months to grow large enough to be noticed. Plantar verruca is treated surgically, though other topical agents may be a preferred method of treatment in order to minimize the loss of training time for the athlete. Dr. Adams emphasized that the best prevention is for athletes to wear sandals in locker rooms and showers and to keep their feet dry.

One of the most common infections in both serious and recreational athletes is tinea pedis, commonly known as athlete's foot. It is often seen in soccer and basketball players, swimmers, and runners, and can be contracted through contact with pool, locker, or shower room floors or as a result of wearing tight or restricting footwear and excessive sweating. The contagious infection is characterized by scaly patches on the skin between the toes or with redness, scaling, or dryness on the foot. In some cases, it can be characterized by pimples or itchy blisters on the feet.

"Anti-fungal creams are an effective treatment and can often relieve symptoms fairly quickly," stated Dr. Adams. "For more severe cases, doctors may need to prescribe antifungal pills." Dr. Adams recommends wearing sandals on wet floors in pool and shower rooms and wearing breathable socks. Drying agents such as foot sprays or powders also can be applied to feet before exercise to help prevent excess moisture.

Sports-related infections can cause serious complications and even epidemics which sideline entire teams. "To reduce risk of infection, athletes should practice basic hygiene, know the infection risks inherent to their sport, recognize signs of infections quickly, and seek proper treatment," said Dr. Adams. "Sports are meant to be enjoyed and treating infections quickly can keep athletes and teams playing at their best."

Endurance Athletes And Moderate Exercisers Could Run Into Trouble With Blisters And Other Skin Problems

When the National Academy of Science's Institute of Medicine recently announced that Americans should exercise an hour a day to fight the country's growing obesity epidemic, collective groans could be heard in big cities and small towns everywhere. However, researchers advise that an exercise program—supplemented by dietary changes—is vital in taking and keeping off weight that is associated with many chronic health problems.

While endurance athletes represent the extreme end of the exercising spectrum, dermatologists are anticipating that the sports-related dermatologic injuries they encounter also will be observed in people who exercise more moderately and those who are just beginning a fitness program.

Speaking in February, 2005, at the 63rd Annual Meeting of the American Academy of Dermatology, dermatologist Scott B. Phillips, M.D., of Chicago, Ill., and commentator for the *Dialogues in Dermatology* article, "Dermatologic Problems of the Endurance Athlete," published in the February 2005 issue of the *Journal of the American Academy of Dermatology*, discussed why healthy skin is important for athletes.

"Even common problems, such as blisters, can be painful and adversely affect athletic participation and performance," stated Dr. Phillips. "If an athlete is unable to compete at their expected level of training or competition, it also can have psychological effects. Recognition of these conditions is important as they are often preventable or treatable."

Blisters form when movement from athletic activity causes the skin to rub against a toe or other object. Heat, moisture, ill-fitting shoes, and excessive or unusual exercises early in training are the most common causes of blisters, which typically occur on the tips of the toes, the balls of the feet, and the heels. For this reason, blisters are the most common complaint of marathon runners—with one study reporting an incidence rate of up to 44 percent by Chicago Marathon runners on race day. Another study that evaluated 81,277 entrants in the Twin Cities Marathon over a 12-year period found that skin problems were noted in 21 percent of the runners treated in the finish line medical area.

✎ What's It Mean?

Sun Protection Factor (SPF): How well a sunscreen work at keeping the sun's burning rays from roasting your skin. (FYI: SPF 45 and higher protects only a bit more than 30 does.) Make sure your sunscreen blocks both UVA and UVB rays (types of light).

Source: From "Sun Proof," BAM! Body and Mind, Centers for Disease Control and Prevention, 2002.

Dermatologists can treat painful blisters by draining the fluid with a sharp, sterile instrument. To prevent blisters, Dr. Phillips recommends wearing moisture-wicking socks of synthetic materials which are thicker at the toe and heel. "Shoes that fit appropriately are essential in preventing blisters," said Dr. Phillips. "We're finding that using drying powders or antiperspirants, petroleum jelly, or adhesive pads also reduce the incidence of blisters."

For athletes who train or participate in outdoor sports, overexposure to the sun—which can lead to skin cancer and premature aging—is a serious threat. The American Academy of Dermatology (Academy) recommends that everyone, including athletes, wear a broad-spectrum sunscreen with a sun protection factor (SPF) of 15 or higher, even on cloudy days. Athletes also should reapply sunscreen every two hours, especially during periods of training and competition, such as a marathon or after the swimming leg of a triathlon. In addition to wearing sunscreen, the Academy advises everyone to wear protective clothing and avoid the midday sun from 10 A.M. to 4 P.M., when the sun's rays are the strongest, whenever possible.

✔ Quick Tip

Oops! I Got Too Much Sun: What Do I Do Now?

- Cool bath
- Unscented moisturizer (lotion, no petroleum jelly)
- Hydrocortisone cream
- Water
- No more sun

An adult may choose to give you medicine that stops pain. When your burn is severe and you have a headache and chills or a fever, too, an adult may need to take you to a doctor.

Source: From "Sun Proof," BAM! Body and Mind, Centers for Disease Control and Prevention, 2002.

Dr. Phillips also noted that athletes are prone to different skin problems, depending on the nature of their sport. For example, runners often experience corns, calluses, chafing, and conditions known as "jogger's toe" and "jogger's nipples." Swimmers may find themselves with allergic reactions to the rubber components of earplugs and goggles. Bicyclists, on the other hand, can be plagued by frictional hair loss and acne from wearing helmets, superficial abrasions or "road rash" after a fall, and "saddle sores" from prolonged riding or an ill-fitting seat.

While exercise is beneficial for everyone, it also has been shown to have positive effects for patients with chronic skin disease, such as psoriasis and atopic dermatitis. Along with increases in quality of life measures, the patients who exercised experienced less depression and emotional disturbances.

"Although the benefits of exercise far outweigh any temporary dermatologic conditions that may result, it is important for athletes and their doctors to recognize these potential problems and take the necessary steps to prevent them in the first place," said Dr. Phillips. "Because some skin problems can be symptoms of serious health conditions, people should not take them for granted. See your dermatologist for proper diagnosis and treatment, especially if your skin looks unusual or if problems continue or worsen."

Chapter 44

Selecting The Right Shoes

Proper-fitting sports shoes can enhance performance and prevent injuries. Follow these specially-designed fitting facts when purchasing a new pair of athletic shoes.

- Try on athletic shoes after a workout or run and at the end of the day. Your feet will be at their largest.

- Wear the same type of sock that you will wear for that sport.

- When the shoe is on your foot, you should be able to freely wiggle all of your toes.

- The shoes should be comfortable as soon as you try them on. There is no break-in period.

- Walk or run a few steps in your shoes. They should be comfortable.

- Always relace the shoes you are trying on. You should begin at the farthest eyelets and apply even pressure as you a crisscross lacing pattern to the top of the shoe.

- There should be a firm grip of the shoe to your heel. Your heel should not slip as you walk or run.

About This Chapter: This chapter begins with "Selecting Athletic Shoes," © 2001 American Orthopaedic Foot and Ankle Society (www.aofas.org). Reprinted with permission. Additional information is from "New Athletic Shoe Components and Design May Enhance Performance," © 2007 American Orthopaedic Foot and Ankle Society (www.aofas.org). Reprinted with permission.

- If you participate in a sport three or more times a week, you need a sports specific shoe.

It can be hard to choose from the many different types of athletic shoes available. There are differences in design and variations in material and weight. These differences have been developed to protect the areas of the feet that encounter the most stress in a particular athletic activity.

Athletic shoes are grouped into seven categories:

- **Running, Training, And Walking:** Includes shoes for hiking, jogging, and exercise walking. Look for a good walking shoe to have a comfortable soft upper, good shock absorption, smooth tread, and a rocker sole design that encourages the natural roll of the foot during the walking motion. The features of a good jogging shoe include cushioning, flexibility, control and stability in the heel counter area, lightness, and good traction.

- **Court Sports:** Includes shoes for tennis, basketball, and volleyball. Most court sports require the body to move forward, backward, and side-to-side. As a result, most athletic shoes used for court sports are subjected to heavy abuse. The key to finding a good court shoe is its sole. Ask a coach or shoes salesman to help you select the best type of sole for the sport you plan on participating in.

- **Field Sports:** Includes shoes for soccer, football, and baseball. These shoes are cleated, studded, or spiked. The spike and stud formations vary from sport to sport, but generally are replaceable or detachable cleats, spikes, or studs affixed into nylon soles.

- **Winter Sports:** Includes footwear for figure skating, ice hockey, alpine skiing, and cross-country skiing. The key to a good winter sports shoe is its ability to provide ample ankle support.

- **Track And Field Sport Shoes:** Because of the specific needs of individual runners, athletic shoe companies produce many models for various foot types, gait patterns, and training styles. It is always best to ask your coach about the type of shoe that should be selected for the event you are participating in.

- **Specialty Sports:** Includes shoes for golf, aerobic dancing, and bicycling.

- **Outdoor Sports:** Includes shoes used for recreational activities such as hunting, fishing, and boating.

New Athletic Shoe Components And Design May Enhance Performance

The desire for improved performance affects all athletes and influences not only training, but also equipment research and design. Shoes are among the most basic equipment for Olympic athletes. Some of the newer features and designs in athletic shoes are outlined below.

Air Soles

First introduced in 1979 by a major athletic shoe manufacturer, this concept utilized encapsulated air units in the midsole to enhance cushioning. Ambient air or Freon also can be used. Depending on the model, the air units may be in the heel, forefoot, or both.

Initial report noted that, although air systems had superior shock absorption and potential energy rebound, stability was poor. Stability in the context of sports refers to the ability of the shoe to resist excessive or unwanted motions of the foot and ankle.

Shoes with very soft well-cushioned midsoles allow significantly more motion than firmer shoes and a poor design can encourage instability. Newer designs addressed the stability problem with success.

Air systems are not as susceptible to compaction as ethylene vinyl acetate (EVA), polyurethane (PU), and other midsole materials and are therefore thought to be more durable.

Energy Return

Compression of a viscoelastic midsole material allows a small amount of strain energy to be stored in the compressed elastic components of the midsole. Theoretically, when weight is released, the elastic components spring back and stored energy is returned to the athlete. It has been suggested that by increasing the energy return of a shoe, the oxygen cost of an activity can be reduced and performance enhanced. There is little evidence to support these claims. The arch of the human foot is also a viscoelastic system and therefore can return energy.

The "Pumps"

The "pumps" are actually inflatable linings in the tongue and other parts of the shoe pumped up by a device built into the top of the shoe. This provides a tight secure fit. Both Nike and Reebok use this fit feature.

Replaceable Plug Systems

A heel plug is found in multi-density outsoles, where the most durable rubber is placed in the high-wear area of the heel. Adidas designed a rear foot plug to be inserted into the heel wedge to improve shock absorption. Brooks marketed a pronation control system which allows pronation to be controlled by inserting medial heel plugs of varying hardness.

Pronation Control Devices

Controlling overpronation in runners and other athletes is a major concern of the sport shoe industry. Most of the motion control features fall into two categories:

A harder density material built into the medial aspect of the midsole and/or heel to counteract pronation.

An added medial component to the inside or outside of the shoe that limits pronation.

In the past, most of the pronation control devices focused on the rear foot. Now more attention is placed on controlling the entire foot.

> ♣ **It's A Fact!!**
> **Women's Shoes**
>
> There has been a lot of recent interest in manufacturing women's athletic shoes, but only a few companies have tried to market shoes for women. In the past most women's models were simply men's models with cosmetic changes. It has been hard to change the common perception that men's shoes are better than women's.
>
> Source: © 2007 American Orthopaedic Foot and Ankle Society.

Chapter 45

Exercise Caution:
Be Aware Of Your Surroundings

The key to a safe workout is to pay attention not only to your body, but also to your environment. Many athletes take unusually high risks regarding their safety. This is contrary to the pursuit of good health and a long life through physical activity.

Man Versus Automobile

The ideal would be to share the road with cars, but since they are bigger and stronger, always give cars the right-of-way.

Avoid exercising on busy roadways, but if these are the only routes to take, time your workout to avoid peak traffic. Run on the shoulder and face traffic (but when possible, run on the outside when going around blind curves). When you cycle, ride with the traffic. Obey traffic laws: you are considered a vehicle with the same rights and responsibilities as an automobile.

Stay in single file, if you exercise in a group. Pedestrians do not have the right-of-way except under certain conditions, such as in walk-ways when crossing at traffic signals. Slow down when you approach an intersection; if necessary, walk across the street. Assume the motorist does not see you. Wave the driver through and try to get eye contact to be sure he or she really knows you are there.

Avoid running or cycling on snow-covered roads. Cars have enough trouble avoiding each other under these conditions.

At dusk or night, wear bright, reflective clothing. Put reflective tape on all moving parts. Carry a light, not so much to see the road, but so others see you. Warn pedestrians and cyclists of your approach. Shout, "on the left," as you pass on that side.

Man Versus Man

When you exercise outdoors, you are put in a vulnerable position—that is, you often are alone, in unpopulated areas, and possibly tired—you are easy prey to muggers, rapists, and other unfavorable characters. Prevent unpleasant and dangerous experiences by trusting your intuition. If you feel uncomfortable in a situation, leave immediately.

Plan you route carefully. Exercise in well-populated, well-lighted places. Avoid running near doorways, alleys, or dense shrubs. Have a variety of routes so that no one can assume you will pass a specific way at a certain time. Familiarize yourself with places along your route where you can get help, especially if you exercise in the dark. Save the safest area for the last part of your workout when you are the most tired. Reserve energy for emergencies.

Act defensively. Carry a light, mace, whistle, or siren device. Some safety devices incorporate a combination of these characteristics. Look confident and strong.

Ignore verbal harassment. Use discretion in acknowledging strangers. If a driver or passerby asks for directions, answer from a distance.

Anger is a good control weapon. When approached, spontaneous anger can intimidate, buy time, and give a potential attacker second thoughts.

Watch for turning cars. If you think a car is trailing you, turn and go in the other direction. If you hear a car or footsteps, look behind you and assess the situation. Many attacks can be prevented if you act on early intuition. Don't wait to be attacked to scream or sound your alarm.

Avoid giving a thief ideas; do not wear conspicuous jewelry when you exercise. A simple theft may become something far worse. If you are attacked make a mental note of the attacker—looks, mannerisms, voice, age, height, and weight—so you can report it to the police.

Man Versus Dog

They say a dog is man's best friend, but that's not necessarily the case when the man is a runner or cyclist. Many dogs instinctively chase, bark, or bite any moving objects.

Never run between a dog and its owner, especially if the owner is a child. The best way to treat a barking dog is to feign indifference, but only feign indifference; actually be alert.

If a dog comes at you, face it. If you act bravely and forcefully yell "go away," usually the dog will retreat. Loud noises or sirens also can scare dogs away. Yet never turn your back on a dog. Dogs like to attack from the rear. Stay alert, even when the dog leaves. It may come back.

♣ It's A Fact!!

If a dog comes at you, you have three choices: 1) Make friends by talking softly and holding your hand out, palm down; 2) Assert your dominance by ordering the dog away, making threatening gestures, and picking up a stick (even an imaginary one can do the trick); or 3) Become submissive so that the dog thinks it has "won." Relax your muscles and glance away. Big dogs often respond to this and walk away.

A dog bite is a serious matter. Dogs transmit diseases through their saliva. If your skin is broken, you will need at least a tetanus shot. Contact the dog's owner and your local police, animal society, or county health department to find out when the dog last had a rabies shot. If the owner does not have written proof, contact the dog's veterinarian.

Man Versus Pollution

Air quality affects not only your performance, but also your health. There is a positive correlation between carbon monoxide exposure, which is found in air pollution, and a high incidence of cardiovascular disease. Since your breathing increases dramatically when you exercise, you will breathe more harmful chemicals when exercising in a polluted environment than when you are still. In one study, athletes had three times the concentration of harmful chemicals in their bloodstream after running in a polluted area. This increase was equivalent to smoking 10 to 20 cigarettes a day.

Air quality is best in the morning. Ozone levels increase soon after dawn and peak at midday. These levels usually drop again after rush hour or around 6 P.M. A midday workout or a hot sunny day is the worst time to exercise in a congested area. Exercising along a busy road or highway also increases your intake of pollutants.

Plan Ahead

Always carry some sort of identification when you exercise. A reflective ID tag is ideal. It should include your name, address, person to contact in case of an emergency, and any pertinent medical information, such as blood type and allergies.

Pay attention to who and what is around you. You can control a number of situations that affect your safety.

Tell someone where you are going to exercise and when you think you will return. Better yet, exercise with a "buddy" so that you can watch out for each other. Run or bike with your head up. Not only does a lowered head hinder breathing, but it also can impair your line of vision.

Chapter 46

Protect Yourself From Weather-Related Risks

Keeping Your Cool

Have you ever spent a hot afternoon playing ball with your friends or running around the park with your dog? Bet you were pretty sweaty and thirsty when you finished playing—maybe even thirsty enough to guzzle an entire gallon of water. That thirst was a sign of dehydration. Dehydration means that your body is losing more fluids than it takes in—and that's not good! Don't depend on your thirst to tell you whether or not your body needs a refill. Make sure you drink water a few hours before gearing up for physical activities, and keep drinking after you're done—be smart and stay hydrated!

Don't Sweat It

When the temperature outside begins to soar, your body heats up faster. To stay cool and beat the heat:

- Play outside during cooler parts of the day—early morning or early evening. The day is usually hottest between 10 A.M. and 4 P.M., so find

About This Chapter: This chapter begins with "Keeping Your Cool," BAM! Body And Mind, Centers for Disease Control and Prevention, 2002. It continues with "Preventing Frostbite and Hypothermia," © 2004 National Safety Council (www.nsc.org). Reprinted with permission. And, "National Athletic Trainers' Association (NATA) Offers Guidelines on How to Prevent Lightning-Related Injuries," September 24, 2004. © National Athletic Trainers' Association (NATA). All rights reserved. Reprinted with permission.

a shady bike path to ride or skate on, plan some indoor activities, take a dip in the pool, or play games under the sprinkler.

- If you do choose to brave the heat, make sure to let your body gradually adjust. Cut back the length and intensity of your activities just for the first two weeks until you get used to the heat.

- Dress cool. Wear clothing that is loose fitting and lightly colored—preferably made of cotton or a sweat-wicking material (designed to pull sweat away from your skin). Stay away from dark-colored clothing like black and dark blue—they soak up sunlight and heat.

♣ It's A Fact!!
Steamy Situation

When your body temperature gets hotter than normal—98.6 degrees Fahrenheit—your brain sends out a distress signal that causes you to sweat, which cools you down. Think of it this way—your body, like an air conditioner, has an internal thermostat that helps control its temperature. Whenever your body heats up from physical activity or the hot weather outside, your internal air conditioner turns on and you begin to sweat. And remember, now that your air conditioner is using its coolant (your sweat), it is important to refill the tank—by drinking lots of H2O.

Source: CDC, 2002.

- Did you know that almost one-fourth of all of your body's sweat glands are in your feet? What does that tell you. To keep your feet cool and blister-free, try wearing shoes that allow your feet to breathe and that don't trap sweat and heat.

- Stay away from drinks that have caffeine, lots of sugar, or carbonation in them—like soda or tea.

- If you're playing center field, practicing your backhand, or ruling the playground for more than 60 minutes, get an extra energy boost from sports drinks. They help to replace the water you've lost during strenuous activity. Sports drinks are great when you're active, but not if you're just chillin'—they have high levels of sugar, salt, and potassium that you don't really need unless you are working your body hard.

✔ Quick Tip
H2O—Guzzle, Gulp, and Chug

Drinking water before, during, and after physical activity is one way to keep your body's air conditioner working. Keep these tips in mind to help your body stay cool:

- Top off your tank a few hours before you hit the court, the field, or your own backyard by drinking about two cups of cold water.

- Keep a water bottle handy to guzzle during water breaks, halftime, or time outs. Try to drink about 10 ounces—that's about 10 large gulps from your water bottle—every 15–20 minutes.

- Did you know that sometimes you can't even see sweat—like when you're swimming? Which means you may not realize you are getting dehydrated. Just another reason to keep your water bottle in plain sight so you'll remember to drink up.

- Even after the game ends, the chugging shouldn't—the more you sweat, the more water you need. Drink bottled water, water flavored with lemon or lime juice or water right from your own sink.

- Eating fruit and other cool snacks is another way to keep your body cool! Pack peaches, oranges, watermelon, and grapes in your cooler—they taste great and re-hydrate!

Source, CDC, 2002.

- Most importantly, listen to your body. If you feel weak, dizzy, or thirsty, take a break in the shade, grab your water bottle, and tell a grown-up.

Now that you know how to beat the heat—get out there, stay active, and keep cool!

Preventing Frostbite And Hypothermia

Prolonged exposure to low temperatures, wind, or moisture—whether it be on a ski slope or in a stranded car—can result in cold-related illnesses such as frostbite and hypothermia. The National Safety Council offers these tips to help you spot and put a halt to these winter hazards.

How To Detect And Treat Cold-Related Illnesses

Frostbite is the most common injury resulting from exposure to severe cold. Superficial frostbite is characterized by white, waxy, or grayish-yellow patches on the affected areas. The skin feels cold and numb. The skin surface feels stiff but underlying tissue feels soft and pliable when depressed. Treat superficial frostbite by taking the victim inside immediately. Remove any constrictive clothing items that could impair circulation. If you notice signs of frostbite, immediately seek medical attention. Place dry, sterile gauze between toes and fingers to absorb moisture and to keep them from sticking together. Slightly elevate the affected part to reduce pain and swelling. If you are more than one hour from a medical facility and you have warm water, place the frostbitten part in the water (102 to 106 degrees Fahrenheit). If you do not have a thermometer, test the water first to see if it is warm, not hot. Rewarming usually takes 20 to 40 minutes or until tissues soften.

Deep frostbite usually affects the feet or hands and is characterized by waxy, pale, solid skin. Blisters may appear. Treat deep frostbite by moving the victim indoors and immediately seek medical attention.

Hypothermia occurs when the body's temperature drops below 95 degrees Fahrenheit. Symptoms of this condition include change in mental status, uncontrollable shivering, cool abdomen, and a low core body temperature. Severe hypothermia may produce rigid muscles, dark and puffy skin, irregular heart and respiratory rates, and unconsciousness.

Treat hypothermia by protecting the victim from further heat loss and calling for immediate medical attention. Get the victim out of the cold. Add insulation such

> ✔ **Quick Tip**
> *How To Prevent Cold-Related Illnesses*
>
> Avoid frostbite and hypothermia when you are exposed to cold temperatures by wearing layered clothing, eating a well-balanced diet, and drinking warm, non-alcoholic, caffeine-free liquids to maintain fluid levels.
>
> Avoid becoming wet, as wet clothing loses 90 percent of its insulating value.
>
> Source: © 2004 National Safety Council.

as blankets, pillows, towels, or newspapers beneath and around the victim. Be sure to cover the victim's head. Replace wet clothing with dry clothing. Handle the victim gently because rough handling can cause cardiac arrest. Keep the victim in a horizontal (flat) position. Give artificial respiration or CPR (if you are trained) as necessary.

National Athletic Trainers' Association (NATA) Offers Guidelines On How To Prevent Lightning-Related Injuries

Every year, millions of lightning flashes strike the ground, causing nearly 100 deaths and 400 injuries in this country alone. Lightning casualties that occur during sports and recreational activities have risen alarmingly in recent decades, many of which could have been prevented.

The National Athletic Trainers' Association (NATA), a not-for-profit organization which represents 30,000 members of the athletic training profession, has issued a position statement on the topic: "Lightning Safety for Athletics and Recreation," which can be read in its entirety at http://www.nata.org/publicinformation/files/lightning.pdf. The statement has been endorsed by the American Academy of Pediatrics and other major health care organizations.

Katie M. Walsh, EdD, ATC [certified athletic trainer], lead author of the position statement, recommends the "flash-to-bang" method in severe weather to avoid lightning danger. "Count seconds between seeing lightning (flash) and hearing the (bang) of thunder," she says. "Then divide by five to determine how far away in miles the lightning activity is occurring. Be inside a safe structure by the time the count approaches 30 seconds (six miles)."

Other Key Recommendations

- Postpone or suspend activity if a thunderstorm appears imminent before or during an activity or contest (regardless of whether lightning is seen or thunder heard) until the hazard has passed. Signs of imminent thunderstorm activity are darkened clouds, high winds, and thunder or lightning activity.

• Designate a safe shelter for each venue, such as inside a residential, office, or school building, but not dug outs or under trees or bleachers where lightning can still strike. An alternate emergency safe shelter is a car (solid roof, not a convertible) with windows rolled up completely.

• Establish a chain of command that identifies who is to make the call to remove individuals from the field.

• Once activities have been suspended, wait at least 30 minutes following the last sound of thunder or lightning flash prior to resuming an activity or returning outdoors.

• Be more wary of the lightning threat than the rain. Lightning or thunder should be the determining factor in postponing or suspending activities—not the amount of rainfall on the playing field. Even a gentle rain can bring lightning.

• Assume the lightning safe position (crouched on the ground, weight on the balls of the feet, feet together, head lowered and ears covered) for individuals who feel their hair stand on end, skin tingle, or hear "cracking" noises. Do not lie flat on the ground.

• Observe the following basic first aid procedures in managing victims of a lightning strike: a) Survey the scene for safety; b) Activate local EMS; c) Lightning victims do not "carry a charge" and are safe to touch; d) If necessary, move the victim with care to a safer location; e) Evaluate airway, breathing and circulation, and begin CPR if necessary; f) Evaluate and treat for hypothermia, shock, fractures, and/or burns.

Also Consider

• There are higher rates of thunderstorm activity (and thus higher lightning casualty rates) in Atlantic seaboard, southwest, southern Rocky Mountains, and southern plain states.

• Three quarters of all lightning injures occur between May and September, with July having the most.

• Nearly four-fifths of lightning casualties occur between 10 A.M. and 7 P.M. (when most athletic or recreational activities occur).

Chapter 47

Safety Tips For Contact Sports

How To Fit Football Equipment

Fitting Football Helmets

For the best fit the athlete should wet down their hair to recreate a practice/game situation. As the athlete sweats the hair becomes wet and the fit of the helmet may change.

The athlete should be instructed to read the WARNING label on the helmet and be sure they understand what is stated on the label.

The athlete's head is next measured with a cloth measuring tape one inch (1") above the eyebrows and around the largest part of the head.

Fit the athlete with the appropriate shell (S, M, or L); have the athlete pull the helmet out by the ear holes and roll the helmet onto their head.

The helmet should sit on the head 1" above the eyebrows and the jawpads should fit snugly against the cheeks. Jawpads come in various sizes and can be interchanged between helmets.

About This Chapter: This chapter begins with "How to Fit Football Equipment" and "Fitting Hockey Equipment," reprinted with permission from Ackland Sports Medicine (www.sportismedicine.com), © 2004. All rights reserved. Excerpts are also included from "Football Activity Card," "Soccer Activity Card," and "Basketball Activity Card," BAM! Body and Mind, Centers for Disease Control and Prevention, 2001.

The chin strap should be fitted next. To do this, place the chin strap on the chin and adjust and attach the front straps. The straps should fit snugly with no slack. Fit the back straps in the same fashion.

Air should be inserted into the bladder(s) of the helmet for fitting purposes via a hand pump. The helmet should fit snugly but comfortably.

At this point the helmet should be rotated. Holding the sides of the helmet, have the athlete hold their head still and rotate the helmet while watching that the helmet does not slide on the athlete, but the skin of the forehead moves with the helmet. Also be sure that the jawpads fit snugly.

The player should inspect their helmet everyday for proper fit and maintenance. Start by looking inside the helmet for any cracking in the air bladders, or padding. Inspect the outside for any loose screws. The athlete should press down on the top of the helmet to be sure there is enough air in the helmet and be sure the helmet does not slide but moves with the athlete. The chin strap should also fit snugly with no slack.

Athletes should ALWAYS wear their mouthguards! Mouthguards are a protective device and should not be altered to decrease their protective properties.

✔ Quick Tip
Football

Be sure to stretch and warm up before every practice and game and always wear your protective gear. To avoid getting hurt, learn from your coaches how to block and tackle correctly. Don't tackle with the top of your head or helmet—not only is it illegal, but it can cause injury to both players. If you play in an organized league, there are lots of rules—and they are there for a reason—to keep you safe. If you break these rules, you risk not only getting hurt, or hurting someone else, but your team will be penalized. If you're playing in the backyard with your friends, stay safe by sticking to touch or flag football, and only play with kids who are around your age and size.

Source: "Football Activity Card," BAM! Body and Mind, Centers for Disease Control and Prevention, 2001.

Fitting Shoulder Pads

Shoulder pads are designed to protect the shoulder joint. The typical point of impact is at the AC joint (acromioclavicular joint). Therefore, the pads should be fitted properly to provide protection for the shoulder.

The athlete should stand facing away from the staff member. The athlete is measured from shoulder to shoulder, the tip of the left humerus to the tip of the right humerus. This measurement is the guide for what size pads the athlete should wear. Sizes go by numbers (number of inches = shoulder pad size). Pick a pair of pads and have the athlete put them on.

Fitting Neck Rolls

Neck rolls should be used for protective purposes not for a look that the athlete is going for. The neck rolls can play a valuable role but should not be relied on to protect the athlete from injury. Safe play and execution of proper technique are the best defenses against injury.

If an athlete has a preexisting condition that would require a neck roll, the athlete should be fitted by a staff member with experience with the fitting and attaching the neck roll to the shoulder pads. The neck rolls should be fitted in their positions.

Fitting Hockey Equipment

When you go out to purchase some hockey equipment there are a few things that you should know. You should never skimp on quality or fit for price, or the thought that you may get an extra season out of it. There are some equipment shops that sell new and used equipment which can prove to be economical when you are a growing child. Remember that properly fitted equipment should be comfortable and also will provide efficient protection from injury. Here are some guidelines to follow for fitting equipment properly.

Helmet: When buying a helmet the athlete should look for protection, comfort, and fit. All helmets must be approved by the HECC (Hockey Equipment Certification Council) or the CSA (Canadian Standard Association); there will be a sticker on the helmet to notify the athlete. The helmet should not be too tight or too loose; you need to have a snug fit; watch that the helmet does not have enough room to crash down on nose. The helmet should rest one to two finger widths above the eyebrows and fit snugly enough so that the helmet does not spin or shift on head. The proper fit will maximize the protection factor of the helmet. The chin strap should be adjusted so it gently makes contact under the chin when fastened.

Cage Versus Shield: Here the choice is up to the athlete. Each individual will have their own preference between the two masks. The basic differences between the two are visibility and ventilation. The cage offers good visibility with excellent ventilation. They are made out of strong durable materials that allow the helmet to take a little bit of a beating. The shield has decreased ventilation and excellent vision. The shields have the tendency to fog up and scratch easily, but when taken care of properly the shield can prove to be the choice face mask. All masks are not made to fit all helmets so be sure that the cage or shield that you choose fits onto the helmet properly leaving no gaps or space at the chin. Shields fog up much more in older rinks that do not have de-humidifiers for ambient air.

Mouthguards: A mouthguard is a must in the older age groups and should not be viewed as a choice to wear one or not. The purpose of a mouthguard is multifaceted. They decrease the risk of mouth/tooth injuries and decrease concussions by dispersing the force and also decrease jaw fractures. Mouthguards are an inexpensive way to protect yourself in a number of ways. They can be bought in a store and molded at home with the use of hot water. Mouthguards can also be custom fit by your dentist to make an exact fit for the athlete. Here each individual will have a personal preference. If the mouthguard is not properly fitted then the ability to communicate can suffer and sometimes breathing is compromised. To insure proper fit, follow package directions for fitting store-bought mouthguards. Be sure to soften the mouthguard using hot water; after 30 seconds or more (read package) insert the mouthguard into the mouth and place on top teeth; press tongue along back of mouthguard and suck all of the air out pulling mouthguard onto teeth. DO NOT double dip—be sure that your first attempt makes the grade—you run the risk of biting through the mouthguard and decreasing the protective qualities of the mouthguard.

Neck Guard: All players have to wear a neck guard. A neck guard will offer protection for the athlete's neck, protection from sharp objects such as skate blades and sticks. When worn properly, the guard will protect the player from potentially dangerous situations.

Shoulder Pads: The center of the shoulder should fit in the center of the shoulder cup of the pads. The pads offer a foam cup that should fit comfortably around the shoulder girdle. Most pads have a universal sizing system, but trying them on will have to be the judgment factor. The athlete should get into their position's stance. A defenseman may benefit from a pair of shoulder pads that cover more area. When on defense players have a greater chance of blocking the puck with their bodies; therefore, a larger chest protector is a good choice. For the forward, they need to be less restricted and tend to wear a smaller pair of shoulder pads. The choice for smaller pads should be for comfort but not for compromising protection. Shoulder pads should offer protection for the shoulder girdle, clavicle (collar bone), chest, ribs, back, and upper arms. The straps that hold shoulder pads in place should fit snugly and hold pads comfortably to the body without restricting movement or breathing. When trying the pads on, athletes should raise their arms up over their heads to be sure that the pads do not move and compromise coverage or decrease cervical range of motion or vision. Move your head around with the helmet on and wear your elbow pads to make sure one does not bind on the other.

Elbow Pads: Elbow pads are to protect the elbow from injury. The pad should fit comfortably around the joint and offer protection from outside hazards. The elbows should fit into the cup shape of the pad and be covered completely to protect the elbow. The pad should fit comfortably but should also fit properly in order to provide the appropriate coverage. The pad should extend to the shoulder pad without compromising or interfering with the gloves to provide additional protection. All pieces of equipment should be tried on in conjunction with their adjacent parts. This will ensure a proper fit. There should not be any discomfort created or any restricted range of motion while providing the protection the hockey payer needs. The player should also put the equipment on and get down in their stance to see if the equipment fits correctly and does not interfere with movements or vision.

Gloves: Gloves are another piece of equipment that should fit comfortably, not too big or too small. Gloves offer protection for the hand, fingers, thumb, and wrist; therefore, a proper fit will provide this protection. The top of the glove should come up to meet the elbow pad leaving little or no gap, to prevent injury. The player's fingers should not go all the way to the end of the finger pockets of the gloves. This will decrease the risk of injuries such as lacerations. Most gloves come standard with a thumb lock feature. This will prevent the thumb from bending backwards causing injury.

Pants: Most people can use their waist size as a guide for fitting pants. Pants come a variety of sizes S-M-L or numerical sizes and also different lengths. The pants should overlap the knee pads/shin pads by one to two inches when standing and still cover while kneeling. Properly fitted pants should cover athletes appropriately leaving no skin or body part exposed to potential injury. Any gap is exactly where you will be hit by a puck.

Shinguards: Shinguards or knee pads provide protection from a number of things: impact with the ice, a puck, a stick, opposing player, the boards... Therefore you want properly fitted pads to provide the most protection possible. The patella or kneecap should fit directly into the center of the patella cup of the pad. The pads are made in a variety of densities. The padding should provide ample protection but not bulkiness that would compromise the fit and protection of the pad. The pad should extend down the length of the leg, making sure that the pad is not too long or not too short. Be sure to try the pads on with skates in order to get the proper fit. If the pad is too long the skates will push the pads out of position and not provide proper protection. The player will develop a personal preference to wear the pads tucked in the skate or outside the skate. Either is acceptable. Be sure that with either choice the pads offer full coverage leaving no area exposed. The older the player, the thicker the pad required to block slapshots. The more expensive pads come as "left and right."

Skates: Skates normally fit 1–1½ sizes smaller than street shoes. They also come in a variety of widths. To assure proper fit the athlete's feet should be measured with a foot measuring device, for length and width. When trying on skates push toes forward to the front of the boot. You should be able to put between one pencil to one finger between the heel and the boot. Before lacing the skate up, slide the heel back into the boot, snugly lace up the first three eyelets, lace the next three loosely, and the rest laced up tight. The eyelets should be 1½–2" apart.

Soccer

Be sure to wear shin guards and appropriate soccer cleats during games as well as practices. Warming up, especially your leg muscles, is very important. To avoid headaches and dizziness, use your head and learn the proper technique for heading a ball in a game. Many leagues have strict rules about wearing jewelry, watches, and barrettes during games. Since any of these items can cause you to get hurt if you're hit with a ball, it's a good idea to not wear them when you play. Also, to protect your mouth from collisions (especially if you have braces), wear a mouthguard.

♣ It's A Fact!!

Soccer: Anterior cruciate ligament (ACL) tears are very common due to the twisting nature of this sport, particularly among female athletes. Other injuries include ankle sprains, patella dislocations, hip strains, and foot injuries.

Source: Excerpted from "Your Sport," reprinted with permission from Jeffrey L. Halbrecht, M.D., Institute for Arthroscopy and Sports Medicine, San Francisco, CA, www.iasm.com. © 2006.

Basketball

Basketball can really make you work, so make sure you stretch and warm up before playing. Because of all of the quick moves and jumping, it can put a lot of wear and tear on your ankles, so protect them by wearing the right pair of shoes—medium or high tops do the best job of supporting your ankles. Protect those knees by learning how to cut, stop, and land a jump safely.

♣ **It's A Fact!!**

Few sports require the combination of twisting, running, cutting, and jumping involved in basketball. Frequent injuries include tears of the anterior cruciate ligament (ACL) and damage to the articular cartilage in the knee. Other common injuries are Achilles tendon tears, patella tendinitis (jumpers knee), and meniscus tears.

Source: Excerpted from "Your Sport," reprinted with permission from Jeffrey L. Halbrecht, M.D., Institute for Arthroscopy and Sports Medicine, San Francisco, CA, www.iasm.com. © 2006.

Be careful not to misuse basketball equipment. It's great if you've got the skills to put up a mean slam dunk, but hanging on the rim is dangerous and could cause you to get hurt. Also, make sure the court and sidelines are clear of any obstacles such as other basketballs or water bottles. If you're playing outside, make sure the baskets and sidelines are not too close to walls, fences, or bleachers and there are no holes on your court.

If you're a serious player, you may want to invest in a mouth guard to keep your teeth safe from flying elbows; knee and elbow pads so you don't get scraped up (especially if you're playing on an outdoor court); and sports glasses to protect your eyes.

Chapter 48

Safety Tips For Non-Contact Team Sports

Baseball

Wear your protective gear during all practices and games, especially if you're a catcher—those fast balls can pack a punch! Don't forget to warm up and stretch before each practice or game. In the infield? Stay behind the base on any throw. You'll avoid hurting yourself—and the base runner. In the outfield? Avoid bloopers with your teammates by calling every fly ball loudly, even if you think nobody else is close by. And in the batters' box, wear a batting helmet and use a batting glove to protect your knuckles from those inside pitches. If you think a pitch is going to hit you, turn away from the ball and take it in the back.

Throwing those fastballs can really take a toll, so if you're a pitcher, make sure to get plenty of rest between games, and don't pitch more than 4–10 innings per week.

Softball

Before you hit the field, WARM UP! Get all of your muscles ready to play by stretching before every game.

About This Chapter: This chapter contains excerpts from "Baseball Activity Card," "Softball Activity Card," "Volleyball Activity Card," "Tennis Activity Card," and "Cheerleading Activity Card," BAM! Body and Mind, Centers for Disease Control and Prevention, 2001.

Whether you're in the field or up to bat, don't forget to wear your safety gear in games and in practices. A helmet is important when batting, waiting to bat, or running the bases. If you're a catcher, make sure you wear your protective gear during all practices and games, and wear it properly—have your coach or a parent check it out for you. Don't wear jewelry like rings, watches, or necklaces—they could cut you (or someone else), or get caught when you're running' the bases.

Did you know that an umpire could call you out for throwing your bat? Well, they can! And, it's not just the out you have to worry about—it's your teammates' safety! Always drop your bat next to your side in the batters box before you head for first base.

Be a team player—always know where your teammates are before throwing the ball or swinging your bat. Make sure they are ready and have their glove up as a target before you throw the ball to them. Call loudly for every fly ball or pop up in the field, even if you don't think any of your teammates are close by. Teams that play together win together!

Volleyball

Be sure to wear knee and elbow pads when you're playing on a hard court to protect you when you dive for the ball. When you go up for the ball, try landing on the balls of your feet with your knees bent and your hips lowered a little. Also, warm up and stretch before you play, and take off any jewelry.

Communicate with your teammates while you're playing to keep from running into each other. Make sure everyone on the team knows to "call" the ball by saying "got it" or "mine" if they plan to go for it.

♣ It's A Fact!!

Volleyball: Jumping and hitting are the main causes of injury. Common injuries are ankle sprains, patella tendonitis and knee ligament tears from jumping, and stretching of the shoulder ligaments or tearing of the rotator cuff from hitting.

Source: Excerpted from "Your Sport," reprinted with permission from Jeffrey L. Halbrecht, M.D., Institute for Arthroscopy and Sports Medicine, San Francisco, CA, www.iasm.com. ©2006.

If you're playing outside, find a soft court made of sand or grass, and clean up any sharp objects that you see. Be sure that there aren't any trees or basketball hoops in your way. And, wear sunscreen and always drink plenty of water. If you're playing inside, the court should be made of wood.

♣ **It's A Fact!!**

Racquet sports frequently cause inflammation of the elbow and shoulder. The most common injuries are rotator cuff tendinitis and tennis elbow. Injury may be prevented by proper equipment, technique, and conditioning.

Source: Excerpted from "Your Sport," reprinted with permission from Jeffrey L. Halbrecht, M.D., Institute for Arthroscopy and Sports Medicine, San Francisco, CA, www.iasm.com. © 2006.

If your volleyball net is held up by wires, make sure they are covered with soft materials. That way you won't get hurt if you accidentally jump or run into the net.

Tennis

Tennis is an activity that forces you to turn your body quickly in many different directions, so make sure you warm up and stretch before playing. Wear tennis shoes with good support to protect your ankles and thick (not cotton) socks that fit well to prevent blisters on your feet. To prevent hand blisters, keep your racquet handle dry by using sawdust or hand chalk. Always bend your arm when you swing, or else it might start to hurt—a problem known as "tennis elbow." Clip your toenails and make sure there is extra room in your shoes because "tennis toe" can be nasty too.

To protect other players, never throw your racquet or tennis balls, and try to keep loose balls off the courts. Be courteous and keep yourself and others safe by staying off courts where other people are playing.

When you're outside waiting to play, sit in the shade and drink lots of water—that way you'll stay cool and won't get sunburned. While you are playing, take a break between games or sets to cool off. And you may want to keep a wet towel around your neck while you wait. Also, you can look and feel cool by wearing a cold, wet bandana on your head while you play. And always wear sunscreen!

Cheerleading

Today's cheerleading is super fun, but it's risky too—especially if you perform stunts. On this team sport, each squad member's position is key to completing the stunts safely and dazzling the crowd.

Make sure you're well conditioned for all those kicks, jumps, and splits—warm up before each practice and game, and do lots of stretching. Focus on stretching your legs and back. If you do stunts and build pyramids, make sure you stretch your arms and shoulders too.

Practice safe stunts. If your squad does lifts, tosses, or builds pyramids, make sure you follow these important safety rules.

♣ It's A Fact!!
Stunt Safety For Cheerleaders

- Always practice stunts on mats or pads.

- Never attempt a stunt unless a coach is there.

- Always use spotters for each and every stunt.

- If you are new to stunting, start with easier stunts and gradually move up to harder ones.

- Remember that if someone in the stunt yells "Down," the stunt should come down immediately.

Source: "Cheerleading Activity Card," BAM! Body and Mind, Centers for Disease Control and Prevention (CDC), 2001.

Chapter 49

Safety Tips For Dancing, Gymnastics, And Other Individual Sports

Ballet

Stretching is one of the most important things a dancer can do. Stretching makes the muscles stronger and more flexible, so make sure you warm up and stay focused while stretching.

To prevent toe trouble, wear toe pads and tape around tender and tight parts of your feet like your toes and heals.

Learn the proper technique. To ensure correct technique, make sure you are being taught by a qualified teacher with proper credentials and that you practice under supervision.

Eat healthy in order to keep your energy and attention levels up so that you can perform at your best. Some dancers confuse healthy eating with not eating enough and develop eating disorders. It's never a good idea to try and make yourself skinny by hurting your body.

About This Chapter: This chapter includes excerpts from "Ballet Activity Card," "Gymnastics Activity Card," "Martial Arts Activity Card," and "Yoga Activity Card," BAM! Body and Mind, Centers for Disease Control and Prevention (CDC), 2001.

Ballet is more than just physical exertion. It's the total process of expressing yourself through creative movement—have confidence in your self expression and in everything else you do.

Simple crunches, lunges, and bike riding are good ways to strengthen back muscles. You can also stretch your back muscles by lying on your stomach, slightly lifting both arms and legs and holding them in place for a few seconds.

Gymnastics

The most important gymnastics rule to remember is to know what you're doing. Never attempt a trick you are not familiar with. Make sure you always have a trained spotter (someone who stands near you in case you need help while doing your tricks) just in case you lose your balance on the beam, or attempt a wobbly handstand.

Before you attempt any trick or stunt, always make sure the equipment is sturdy and has been set up properly (always ask a coach or another grown-up for help). Floors should be padded with mats that are secured under every piece of equipment. Also, make sure there is enough distance between each piece of equipment before you start swinging. Collisions can cause you, or others around you, to get hurt if you don't watch out. Use your head. Pay attention and be serious about your practice—horseplay and goofing around can get you into trouble. Always know what your teammates are doing and where they are.

And last but not least, never eat or chew gum while doing gymnastics—the moment you become unaware of what is in your mouth, it can easily become lodged in your throat and you could choke.

Martial Arts

Look for an instructor who's into respect and discipline, but still has plenty of patience. The class area should have lots of space and a smooth, flat floor with padding. The fewer students the better—more attention for you.

Wear all the right gear. Warm up and stretch so you're loose and ready to go. You need good instruction before launching into any moves. And when you do learn the moves, remember your limits. For example, white belt students shouldn't spar (practice fight).

When you are ready for matches, you've got to have an instructor around to regulate. Some martial artists use special weapons (like swords), but it's almost a sure thing that you'll get hurt with them unless you're totally advanced...so, no weapons. During your match, make sure that your partner knows when you're ready to stop. If you let your guard down, your partner may think it's a good chance to take you down.

Yoga

It's important to make sure your muscles are warmed up before you begin your yoga routine. Never force your body into a posture or try to go beyond your limits—you could strain your muscles. Using the correct form is also key to getting the most out of your yoga experience, so get into a class that's right for you (whether you're a beginner or an expert). And, don't be afraid to ask your teacher for help. Learning the correct way to do each pose is important for overall mind and body development.

Feeling stiff or sore? If you are, you've overdone it. If you're just getting into yoga, it's important to start off slowly. Since yoga is not a competitive sport, your progress may be slow, but with time your body will become more flexible and you'll be able to achieve more difficult poses.

Interested in giving yoga a try, but not sure where to find classes in your area? It's important to find a class that you feel comfortable in, and has an experienced teacher. Try asking friends and family members if they know of a good place, or check out your local YMCA, county recreation centers, and fitness clubs—they sometimes have classes for all ages and skill levels. Also, don't forget about your local library—there you can find more information on yoga itself, as well as magazines or books that may have a listing of classes in your area.

♣ It's A Fact!!
One of the most important things you will need is a yoga or exercise mat to use during seated or floor postures. Don't worry if you don't have a special mat, use a firm pillow or folded up blanket—they work just as well.

Source: "Yoga Activity Card," BAM! Body and Mind, Centers for Disease Control and Prevention (CDC), 2001.

Chapter 50

Safety Tips For Skaters And Skateboarders

Inline Skating

No matter what kind of skates you wear, always wear a helmet, as well as wrist guards, elbow pads, and knee pads.

Play It Safe

Avoid getting hurt by making sure your helmet and pads are on correctly. Your helmet should be tightly buckled, with the front coming down to right over your eyebrow, and your pads should be on tight, so they don't slip while you are skating. It's also important that your helmet is approved by one of the groups who test helmets to see which ones are the best: the Consumer Product Safety Commission (CPSC), or Snell B-95 standards are best for inline skating helmets. Make sure you are always in control of your speed, turns, and stops, and be careful of cracks in the pavement where you are skating—they can be dangerous if your wheels get caught in them. It's best to go skating out of the way of traffic and other people (skating rinks are great places to skate).

About This Chapter: This chapter includes excerpts from "Inline Skating Activity Card" and "Skateboarding Activity Card," BAM! Body and Mind, Centers for Disease Control and Prevention, 2001.

Skateboarding

Before you ride, make sure you give your board a safety check to make sure everything is put together right. Always wear all of your protective gear including a helmet, knee and elbow pads, and wrist guards. If you do tricks with your board, you may also want to wear gloves to protect your hands from the pavement. If you're just starting out, skate on a smooth, flat surface so you can practice keeping control of your board. And no matter how experienced you are—never hold on to the back of a moving vehicle! It's best to skate out of the way of traffic and other people (skate parks are great places to skate). But if you are skating in streets near your house, be aware of cars and people around you, and stay out of their way. Also, once the sun sets, it's a good idea to put up your board for the night, since skating in the dark can be dangerous.

> ✔ **Quick Tip**
>
> It's important that your helmet is approved by one of the groups who test helmets to see which ones are the best: the Snell B-95 standard is best for skateboarding helmets. Non-slippery shoes are a good idea too, so you can have better control of your board.
>
> Source: "Skateboarding Activity Card," CDC, 2001.

Chapter 51

Safety Tips For Winter Sports

Getting Ready For That Ski Trip

Some Exercises To Do Before Hitting The Slopes

Unless you are a person given to using your legs vigorously through daily exercise or by virtue of your occupation, before going away on that ski trip you should consider these recommendations. The exercises are best begun at least three weeks before the trip.

Stretching Exercises

Trunk Rotation Stretch: Bend left knee, cross over and lock ankle under right leg. Left knee should be in contact with floor. Right hand holds left knee down and left arm extends across to the left on a diagonal. Hold for 45 seconds. Repeat in opposite direction. One in each direction. This is not only a pre-conditioning stretch but stretch that could be done in the morning before skiing. If you have known or possible disk pathology do not perform this exercise.

Modification Of Trunk Rotation Stretch: Sit on the floor or table with left leg straight, right leg bent with foot crossed over left leg. Lock left elbow

✔ **Quick Tip**

Play It Safe

- Always check the snow conditions of the slope before you go up—you'll need to ski differently in icy conditions than you would if you were on wet snow or in deep powder.

- Altitude can zap your energy. Don't push it. Ski the easier runs later in the day when you are tired. Most importantly—know when to quit.

- While on the slopes, set a meeting time and place to check in with your parents or friends. And always ski with a buddy. And wear plenty of Sunblock, because those rays are strong on the mountain due to high altitude and reflection off the snow.

Stay Warm On The Slopes

- Long underwear to keep you warm and absorb sweat.

- Insulated tops and pants such as sweaters and leggings—this layer should be warm, but not baggy.

- Ski pants and jackets to protect you from snow and wetness.

- A hat, because 60 percent of heat loss is through the head.

Source: Excerpted from "Snow Skiing Activity Card," BAM! Body and Mind, Centers for Disease Control and Prevention, 2001.

across outside of right knee. Rotate to the right. Hold for 45 seconds and repeat for other side.

Rectus Femoris/Quadriceps Stretch: Place right knee on chair or table, step forward of right knee with left foot. Grab right ankle with left hand and lean forward. Hold for 45 seconds and repeat for other leg. This stretch should be felt in the thigh and not in the knee.

Soleus Stretch: Place hands against wall and right foot forward. Left calf (to be stretched) placed back with the knee bent. Keep left heel in contact with floor and lean hips forward. Stretch should be felt in left calf. Hold for 45 seconds and repeat for other leg.

Strengthening Exercises

Wall Sit: This is an isometric strengthening exercise for the quadriceps. Bend knees to 90 degrees placing back flat against wall. Lower leg should be perpendicular to floor. Hold 30 seconds, repeat three times following 30 seconds rest between sets. Progress by increasing five seconds per session. To decrease difficulty, decrease knee angle to 45 degrees but keep back flat against wall and lower leg perpendicular to the floor. Discomfort should be felt in quadriceps and not in the knee cap.

Dynamic Double Leg Jump-Overs: Initially, jump over a ruler not a higher obstacle until you have progressed through lower obstacles. Standing with feet together to left of obstacle, jump sideways to right of obstacle and return in opposite manner. Continue for 30 seconds. Progress by 5 seconds each session. Emphasize smooth landing by taking shock with the thigh muscles and knees bent. Take off and landing should be nearly simultaneous for both feet.

Hamstring Strengthening Exercise: This is best done with a partner but can be performed with heels firmly locked under an immovable object. Place

♣ It's A Fact!!

The most common injuries in downhill skiing are to the knee, shoulder, and thumb. Because of the long twisting lever arm of the ski, tears of the anterior cruciate ligament (ACL) and medial collateral ligament are the most common knee injuries. Impact from moguls or jumps can cause chipping of the surface of the knee (articular cartilage). Shoulder injuries occur with tumbling falls, causing either dislocations or rotator cuff tears. If the pole gets caught between the thumb and forefinger, a tear of the ulna collateral ligament of the thumb may occur. Ski injuries may be prevented by proper preseason conditioning and proper falling technique.

Source: Excerpted from "Your Sport," reprinted with permission from Jeffrey L. Halbrecht, M.D., Institute for Arthroscopy and Sports Medicine, San Francisco, CA, www.iasm.com. © 2006.

soft cushion under knees, heels locked. Lean forward to count of five and return, repeat 10 times. This can be a strenuous exercise so lean only slightly forward the first time you perform it. The hamstrings are an important muscle to help stabilize the knee.

Trunk Rotation Strengthening: Begin with right leg bent, left leg straight and approximately 12 inches above floor at the foot. Hands loosely touching ears, reach for right knee with left elbow and be sure to exhale at the same time. The loose hands should prevent you from pulling the head and neck forward. Repeat in opposite manner without contacting floor with upper back. In essence, this is a continuous cycling motion. Try for 20 repetitions and increase as tolerated. Be sure to breath rhythmically, exhaling with each cross-over.

A Note About Delayed Onset Muscle Soreness (DOMS)

If you have not exercised a group of muscles vigorously and do so (say on a skiing trip), it is not uncommon to experience pain in those muscles some 24 to 48 hours after that bout of exercise. The muscles will actually be tender to the touch and you will experience real loss of strength. This condition is known as delayed onset muscle soreness (DOMS).

DOMS occurs to a much greater extent in muscles that are exercised "eccentrically." In this type of contraction, the muscles are contracting to keep a joint from moving in a direction opposite to prevailing forces. An example of this is the work of the quadriceps (front thigh muscles) when you land with slightly flexed knees from a jump. Even though the muscles are firing, the muscles still lengthen.

It is virtually impossible to prevent DOMS in muscles that have not been trained to experience eccentric contraction. Therefore, if you have skied before, and know the muscles in which you experience DOMS, try to get through the pain and strength loss by inducing the condition about one to two weeks before you go skiing. Some of the above exercises will induce DOMS in those muscles. At present, there is no other way of avoiding this occurrence while on vacation, or following introduction of a new form of physical activity.

DOMS is not caused by lactate accumulation. There is actual microscopic damage to the muscle fibers with inflammation. Muscles so affected will be weaker while they are sore and this may increase your risk of injury. Do not ski as hard as you normally would if you are experiencing DOMS. Over-the-counter pain medication is purely palliative and will not prevent the condition from occurring. It is extremely important that when you experience DOMS you should consume plenty of non-alcoholic, non-caffeinated beverages, a good rule of thumb any time you are visiting altitudes greater than 5000 feet.

✔ **Quick Tip**
Figure Skating

Be a courteous skater—always be aware of other skaters and follow the traffic flow of the rink. Be careful not to get too close to other skaters with your exposed blades. And keep your skate laces tied tightly so that you don't trip yourself or anyone else up.

If you feel yourself beginning to fall, bring your hands, arms, and head into your body to absorb the shock of hitting the ice. And make sure you hop up quickly so that you are not in the way of other skaters.

Skating can be hard work, and puts a lot of stress on your leg and back muscles, so be sure to warm up before you skate and stretch those muscles well.

Source: Excerpted from "Figure Skating Activity Card," BAM! Body and Mind, Centers for Disease Control and Prevention, 2001.

Snowboarding Injuries And General Conditioning

The ski industry was reluctant at first to embrace snowboarding as a sport because of concerns over safety and injury rates. Despite these concerns, snowboarding has dramatically increased in popularity over the past ten years in younger as well as older populations. Beginner snowboarders are predisposed to injury due to their lack of balance when first learning the sport. Snowboarding injuries may vary from the simple abrasions, cuts and contusions to the more complex sprains, fractures, and dislocations.

Common Snowboarding Injuries

- **Wrist Fractures And/Or Sprains:** Falls are the most common mechanism of injury in snowboarding, often resulting in wrist fractures and/or sprains. These injuries are sustained when a snowboarder loses his or her balance or catches an edge and attempts to break the fall with his or her hands.

- **Ankle Sprains:** Ankle sprains occur more frequently in snowboarders than in skiers mainly due to equipment differences. Ski boots are solid and prevent motion at the ankle, where snowboarders have a choice between a variety of types of boots. Soft-shell boots allow the most motion at the ankle and have been thought to contribute to an increase in ankle sprains. Hard shell boots are more similar to ski boots and have been thought to decrease the possibility of ankle sprains. Finally there are hybrid boots, which are basically a combination of the soft and hard shell boots.

- **Ankle Fractures:** Similar to ankle sprains, ankle fractures are more common in snowboarders than in skiers due to the equipment differences. Although not very common, a fracture of the lateral process of the talus is unique to snowboarders and can be disguised as a lateral ankle sprain. A computed tomography (CT) scan is often needed to diagnose this fracture because a normal x-ray usually does not pick up this fracture. The diagnosis and proper treatment of these fractures are of paramount importance because an untreated talus fracture has the possibility to lead to significant disability.

Prevention Of Snowboarding Injuries

- Maintain physical condition which matches the physical demands of snowboarding (refer to stretching and exercises below).

- Wear protective equipment: Wrist guards help decrease the possibility of wrist injuries; helmets; knee pads and elbow pads.

- Snowboarding lessons from a knowledgeable instructor: instructors teach proper snowboarding techniques, as well as safer techniques on how to fall which decrease the possibility of upper extremity injury.

Stretches To Maintain Flexibility Necessary For Snowboarding

Stretches should be held for a minimum of 30 seconds.

Quad Stretch: Stand with one hand holding onto the back of a chair to maintain balance. With the free hand, reach behind and grasp the instep of the lower extremity you want to stretch and bring it up toward your buttocks. You should feel a stretch in the front of your thigh.

Hamstring Stretch: Place the foot of the lower extremity you want to stretch on a chair. Lean forward slowly reaching down your leg until a stretch is felt in the back of your thigh.

Calf Stretch: Stand two to three feet away from a wall. Put your hands against the wall at about shoulder level to support your weight. Lean in toward the wall by bending your elbows until you feel a stretch in the back of your calves. Keep your body erect, your knees straight, and your hips forward. DO NOT bend at the waist. Make sure your heels remain on the ground. Alternate foot position by turning the feet outward, stretching, then inward, and repeating the stretch. To increase stretch, a book can be placed under the "ball" of the foot, letting the heels hang down.

Exercises For Muscle Groups Used While Snowboarding

Aerobic Exercise: Aerobic exercise, such as jogging or bicycling, is necessary to maintain overall physical endurance to prevent injury secondary to fatigue. Aerobic exercise should be done for 20–30 minutes at least three times a week.

Squats: Squats are a good exercise for the multiple muscle groups that are used during snowboarding. Squats are performed from a standing position with feet shoulder width apart. The exercise begins by flexing the hips, knees, and ankles until thighs are parallel to the floor. At that point, return to the standing position. Start with three sets of 10 repetitions and progress as appropriate.

Toe Raises: Calf strength is necessary in snowboarding for performing turns as well as maintaining overall balance while snowboarding. Calf raises can be performed by standing on a step with heels hanging off the edge; slowly lower the heels then raise the heels until up on toes. Start with three sets of 20 repetitions and progress as appropriate.

✔ **Quick Tip**

Tips For Safer Sledding And Tobogganing

Sliding downhill is an exhilarating winter sport. People of all ages can participate, and use all kinds of containers, from large toboggans to plastic disks or even cardboard boxes. But sledding unintentional injuries are surprisingly common despite snow's cushioning effect. Estimates of the number of injuries treated in hospital emergency rooms every year show about 33,000 sledding injuries and 1,500 from tobogganing.

Sledding injuries often include facial lacerations or skull fractures. Tobogganing injuries almost always involve the lower half of the body.

Children ages 5 to 9 are most susceptible to injury. Parents of young children should not let them sled alone. Older children should be taught to check for hazards.

The National Safety Council offers these guidelines for safe and fun sledding and tobogganing:

- Keep all equipment in good condition. Broken parts, sharp edges, cracks, and split wood invite injuries.

- Dress warmly enough for conditions.

- Sled on spacious, gently sloping hills which have a level run-off at the end so that the sled can come to a halt safely. Avoid steep slopes and slopes located near streets and roadways.

- Check slopes for bare spots, holes, and other obstructions which might cause injury. Bypass these areas or wait until conditions are better.

- Make sure the sledding path does not cross traffic and is free from hazards such as large trees, fences, rocks, or telephone poles.

- Do not sled on or around frozen lakes, streams, or ponds because the ice may be unstable.

- The proper position for sledding is to sit or lay on your back on the top of the sled, with your feet pointing downhill. Sledding head first increases the risk of head injury and should be avoided.

- Sledders should wear thick gloves or mittens and protective boots to protect against frostbite as well as potential injury.

Source: "Tips for Safer Sledding and Tobogganing," © 2004 National Safety Council (www.nsc.org). Reprinted with permission.

Ankle Exercise With An Elastic Band: Ankle dorsiflexor strength is also necessary in snowboarding for performing turns as well as maintaining overall balance. This exercise can be performed while sitting on the floor facing a door. The elastic band should be looped around the instep of the foot and anchored at the other end in the door jamb. After the elastic band is secured, the exercise is done by moving the ankle up toward the thigh against the resistance of the band. Start with three sets of 20 repetitions and progress as appropriate.

Abdominal crunches: Abdominal strength is important in snowboarding for both maintaining balance as well as performing turns. This exercise is performed by crossing both arms across your chest and curling up your upper trunk so that your shoulder blades are raised off the floor. Start with three sets of 15 repetitions and progress as appropriate.

Chapter 52

Safety Tips For Water Sports

H2O Smarts

What do surfing, fishing, water skiing, and swimming have in common? They are all lots of fun... and they all take place in, on, or around the water. Water activities are a great way to stay cool and have a good time with your friends or your family. Take along these tips—and your common sense—to get wet, make waves, and have a blast.

Top Ten Tips

- DO learn to swim. If you like to have a good time doing water activities, being a strong swimmer is a must.

- DO take a friend along. Even though you may be a good swimmer, you never know when you may need help. Having friends around is safer and just more fun.

- DO know your limits. Watch out for the "too's" —too tired, too cold, too far from safety, too much sun, too much hard activity.

About This Chapter: This chapter includes excerpts from "H2O Smarts," "Swimming Activity Card," "Fishing Activity Card," "Snorkeling Activity Card," "Diving Activity Card," "Canoeing/Kayaking Activity Card," "Surfing Activity Card," "Water Skiing Activity Card," and "White-Water Rafting Activity Card," BAM! Body and Mind, Centers for Disease Control and Prevention, 2002.

- DO swim in supervised (watched) areas only, and follow all signs and warnings.

- DO wear a life jacket when boating, jet skiing, water skiing, rafting, or fishing.

- DO stay alert to currents. They can change quickly. If you get caught in a strong current, don't fight it. Swim parallel to the shore until you have passed through it. Near piers, jetties (lines of big rocks), small dams, and docks, the current gets unpredictable and could knock you around. If you find it hard to move around, head to shore. Learn to recognize and watch for dangerous waves and signs of rip currents—water that is a weird color, really choppy, foamy, or filled with pieces of stuff.

- DO keep an eye on the weather. If you spot bad weather (dark clouds, lighting), pack up and take the fun inside.

- DON'T mess around in the water. Pushing or dunking your friends can get easily out of hand.

- DON'T dive into shallow water. If you don't know how deep the water is, don't dive.

✔ Quick Tip
The Deal On Water Parks

Read all the signs before going on a ride. Make sure you are tall enough and old enough. Ask questions if you are not sure about how you're supposed to go on the ride. (On most water slides, you should go down face up, arms crossed behind your head, and feet first with your ankles crossed.)

When you go from ride to ride, don't run. It's slippery!

Bumping into others on a slide can hurt. That's why no "chains" of people are allowed on water rides. So, count five seconds after the rider ahead of you has gone before you take your turn.

Wear a life preserver—the park supplies it for a reason.

Source: "H2O Smarts," CDC, 2002.

• DON'T float where you can't swim. Keep checking to see if the water is too deep or if you are too far away from the shore or the poolside.

Watch Out For Mother Nature

Look out for signs warning you that the water is not clean, because polluted water could make you sick. (And even if it is clean, try not to swallow it.)

It's also smart to keep clear of objects in the water like water plants and animals. They can cause problems for you so, if you see them—go the other way. (You've heard about what jellyfish and snapping turtles can do, right?)

Finally, if you're outside, you need to guard against the sun. Those burning rays reflect off the water and sand onto you... and they can really spoil the fun. So, rub on some sunscreen to get sun proof.

Swimming

Learn to swim and always swim with a friend. It's more fun and having a friend there if you need one is just plain smart.

Make sure to respect rules and lifeguards. Pool rules like "no running" or beach rules like "no swimming outside the flags" are there to protect you. (And lifeguards enforce them so that you can stay safe, not to ruin your fun.) Make sure a lifeguard or an adult can see you just in case you need help.

♣ It's A Fact!! Lifeline

If you see someone struggling in the water, go get help. You can also throw out a life preserver or other object that floats, BUT DO NOT JUMP IN YOURSELF!

If you jump in without anyone else around, who will help save YOU if there is a problem?

Source: "H2O Smarts," CDC, 2002.

Don't try to keep up with stronger or more experienced swimmers, especially if they swim out further than you think you can swim back.

Swimming is a real workout. So, take breaks. If you get tired while you're in the water, float on your back for a few minutes until you get your power back.

Make sure to keep an eye on mother nature. If you spot bad weather (dark clouds, lightening), it's time to take the fun inside.

And when you get out of the water, tilt and shake your head to let all of the water drain out of your ears—"swimmers ear" can be a real pain.

Diving makes a splash, but make sure you know how deep the water is before you leap.

Fishing

Make sure someone knows where you are and how long you will be gone. Check out all the signs where you'll be fishing and stick to what they say. Pick the right spot—stay away from tree branches that hang over the water, power lines, or strong currents. Look before you sit, step, or touch—you don't want to get near animals or slip on wet rocks. Be careful if you're fishing off a dock or pier so you don't fall in. Check the weather report before going fishing and if a storm sneaks up on you, head for home.

Wear a life jacket if you are anywhere near deep water, running water, or on the ice. Wear a hat and sunscreen to shield you from the rays, and make sure you have your shades on to fight the glare off the water.

Fishing hooks are sharp, so be careful not to hook yourself or someone else. Keep a first aid kit handy in case you get stuck. Carry a whistle to get help if you need it.

If you want to ice fish (fishing through a hole drilled in the ice), wait until the ice is at least 4 inches thick. For fly fishing (special type of fishing in moving water with bait handmade to look like bugs), shuffle into the flowing current sideways. If you're fishing in the waves, shuffle your feet along to scare away fish and other sea creatures.

Snorkeling

Always make sure your snorkel, fins, and mask are in good working order before taking the plunge. It's also important to know the basics like how to clear water from your snorkel (blasting) and how to put your mask back on while treading water. Until you get more experienced, you may want to wear a life jacket—it will help you stay afloat if you need a rest or if you get into trouble in the water.

Most importantly, never snorkel alone. Always swim with a buddy and keep them close by so you can help each other out—and, it's more fun with a friend.

Use your noggin'—check out the weather forecast and the water's visibility before you jump in. And don't forget, coral reefs are fun to explore, but don't go too close to them until you've learned how to steer your body in the water. Never touch a reef—they are sharp and some have ocean life that may be poisonous. Always be considerate of the places you are snorkeling in, they may be another animal's home.

Finally, watch out for the sun. Wear a T-shirt and sunscreen to make sure you don't get sunburned.

Diving

Here's the deal: Know how to swim well before stepping on the board. Always dive with someone else. And...protect your noggin. You've got to know the water depth before you dive, and never ever dive into shallow water. Check

❖ It's A Fact!!

Alcohol use is involved in about 25% to 50% of adolescent and adult deaths associated with water recreation. Alcohol influences balance, coordination, and judgment, and its effects are heightened by sun exposure and heat. Alcohol was involved in about one-third of all reported boating fatalities.

Source: Excerpted from "Water-Related Injuries Fact Sheet," Centers for Disease Control and Prevention, April 2007.

around for signs or ask a lifeguard. Diving areas are usually marked. In case you haven't figured this out yet, above-ground pools are not designed for diving. They're way too shallow. (Lots of in-ground pools aren't deep enough either, so check out the water before you dive.)

When you are on the board, enter the water straight on and make sure there's nothing in your way before you leap. If people come into the diving area from other parts of the pool, wait until they're gone, or just ask the lifeguard to clear the area for you. If you jump when there is someone else in the diving area, or even just mess around while diving, you could land on top of someone and get hurt.

Don't run up to a dive. Always stand at the edge of the board or pool and then dive. And dive straight ahead—not off to the side.

It's also important to warm-up and stretch before diving, and then cool down after your plunge session.

Most of all, only try dives that are in your comfort zone. Leave those fancy or stunt leaps to experienced divers. An adult can help you decide which dives are safe to try.

Canoeing/Kayaking

You need to be a strong swimmer because you might have to swim underwater, or in moving water. Always go paddling with another person—not just for times of trouble, but because someone should help you carry, load, and launch your boat, right?

Make sure your life jacket fits. Since paddling is an activity that you can do all through the year, leave enough room to put clothes under it when it is cold out. Be prepared to get wet. Take along extra dry clothing, just in case. Remember to keep sun proof with sunscreen.

Save paddling for good weather days. Since you don't know what mother nature will throw at you, know where your float trip will take you, spots where you can get out or camp for the night, and different ways to go in case unexpected trouble strikes your route. Avoid whitewater rapids, dams, and falls—only experienced whitewater paddlers should take these on.

Sure, you want all your friends and their stuff to come along, but don't put too much weight in the boat—you should have more than six inches of side between the top of the fully loaded boat and the water. Spread out the weight (including people) so the boat will stay balanced.

Take lessons to help you learn ways to get yourself back in your boat if it tips over—before you take your first trip. And then practice them. The main thing to remember is...don't panic. If you can't get back in, stay with your boat and flip it back over—it'll float—and try to swim the boat to shore. (Remember, you're wearing a life jacket, right?!)

Surfing

First things first ...you've got to be a strong swimmer. As a beginner, you are going to be in the water more than riding your board. And always surf with someone else.

While you're a beginner, stick to waves no bigger than three feet. If you are a real beginner, surf only broken (white) waves. Never paddle out farther than you can swim back with your board. Most of all, if it doesn't feel right or you are too scared, just don't go.

Always leash your board to control it. When you begin the wipeout (fall at the end of a ride), kick your board out and away from you.

Bad weather = No surfing.

Did you know that surfers have rules for who "owns" a wave? Surfers riding waves have to get out of the way of those paddling out, and everyone has to stay clear of swimmers. A surfer who is standing and riding a wave gets to keep it—no one should "drop in" (try to catch the same wave).

Finally, make sure to wear sunscreen.

✤ It's A Fact!!

Windsurfing: Most windsurfing injuries are overuse injuries related to gripping the boom. Typical problems are rotator cuff impingement, carpal tunnel syndrome, and elbow tendinitis. Foot injuries may occur with use of footstraps. Many injuries can be prevented by equipment or technique modification.

Source: Excerpted from "Your Sport," reprinted with permission from Jeffrey L. Halbrecht, M.D., Institute for Arthroscopy and Sports Medicine, San Francisco, CA, www.iasm.com. © 2006.

Water Skiing

Water skiers need to be good swimmers and always wear a life jacket that fits properly.

Safe water skiing requires three people: the skier, an experienced boat driver, and the spotter to look out for the skier's signals. Since the noise from the boat is so loud, it's important that everyone agrees on and understands the hand signals to use so you can talk without saying a word. Remember, you need to master hand signals before you begin cutting across the water on your skis.

When you're out on the water, be sure you're in a safe area to ski. Don't ski near docks, boats, rocks, or in shallow water. The only place to start is in the water—dock or land starts should be left to the pros.

If you start to lose your balance while skiing, just bend your knees and crouch down so you don't fall. If you do fall—and everyone does—remember to let go of the rope. Then, find your skis and hold one of them up to signal you're okay and to let other boaters know you're in the water.

Before you start, get H2O smart about what to do on and in the water.

White-Water Rafting

Before jumping into that raft, it's important to know how to swim. Even if you're a strong swimmer, always wear a life jacket. It should fit snugly and have back and shoulder protection as well as floatation to help you swim safely in white water. Also, don't forget to wear your helmet—it should be designed for water sports, fit properly and snugly on your head, and allow for water to drain from the helmet. It should also cover your ears, temples, and the back of your neck. Once you have the proper gear and are sure it's all in working order, you're ready to run the river.

It's also really helpful if you've done a little exploring first. Make sure you know the river you are rafting on—check out the rating of the rapids and what the current is like. It's best to a have a trained, experienced guide on your team and in your raft. The guide will know the best course and the safest passage. Don't enter a rapid unless you're sure you can run it safely or swim it without getting hurt. If you fall out of the raft, position your body so that you are on your back with your feet facing down river—try to keep your feet and legs up.

Usually a group of three boats is the minimum on a river—but only one boat should run the rapids at a time. Safe rafting is all about teamwork, so pick a captain to call out directions so everyone can work together.

Most importantly, be prepared. Get a first aid and survival kit, and include extra ropes, a raft repair kit, and extra life vests. Better safe than stranded.

Chapter 53

Safety Tips For Hiking, Biking, And Other Recreational Pursuits

Hiking

Get in shape before you head out on your hike. Try walking around your neighborhood with your pack loaded with five pounds more gear than you'll actually carry on your hike. If that goes well, plan a short hike to test your abilities on the trail.

Take a friend and an adult along on your hike. That way you can look out for each other and you'll have people to talk to. Also, be sure to let someone who's not going know where you'll be hiking and what time you'll be back.

Carry lots of water even if you are only planning a short hike. For warm-weather hikes, bring six to eight quarts of water per day. In the cold weather or higher elevations, you can be safe with half that amount. Whenever you are near water, make sure you wet yourself down. Dampen a bandana and wipe your face, neck, and arms or wrap it around your head while you hike.

To prevent blisters, try spraying your feet with an antiperspirant before heading out. Bring extra pairs of socks that you can change into if your feet

About This Chapter: This chapter includes excerpts from "Hiking Activity Card," 2002, "Walking Activity Card," 2002, "Bicycling Activity Card," 2001, "Golf Activity Card," 2002, "Frisbee Activity Card," 2001, "Jump Rope Activity Card," 2002, and "Table Tennis Activity Card," 2007, BAM! Body and Mind, Centers for Disease Control and Prevention get wet or sweaty—if they aren't made of cotton, they'll keep your feet drier. Once you're on the trail, stop as soon as you feel a "hot spot" on your feet and apply special type of bandage called "moleskin" to the sore area. Also, try using a hiking stick to keep some pressure off of your legs and knees.

Don't get bugged by bugs. Protect yourself from bites and stings by using a bug repellant that includes DEET. Repellents that contain DEET are the most effective, but make sure you rub them on according to the directions. A good rule of thumb from the experts is that kids should use repellents with less than 10% DEET. Get your parents to help you put it on your face so you don't get it in your mouth or eyes. And wash your hands after you apply it. Remember that stuff that smells good to you smells good to bugs too, so don't use scented shampoos or lotions before hiking.

When it's hot, pick trails that are shaded and run near streams. If you need to hike uphill in the sun, first soak yourself down to stay cool. You can also try wearing a wet bandana around your head or neck. Also, try to stay out of cotton clothes. Keep yourself out of bad weather by checking forecasts before you hike and watching the skies once you're out on the trail. During lightening storms, head downhill and away from the direction of the storm, and then squat down and keep your head low.

To stay healthy on your hike, you'll need to know how to keep your food and water safe. Remember the four C's: contain, clean, cook, and chill.

♣ It's A Fact!!

Running: Subtle malalignment can cause a multitude of problems for the runner. Common injuries include iliotibial band syndrome, chondromalacia patella, plica syndrome, and popliteal cysts. Many problems can be treated with orthotics to control alignment, rotation, and leg length and with the use of proper stretching, training techniques, and running shoes.

Source: Excerpted from "Your Sport," reprinted with permission from Jeffrey L. Halbrecht, M.D., Institute for Arthroscopy and Sports Medicine, San Francisco, CA, www.iasm.com. © 2006.

Walking

Before you walk out the door, talk about the best walking routes with your parents so you know your safety zones and how to avoid traffic. And, only walk in those areas so your parents will know where you are.

It's always best to walk where you can avoid traffic—like parks or even the mall. Or try to find an area where there are sidewalks. If you have to walk on a street without sidewalks, walk close to the curb facing traffic. Remember to cross the street only at marked crosswalks or at corners, keep your ears and eyes open, and watch out for traffic in front and back of you. Wear bright-colored clothing or reflectors so drivers can see you. If you are walking alone, don't wear headphones—if they are too loud, they can keep you from hearing any oncoming traffic.

Water, water, water. It's a good idea to drink some water before you head out to walk, while you are walking, and when you get back—even if it's cold outside or you don't feel thirsty. In the summer, late afternoons (not nights) and mornings are the best times to walk to avoid the midday heat and humidity.

☞ Remember!!

Start out slowly and gradually increase the speed and distance you walk—don't try walking a marathon your first time out. And no matter where you are walking, be aware of what is going on around you.

Source: "Walking," CDC, 2002.

It is best to warm up your muscles before stretching them, so warm up for 5 minutes at an easy walking pace before stretching. Then stretch by starting at the top of your body and working your way down. Make sure to cool down and stretch after your walk too.

Bicycling

Use your head and wear a helmet. You should always wear a helmet when you ride—plus, it's the law in many states. It's also important that your helmet is approved by one of the groups who test helmets to see which ones are the best: the Consumer Product Safety Commission (CPSC) or Snell B-95 standards are best for bicycling helmets. Try not to ride at night or in bad weather, and wear brightly colored, or reflective clothes whenever you ride

---

♣ It's A Fact!!
Bike + Mountains = Excitement And Challenge

Tired of paved roads? Want to go where there aren't any speed limits?

If you answered yes, then your vehicle of choice could very well be a mountain bike. Ever since a group of friends took a fast-paced ride down a steep incline in Northern California, mountain biking has been an exciting challenge to off-road riders.

Its inclusion as an event in the 1996 Olympics confirmed what riders already know: Mountain biking is one of the fastest growing sports in the world, both in popularity and participation.

If you've never been on a mountain bike you might wonder what all the fuss is about. Many riders say it's the freedom. After all, destinations are unlimited on these machines built for rough terrain.

The Right Equipment: Mountain bikes are sturdier than your average 10-speed or hybrid bicycle so they can withstand rough roads. They have wide tires that grip the trail and cantilever brakes, similar to those found on a motorcycle.

When purchasing a mountain bike, be sure that it isn't too large. You should always be able to put a foot on the ground to steady yourself. A helmet is a must, and knee and elbow pads are sure-fire scar preventers.

Your Body On A Bike: Riding a bike is one of the best cardiovascular exercises around. Not only does it provide an aerobic workout, but it strengthens the large muscles of the lower body, including the thighs, hips, and buttocks, without putting a lot of stress on the joints. The upper body and arms come into play when climbing hills.

Always warm up before you begin your ride. Pedal in a low gear over flat terrain until you begin to sweat or feel warm.

so you can be seen. You can even put reflectors or funky reflective stickers on your bike—who knew being safe could look so cool? Also, watch out for loose pant legs and shoe laces that could get caught in your bike chain.

This usually takes about five to 10 minutes. And don't neglect to cool down when you come to the end of your ride. Gradually lowering your heart rate can help prevent the pooling of lactic acid in the muscles. Again, pedal slowly in a low gear.

On The Trail: Practice makes perfect isn't a cliché when it comes to handling a mountain bike. Once you start heading up hills and mountains and over rocks and steep falls, you'll need to rely on your instincts, which, if they don't come naturally, develop through practice.

One of the first things to do is to get a feel for how the brakes work. The front brake on a mountain bike usually has more power than the back, and pulling it alone may send you flying over the handlebars. Practice quick stops before you hit the trail so you can feel how your weight may affect how you stop.

Cantilever brakes are stronger than those on other bikes, allowing riders to control factors such as their rate of decline. When descending a hill, lightly squeeze and release the brakes—a technique called feathering—to prevent the wheels from locking.

Change gears as it becomes necessary in order to keep a steady cadence. Use a low gear when you need power and a high gear when you want speed.

Climbing requires a shift in your weight that will control the tires' grip on the ground. Short, steep hills may require out-of-the-seat pedaling to garner more power.

If you try this on a long climb, however, you'll likely tire before you reach the top. Shift your weight forward, off the seat if necessary, to gain the power you need.

Get Pedaling: You can obtain information about trails in your area from your local library or mountain-biking group. The sooner you start pedaling, the sooner you can test your limits—those set by both your body and your mind.

Source: "Bike + Mountains = Excitement And Challenge," reprinted with permission from the American Council on Exercise, © 2007. All rights reserved.

✔ **Quick Tip**
Pre-Golf Stretches

Golf is a popular sport of all ages played year-round. Range of motion of the trunk and upper extremities is key to a successful golf swing. Unfortunately, as one gets older, flexibility (or range of motion) is likely to decrease, predisposing one to injury. Golf is a game of repetitive twisting and rotation of the trunk. Excessive rotation puts a shear stress of the spine which may increase risk of injury. In addition, most participants who play on the average of once or twice a week do not bother warming up beforehand.

Flexibility exercises not only have the potential to prevent injury but also to improve golf performance. To help prepare oneself for the game, here are a few exercises to do before golfing:

Side Bending: Stand up straight with your feet shoulder width apart and arms at your sides. Bend to the right (keeping your hips facing forward) letting your right arm slide down along the outside of your thigh. Your left arm leaning overhead to the right. Feel a stretch along the left side of your trunk/torso. Hold each stretch for a count of 10. Repeat three times. Reverse arm positions bending to the left.

Upper Body Trunk Rotation: Stand up straight with your feet shoulder width apart and arms bent at elbows grasping golf club behind your head. Twist your upper body toward the right keeping your hips facing forward. Hold for a count of 10. Now twist your body toward the left and hold. Repeat each stretch three times.

Be street smart. Ride on the right side of the road, moving with traffic, and obey all traffic signs and signals. Discuss the best riding routes with your parents—they'll help you determine safe places to ride near your home.

When you reach an intersection, be sure to stop and look left, right, and then left again to check for cars—then go. Use hand signals to show when you're going to turn, and be sure to keep an eye out for rough pavement ahead so you can avoid it. And although you may think you can't go out without your favorite tunes, never wear headphones when you're on your bike.

Shoulder Stretch: Grasp your club in front of you with your hands crossed. The bottom hand palm up and top hand palm down. With the bottom hand push the club in the direction of the top hand. Feel a stretch in the back of your shoulder. Hold each stretch for a count of 10 and repeat three times. Now switch hand positions and repeat the stretch on that side.

ITB Stretch: Sit on the floor with your legs out in front. Keeping your left leg straight, bend your right knee and place your right foot flat on the floor on the outside of your left knee. Then turn your body toward the right so your left elbow is on the outside of your right knee. Also, turn your head to look over your right shoulder. Keep your hips flat on the floor at all times. Now switch sides and turn toward the left. Hold each stretch for a count of 10 and repeat three times on each side.

Hamstring Stretch: Sit with your right leg out in front and your left leg bent so the outside of your left leg is resting on the floor and your left foot touches your right knee. Slowly reach down the right leg until you feel a stretch in the back of your thigh. Grasp onto your leg to maintain the stretch. Now switch sides. Hold each stretch for a count of 10 and repeat each side three times.

Quadriceps Stretch: Stand with one arm holding onto a wall or your golf partner. With the other hand grasp your ankle and pull your foot behind you toward your buttocks. Keep your knee back—don't let it come forward. Feel a stretch in the front of your thigh. Hold for a count of 10 and repeat three times on each leg.

Source: "Pre-Golf Stretches," reprinted with permission from the Nicholas Institute of Sports Medicine and Athletic Trauma, © 2007. All rights reserved.

Golf

It's important to warm-up and stretch before you step onto your local golf course. Before swinging, make sure that no one is standing too close— it's a good rule of thumb to stand at least four club lengths away from the person swinging the club. Don't play until the group in front of you is out of the way. Stand still and stay quiet while others are in play. If your ball lands in the rough of the course (in high grass, brush, or trees), watch out for creepy, crawly animals, and poisonous plants.

Check the weather forecast before going out onto the course. The general rule for avoiding storms is: If you can see lightning, flee it, if you can hear thunder, clear it. Get away from small metal vehicles like golf carts, and put your clubs away. Stay away from trees because they attract lightning, and avoid small on-course shelters—they are made to protect you from rain showers and provide shade.

Whether you're walking the course or riding in a cart, don't forget your water bottle. It's important to drink plenty of water before, during, and after your round. Need a rest? Sit down in a shady area or under a tree—put a cold towel around your neck to keep you cool.

Frisbee

When playing a game of Frisbee, just make sure that you don't throw too hard and always try and stay on your feet while playing. If you are playing a more intense game of Ultimate also make sure to avoid diving for the Frisbee.

It's important to warm up and stretch before any game. Listen to your body. Don't play through any pain. If you are injured, wait until you've healed before starting to play again. And if you have glasses or braces, wear protective eye or mouth guards.

Whether you're just tossing the Frisbee with friends or playing a competitive game of Ultimate, make sure to drink plenty off water before, during, and after your game. It's also a good idea to wear sunscreen to keep from burning and bug repellent to keep the bugs where they belong—off of you.

Jump Rope

Avoid spills—set the right length for your rope. To find out what that is, stand on the center of the cord and pull the handles up so they fit right under your arms. When you jump over the rope, the rope should just brush the floor under your feet. If it doesn't touch the floor, it's too short. If it hits the floor in front of your feet, it's too long.

Table Tennis

During any physical activity, it's always important to play it safe. Understanding the rules of a game always helps, and you should do things like stretching to help prevent injuries. So when playing table tennis, make sure you play by the rules and stay alert. It's also a good idea to rest in between training sessions so that your body can relax and your muscles can recover from the workout.

Part Four

If You Need More Information

Chapter 54

Hazard Screening Reports For Team Sports, Sports Activities, And Equipment

Team Sports

Basketball, Football, Baseball, Softball, Lacrosse, Volleyball, Soccer, Ice Hockey, Field Hockey, Rugby, Roller Hockey, Street Hockey, Other Ball Sports

- ER Treated Injuries (2002): 1,695,790

- Medically Treated Injuries (2002): 4,477,950

- Percent Of ER Treated Hospitalized: 1.49%

- Deaths (2000): 28

- Death Costs (Millions): $140.0

- Cost Of Medically Treated Injuries (Millions): $69,504.0

- Total Known Costs (Millions): $69,644.0

About This Chapter: This chapter includes excerpts from "Hazard Screening Report: Team Sports," July 2004, and "Hazard Screening Report: Sports Activities and Equipment (Excluding Major Team Sports," May 2005, both produced by the U.S. Consumer Product Safety Commission. The full text is available online at http://www.cpsc.gov/library.

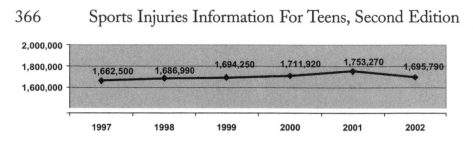

Figure 54.1. Estimated Number Of Emergency Room Treated Injuries Associated With 15 Team Sports, by Year, 1997–2002

Addressability: Injuries

[Addressability refers items that could possibly be addressed by some action the Consumer Product Safety Commission could, at least in theory, take.] For example, if a boy trips over a rake in the driveway, any injury he suffers could be associated with the category of Yard and Garden Equipment. But it is very unlikely that such injuries could be prevented by changing the design of rakes.

- Basketball: protruding bolts, goal collapse, net entrapment, collision with basketball pole

- Football: head injuries, helmet to helmet collision, collision with goal post

- Baseball: sliding/base failure, bat breakage, ball to head contact

- Softball: sliding/base failure, ball to head contact, mask failure

- Lacrosse: ball and stick injuries to head/facial area

- Volleyball: none determined to be addressable

- Soccer: kicked in leg, pole/goal contact

- Ice Hockey: puck/stick injuries to head/facial area

- Field Hockey: puck/stick/ball injuries to head/facial area

- Rugby: equipment failure (helmet/head injuries)

- Roller Hockey: puck/stick injuries to head/facial area

- Street Hockey: puck/stick injuries to head/facial area

- Other Ball Sports: none determined to be addressable

Addressability: Deaths

- Basketball: goal collapse, net entrapment, collision with basketball pole

- Football: head/chest injuries, helmet to helmet collision

- Baseball: death of participant in organized game, death of player under 15 years old, struck by ball or bat

- Softball: death of participant in organized game, death of player under 15 years old, struck by ball or bat

- Lacrosse: struck by ball to chest area

- Volleyball: none reported

- Soccer: soccer goal tip-over

- Ice Hockey: puck to head

- Field Hockey: none reported

- Rugby: none reported

- Roller Hockey: none reported

- Street Hockey: none reported

- Other Ball Sports: none reported

Sports Activities And Equipment

Individual Product Categories: All-terrain vehicles; Exercise activity and equipment; Swimming activities; Snow sports; Other sports; Gymnastics/ Cheering, etc.; Other off-road vehicles; Fighting sports; Golf; Water sports; Racquet/Volleying sports; Miscellaneous sports activities; Low impact sports; Shooting sports; Indoor activities

- ER Treated Injuries (2003): 1,273,630

- Medically Treated Injuries (2003): 3,454,800

- Percent Of ER Treated Hospitalized: 4.81%

- Deaths (2000): 3,326

- Death Costs (Millions): $16,630

- Cost Of Medically Treated Injuries (Millions): $73,132.3

- Total Known Costs (Millions):* $89,762.3

*This total represents an index rather than an actual single year estimate of costs, because injury costs are based on 2003 and death costs are based on 2000. These are the most recent years for which each of these cost items was available.

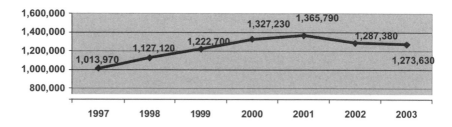

Figure 54.2. Estimated Emergency Room Treated Injuries Associated With Sports Activities And Equipment, Not Including Major Team Sports, 1997–2003, Source: National Electronic Injury Surveillance System (NEISS), 1997–2003.

Addressability: Injuries

- Exercise activity and equipment: caught in exercise machinery, other exercise machine related injuries, mat burn, insufficient mat coverage, pull up bar related head injuries, sharp edges, preventable spotter failures, falls from treadmills

- Swimming activities: slips and falls on ladders or stairs in pools, collisions with lane markers, injuries from drain suction, submersion injuries, sharp edges

- Snow sports: head injuries, binding release failures

- Other sports: head injuries, sharp edges

- Gymnastics/Cheering, etc.: No addressable injuries identified

- Other off- road vehicles: tire blow outs, brake failures, falling out of the vehicle, vehicles flipping or rolling, head injuries

- Fighting sports: concussions, other head injuries, collisions with walls

- Golf: falling out of a golf cart, golf carts tipping over

- Water sports: dizziness, numbness, and other injuries that should have been prevented by scuba gear

- Racquet/Volleying sports: ball injuries to the eyes or face, accidental self inflicted racquet injuries

- Miscellaneous Sports Activities: falls from bleachers, entrapment in bleachers, head injuries, injuries related to equipment, self standing products falling over, sharp edges

- Low impact sports: hit by bowling ball, tripped on boundary marker, finger stuck in bowling ball, gutter related injuries, caught between bowling balls, cuts from horseshoe stakes

- Shooting sports: paintball injuries to the eyes, firing after a jam, firing after impact, shots during repair or cleaning, shots while the safety was on, sharp edges, injuries from springs, shots from apparently unloaded weapons

- Indoor activities: table collapse, sharp edges, splinters

Addressability: Deaths

- Exercise activity and equipment: strangled on exercise machine

- Swimming activities: submersions

- Snow sports: head injuries, deaths related to sports equipment

- Other sports: head injuries, electrocutions

- Other off-road vehicles: some head injuries, ejections from vehicle

- Fighting sports: head injuries

- Golf: falling out of a moving golf cart, choking hazards

- Water sports: head injuries, pressure related scuba injuries

- Miscellaneous sports activities and equipment: head injuries, deaths related to sports equipment

Chapter 55

National Collegiate Athletic Association's Injury Surveillance System

The National Collegiate Athletic Association (NCAA)'s Injury Surveillance System (ISS) was developed in 1982 to provide current and reliable data on injury trends in intercollegiate athletics. Injury data are collected yearly from a sample of NCAA member institutions, and the resulting data summaries are reviewed by the NCAA Committee on Competitive Safeguards and Medical Aspects of Sports. The committee's goal continues to be to reduce injury rates through suggested changes in rules, protective equipment or coaching techniques, based on data provided by the ISS.

Sampling: Participation in the ISS is voluntary and limited to NCAA member institutions. ISS participation is available to the population of institutions sponsoring a given sport. Schools qualifying for inclusion in the final ISS sample are selected from the total participating schools for each ISS sport, with the goal of a minimum 10 percent representation of all three NCAA divisions. A school is selected as qualifying for the sample if they meet the minimum standards for data collection set forth by the ISS staff. For a more detailed explanation of ISS sampling methodology, see: National Collegiate Athletic Association Injury Surveillance Summary for 15 Sports, 1988-1989 Through 2003-2004. *J Athl Train.* 2007;42(2).

It is important to recognize that this system does not identify every injury that occurs at NCAA institutions in a particular sport. Rather, the emphasis is collecting all injuries and exposures from schools that voluntarily participate in the ISS. The ISS attempts to balance the dual needs of maintaining a reasonably representative cross-section of NCAA institutions while accommodating the needs of the voluntary participants.

Injuries: A reportable injury in the ISS is defined as one that:

1. Occurs as a result of participation in an organized intercollegiate practice or competition;

2. Requires medical attention by a team athletic trainer or physician; and

3. Results in restriction of the student-athlete's participation or performance for one or more days beyond the day of injury.

Exposures: An athlete exposure (A-E), the unit of risk in the ISS, is defined as one athlete participating in one practice or competition in which he or she is exposed to the possibility of athletics injury.

Injury Rate: An injury rate is simply a ratio of the number of injuries in a particular category to the number of athlete exposures in that category. In the ISS, this value is expressed as injuries per 1,000 athlete exposures.

All Sports Figures: The following figures outline selected information from the 16 sports currently monitored by the ISS.

Figure numbers 55.1 and 55.2 compare the practice and competition injury rates across 16 sports without regard to severity. Comparisons of injury rates between sports are difficult because each sport has its own unique schedule and activities. If such comparisons are necessary, it may be best to use the game data for which the intensity variable is most consistent.

Figure numbers 55.3 through 55.6 examine two measures of severity found in the ISS—time loss and injuries that required surgery. These combined practice and game data are presented to assist in decisions regarding appropriate medical coverage for a sport; however, each severity category has some limitations that should be considered.

1. **Time loss:** Figure numbers 55.3 through 55.5 evaluate the rate of reported injuries that caused restricted or loss of participation of seven days or more. Limitations to this type of severity evaluation include: a) An injury that restricts participation in one sport may not restrict participation in another

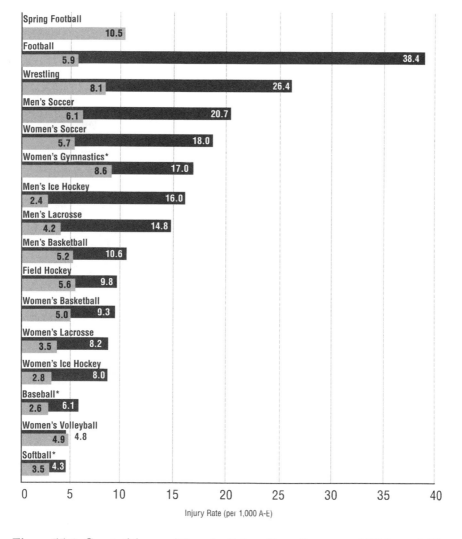

Figure 55.1. Competition and Practice Injury Rates Summary (All Sports). Figure 55.1 represents the average competition (black) and practice (grey) injury rates (expressed as injuries per 1,000 athlete-exposures) for all sports analyzed in the ISS for the 2004–05, 2005–06 and 2006–07 seasons.

sport; and b) Injuries that occur at the end of a season can only be estimated with regard to time loss.

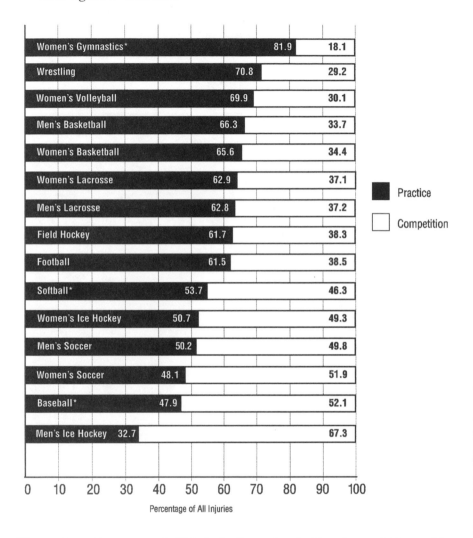

*Figure 55.2. Percentage of All Injuries Occurring in Practices and Competition. Figure 55.2 represents the average percentage of all injuries that occurred in practices and in competition in the 2004–05, 2005–06, and 2006–07 seasons. The relatively few injuries that occurred in the weight room were not included in the practice and competition percentages. It should be noted that these calculations are based only on the absolute number of injuries and do not take exposures into consideration. (*Two-season average.)*

2. **Injuries that require surgery:** Figure numbers 55.3, 55.4 and 55.6 evaluate the rate of reported injuries that required either immediate or postseason surgery. Limitations to this severity evaluation include: a)

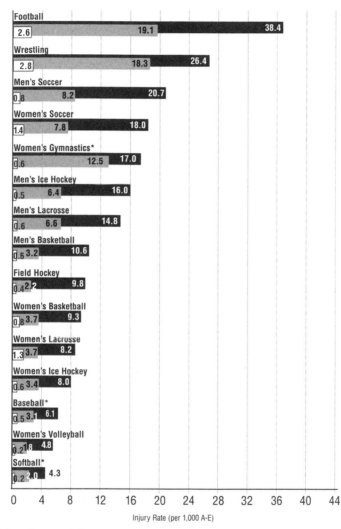

*Figure 55.3. Competition Injury Rates Summary (All Sports). Figure 55.3 represents the average overall competition injury rate (black), the game rate of injuries that caused reduced or missed participation for seven or more days (grey) and the game rate of reported injuries that required surgery (clear). The rates are expressed as injuries per 1,000 athlete-exposures for all sports analyzed in the ISS for the 2004–05, 2005–06, and 2006–07 seasons. *Two-season average.*

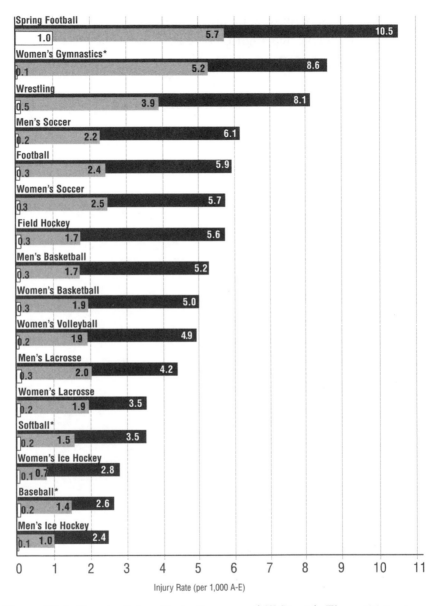

*Figure 55.4. Practice Injury Rates Summary (All Sports). Figure 55.4 represents the average overall practice injury rate (black), the practice rate of injuries that caused reduced or missed participation for seven or more days (grey) and the practice rate of reported injuries that required surgery (white). The rates are expressed as injuries per 1,000 athlete-exposures for all sports analyzed in the ISS for the 2004–05, 2005–06, and 2006–07 seasons. *Two-season average.*

The changing nature of surgical techniques and how they are applied; b) The assumption that all sports had access to the same quality of medical evaluation; and c) Injuries can occur that may be categorized as severe, such as concussions, that may not require surgery.

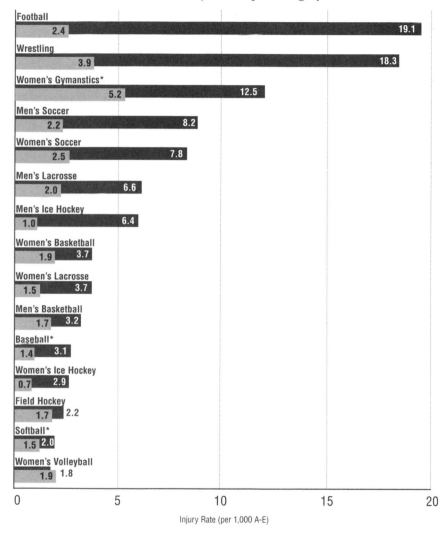

Sport	Practice (grey)	Competition (black)
Football	2.4	19.1
Wrestling	3.9	18.3
Women's Gymanstics*	5.2	12.5
Men's Soccer	2.2	8.2
Women's Soccer	2.5	7.8
Men's Lacrosse	2.0	6.6
Men's Ice Hockey	1.0	6.4
Women's Basketball	1.9	3.7
Women's Lacrosse	1.5	3.7
Men's Basketball	1.7	3.2
Baseball*	1.4	3.1
Women's Ice Hockey	0.7	2.9
Field Hockey	1.7	2.2
Softball*	1.5	2.0
Women's Volleyball	1.9	1.8

Injury Rate (per 1,000 A-E)

*Figure 55.5. Competition and Practice 7+ Days Time Loss Injury Rates Summary (All Sports). Figure 55.5 represents the average rate of injuries that caused reduced or missed participation for seven or more days, suffered either in competition (black) or in practice (grey). The rates are expressed as injuries per 1,000 athlete-exposures for all sports analyzed in the ISS for the 2004–05, 2005–06, and 2006–07 seasons. *Two-season average.*

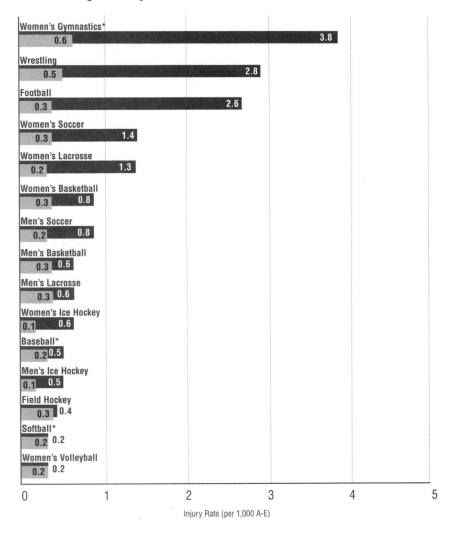

*Figure 55.6. Competition and Practice Injuries Requiring Surgery Rate Summary (All Sports). Figure 55.6 represents the average rate of reported injuries that required surgery, suffered either in competition (black) or in practice (white). The rates are expressed as injuries per 1,000 athlete-exposures for all sports analyzed in the ISS for the 2004–05, 2005–06, and 2006–07 seasons. *Two-season average.*

Chapter 56

Resources For More Information About Traumatic And Chronic Sports-Related Injuries

General Sports Medicine Resources

Ackland Sports Medicine
449 Route 130, Suite 8
Sandwich, MA 02563
Phone: 508-888-6907
Website: http://www.sportismedicine.com

American Academy of Orthopaedic Surgeons
6300 North River Road
Rosemont, IL 60018-4262
Toll-Free: 800-346-AAOS
(346-2267)
Phone: 847-823-7186
Fax: 847-823-8125
Website: http://www.aaos.org
E-mail: pemr@aaos.org

American Academy of Physical Medicine and Rehabilitation
330 North Wabash Ave.
Suite 2500
Chicago, IL 60611-7617
Phone: 312-464-9700
Fax: 312-464-0227
Website: http://aapmr.org
E-mail: info@aapmr.org

About This Chapter: Information in this chapter was compiled from many sources deemed reliable. Inclusion does not constitute endorsement, and there is no implication associated with omission. All contact information was verified in December 2007.

American Board for Certification in Orthotics and Prosthetics
Website: http://www.oandpcare.org

American College of Sports Medicine
P.O. Box 1440
Indianapolis, IN 46206-1440
Phone: 317-637-9200
Fax: 317-634-7817
Website: http://www.acsm.org

American Orthopaedic Society for Sports Medicine
6300 N. River Road
Suite 500
Rosemont, IL 60018
Phone: 847-292-4900
Fax: 847-292-4905
Website: http://www.sportsmed.org
E-mail: aossm@aossm.org

American Osteopathic Academy of Sports Medicine
2810 Crossroads Drive
Suite 3800
Madison, WI 53718
Phone: 608-443-2477
Fax: 608-443-2474
Website: http://www.aoasm.org

American Physical Therapy Association
1111 North Fairfax Street
Alexandria, VA 22314-1488
Toll-Free: 800-999-2782
Phone: 703-684-APTA (684-2782)
Fax: 703-684-7343
TDD: 703-683-6748
Website: http://www.apta.org

American Shoulder and Elbow Surgeons
6300 North River Road, Suite 727
Rosemont, IL 60018-4226
Phone: 847-698-1629
Website: http://www.ases-assn.org

American Sports Medicine Institute
2660 10th Avenue South, Suite 505
Birmingham, AL 35205
Phone: 205-918-0000
Fax: 205-918-0800
Website: http://www.asmi.org

Center for Orthopaedics and Sports Medicine
1211 Johnson Ferry Road
Marietta, GA 30068
Phone: 770-565-0011
Website:
http://www.arthroscopy.com

Clinical Sports Medicine

Website: http://
www.clinicalsportsmedicine.com
E-mail:
info@clinicalsportsmedicine.com

Geisinger Sports Medicine

115 Woodpile Lane
Danville, PA 17822
Phone: 866-414-4988;
800-921-1467
Website: http://
www.geisingersportsmed.com

Hospital for Special Surgery

535 East 70th Street
New York, NY 10021
Phone: 212-606-1000
Website: http://www.hss.edu

Hughston Sports Medicine Foundation

6262 Veterans Parkway
Columbus, GA 31908-9517
Toll-Free: 800-331-2910
Phone: 706-324-6661
Website: http://www.hughston.com

Institute for Arthroscopy and Sports Medicine

2100 Webster St., Suite 331
San Francisco, CA 94115
Phone: 415-923-0944
Fax: 415-923-5896
Website: http://www.iasm.com

Institute for Preventative Sports Medicine

P.O. Box 7032
Ann Arbor, MI 48107
Phone: 734-572-4577
Fax: 734-459-0814
Website: http://www.ipsm.org
E-mail: info@ipsm.org

National Academy of Sports Medicine

26632 Agoura Road
Calabasas, CA 91302
Toll-Free: 800-460-NASM
(460-6276)
Phone: 818-595-1200
Fax: 818-878-9511
Website: http://www.nasm.org

National Center for Injury Prevention and Control

Centers for Disease Control and
Prevention (CDC)
Mailstop K65
4770 Buford Highway NE
Atlanta, GA 30341-3724
Phone: 770-488-1506
Fax: 770-488-1667
Website: http://www.cdc.gov/ncipc
E-mail: CDCINFO@cdc.gov

National Center for Sports Safety

2301 Morris Avenue, Suite 105
Birmingham, AL 35203
Toll-Free: 866-508-NCSS
Phone: 205-329-7535
Fax: 205-329-7526
Website: http://
www.sportssafety.org
E-mail: info@sportssafety.org

National Institute of Arthritis and Musculoskeletal and Skin Diseases

1 AMS Circle
Bethesda, Maryland 20892-3675
Toll-Free: 877-22-NIAMS
(226-4267)
Phone: 301-495-4484
Fax: 301-718-6366
TTY: 301-565-2966
Website: http://www.niams.nih.gov
E-mail: niamsinfo@mail.nih.gov

Newport Orthopedic Institute

22 Corporate Plaza Drive
Newport Beach, CA 92660
Phone: 949-722-7038
Fax: 949-630-4900
Website: http://
www.newportortho.com

Nicholas Institute of Sports Medicine and Athletic Trauma

130 East 77th Street, 10th Floor
New York, NY 10021
Phone: 212-434-2700
Website: http://www.nismat.org
E-mail: info@nismat.org

Orthosports

3251 McMullen Booth Road
Suite 201
Clearwater, FL 33761
Phone: 727-725-6231
Fax: 727-791-4563
Website: http://
www.orthosports.com

Sports Injury Clinic

Website: http://
www.sportsinjuryclinic.net

Southern California Orthopedic Institute

6815 Noble Avenue
Van Nuys, CA 91405
Phone: 818-901-6600
Website: http://www.scoi.com

Sports Science Orthopaedic Clinic

Website: http://www.ssoc.co.za
E-mail: dion@grucox.com

University of North Carolina Orthopaedics

CB #7055, Bioinformatics Building
University of North Carolina
School of Medicine
Chapel Hill, NC 27599-7055
Website: http://www.med.unc.edu/ortho

University of Pittsburgh Medical Center Sports Medicine

200 Lothrop Street
Pittsburgh, PA 15213-2582
Toll-Free: 800-533-UPMC (8762)
Phone: 412-647-UPMC (8762)
Website: http://www.upmc.com

Brain Injuries

Brain Injury Association of America

8201 Greensburro 611
 McLane, VA 22102
Phone: 703-761-0750
Fax: 703-761-0755
Website: http://www.biausa.org

Dental Injuries

American Dental Association

211 East Chicago Ave.
Chicago, IL 60611-2678
Phone: 312-440-2500
Website: http://www.ada.org

Eating Disorders

National Association of Anorexia Nervosa and Associated Disorders, Inc.

Box 7
Highland Park, IL 60035
Phone: 847-831-3438
Fax: 847-433-4632
Website: http://www.anad.org

Emergency Medicine

American College of Emergency Physicians

Mail: P.O. Box 619911
Dallas, TX 75261-9911
Location: 1125 Executive Circle
Irving, TX 75038-2522
Phone: 800-798-1822;
972-550-0911
Fax: 972-580-2816
Website: http://www.acep.org
E-Mail:membership@acep.org

Exercise-Induced Asthma

American Lung Association

61 Broadway, 6th Floor
New York, NY 10006
Toll-Free: 800-LUNGUSA
Phone: 212-315-8700
Website: http://www.lungusa.org

Eye Injuries

Coalition to Prevent Sports Eye Injuries
5 Summit Avenue
Hackensack, NJ 07601
Phone: 866-265-3582
Fax: 201-621-4352
Website: http://www.sportseyeinjuries.com

Prevent Blindness America
211 West Wacker Drive
Suite 1700
Chicago, IL 60606
Toll-Free: 800-331-2020
Website: http://www.preventblindness.org
E-mail: info@preventblindness.org

Unite for Sight, Inc.
Website: http://www.uniteforsight.org

Facial Injuries

American Academy of Otolaryngology–Head and Neck Surgery
One Prince Street
Alexandria, VA 22314-3357
Phone: 703-836-4444
Website: http://www.entnet.org

American Association of Oral and Maxillofacial Surgeons
9700 W. Bryn Mawr Avenue
Rosemont, IL 60018-5701
Phone: 847-678-6200
Fax: 847-678-6286
Website: http://www.aaoms.org

Female Athlete Triad

Female Athlete Triad Coalition
American College of Sports Medicine
401 W. Michigan St.
Indianapolis, IN 46202
Phone: 317-637-9200
Fax: 317-634-7817
Website: http://www.femaleathletetriad.org
E-mail: info@femaleathletetriad.org

Foot Injuries

American Academy of Podiatric Sports Medicine
P.O. Box 723
Rockville, MD 20848-0723
Phone: 888-854-FEET (3338)
Fax: 301-962-3850
Website: www.aapsm.org
E-mail: info@aapsm.org

American College of Foot and Ankle Surgeons

Website: http://
www.footphysicians.com

American Podiatric Medical Association

9312 Old Georgetown Road
Bethesda, MD 20814-1621
Phone: 301-571-9200
Fax: 301-530-2752
Website: http://www.apma.org
E-mail: askapma@apma.org

American Orthopaedic Foot and Ankle Society

6300 N. River Road, Suite 510
Rosemont, IL 60018
Toll-Free: 800-235-4855
Phone: 847-698-4654
Website: http://www.aofas.org
E-mail: aofasinfo@aofas.org

ePodiatry.com

Website: http://www.epodiatry.com

Hand Injuries

American Society for Surgery of the Hand

6300 North River Road, Suite 600
Rosemont, IL 60018
Phone: 847-384-8300
Fax: 847-384-1435
Website: http://www.assh.org
E-mail: info@assh.org

Heat-Related Injuries

Gatorade Sports Science Institute

617 West Main Street
Barrington, IL 60010
Toll-Free: 800-616-GSSI (4774)
Website: http://www.gssiweb.com

Skin Conditions

American Academy of Dermatology

P.O. Box 4014
Schaumburg, IL 60618-4014
Toll-Free: 866-503-7546
Phone: 847-240-1280
Website: http://www.aad.org

National Institute of Arthritis and Musculoskeletal and Skin Diseases

National Institutes of Health
1 AMS Circle
Bethesda, MD 20892-3675
Toll-Free: 877-22-NIAMS
(266-4267)
Phone: 301-495-4484
Fax: 301-718-6366
TTY: 301-565-2966
Website: http://www.niams.nih.gov
E-mail: niamsinfo@mail.nih.gov

Spinal Cord Injuries

Christopher Reeve Foundation and Resource Center
636 Morris Turnpike, Suite 3A
Short Hills, NJ 07078
Toll-Free: 800-225-0292
Phone: 973-379-2690
Fax: 973-912-9433
Website: http://
www.christopherreeve.org
E-mail: info@paralysis.org

North American Spine Society
7075 Veterans Blvd.
Burr Ridge, IL 60527
Phone: 630-230-3600
Fax: 630-230-3742
Website: http://www.spine.org

Paralyzed Veterans of America (PVA)
801 18th Street, NW
Washington, DC 20006-3517
Toll-Free: 800-424-8200
Phone: 202-872-1300
Fax: 202-785-4452
Website: http://www.pva.org
E-mail: info@pva.org

Spine University
Website: http://
www.spineuniversity.com

Spinal Cord Society
19051 County Highway 1
Fergus Falls, MN 56537
Phone: 218-739-5252;
 218-739-5261
Fax: 218-739-5262
Website: http://members.aol.com/
scsweb

University of Southern California-Center for Spinal Surgery
1520 San Pablo Street
Suite 2000
Los Angeles, CA 90033
Phone: 323-442-5300
Fax: 323-442-5301
Website: http://uscspine.com

Steroids

National Institute on Drug Abuse
National Institutes of Health
6001 Executive Boulevard,
Room 5213
Bethesda, MD 20892-9561
Phone: 301-443-1124
Website: http://www.nida.nih.gov;
www.drugabuse.gov

Chapter 57

Resources For More Information About Fitness and Exercise

General Information About Fitness, Exercise, And Sports

Action for Healthy Kids
4711 West Golf Road, Suite 625
Skokie, IL 60076
Toll-Free: 800-416-5136
Website: http://
www.actionforhealthykids.org
E-mail:
info@actionforhealthykids.org

Amateur Athletic Union
Mail: P.O. Box 22409
Location: 1910 Hotel Plaza Blvd.
Lake Buena Vista, FL 32830
Toll-Free: 800-AAU-4USA
Phone: 407-934-7200
Fax: 407-934-7242
Website: http://www.aausports.org

American Alliance for Health, Physical Education, Recreation and Dance
1900 Association Drive
Reston, VA 20191
Toll-Free: 800-213-7193
Website: http://www.aahperd.org
E-mail: info@aahperd.org

About This Chapter: Information in this chapter was compiled from many sources deemed reliable. Inclusion does not constitute endorsement, and there is no implication associated with omission. All contact information was verified in December 2007.

American Council on Exercise

4851 Paramount Drive
San Diego, CA 92123
Toll-Free: 800-825-3636
Phone: 858-279-8227
Fax: 858-279-8064
Website: http://www.acefitness.org
E-mail: support@acefitness.org

American Fitness Professionals and Associates

P.O. Box 214
Ship Bottom, NJ 08008
Toll-Free: 800-494-7782
Phone: 609-978-7583
Website: http://
www.afpafitness.com
E-mail: afpa@afpafitness.com

BAM! (Body And Mind)

Centers for Disease Control and
Prevention
1600 Clifton Road, MS C-04
Atlanta, GA 30333
Phone: 404-639-3534
Website: http://www.bam.gov
E-mail: bam@cdc.gov

Center for the Study of Sport in Society

360 Huntington Ave.
Richards Hall, Suite 350
Boston, MA 02115
Phone: 617-373-4025
Fax: 617-373-4566
Website: http://
www.sportinsociety.org
E-mail: sportinsociety@neu.edu

Cooper Institute

12330 Preston Road
Dallas, TX 75230
Phone: 972-341-3200
Fax: 972-341-3224
Website:
http://www.cooperinst.org

Exrx.net

Website: http://www.exrx.net

Human Kinetics

P.O. Box 5076
Champaign, IL 61825-5076
Toll-Free: 800-747-4457
Fax: 217-351-2674
Website: http://
www.humankinetics.com
E-mail: info@hkusa.com

IDEA Health and Fitness Association

10455 Pacific Center Court
San Diego, CA 92121-4339
Toll-Free: 800-999-4332
Fax: 858-535-8234
Website: http://www.ideafit.com
E-mail: contact@ideafit.com

iEmily.com

Website: http://www.iemily.com

International Health, Racquet and Sportsclub Association

263 Summer Street
Boston, MA 02210
Toll-Free: 800-228-4772
Phone: 617-951-0055
Fax: 617-951-0056
Website: http://cms.ihrsa.org
E-mail: info@ihrsa.org

International Sports Sciences Association

1015 Mark Avenue
Carpinteria, CA 93013
Toll-Free: 800-892-4772
Phone: 805-745-8111
Fax: 805-745-8119
Website: http://
www.issaonline.com
E-mail: info@issaonline.com

National Alliance for Youth Sports

2050 Vista Parkway
West Palm Beach, FL 33411
Toll-Free: 800-688-KIDS
(688-5437)
Phone: 561-684-1141
Fax: 561-684-2546
Website: http://www.nays.org
E-mail: nays@nays.org

National Association for Fitness Certification

P.O. Box 67
Sierra Vista, AZ 85636
Toll-Free: 800-324-8315
Phone: 520-452-8712
Website:
http://www.body-basics.com
E-mail:
bodybasics@body-basics.com

National Athletic Trainers Association

2952 Stemmons Freeway
Dallas, TX 75247-6196
Phone: 214-637-6282
Fax: 214-637-2206
Website: http://www.nata.org

National Center on Physical Activity and Disability

1640 W. Roosevelt Road, Suite 711
Chicago, IL 60608-6904
Toll-Free: 800-900-8086
Fax: 312-355-4058
Website: http://www.ncpad.org
E-mail: ncpad@uic.edu

National Coalition for Promoting Physical Activity

1100 H Street NW, Suite 510
Washington, DC 20005
Phone: 202-454-7521
Fax: 202-454-7598
Website: http://www.ncppa.org
E-mail: info@ncppa.org

National Collegiate Athletic Association (NCAA)

P.O. Box 6222
Indianapolis, IN 46206-6222
Phone: 317-917-6222
Fax: 317-917-6888
Website: http://www.ncaa.org

National Exercise Trainers Association

5955 Golden Valley Road, Suite 240
Minneapolis, MN 55422
Toll-Free: 800-AEROBIC (237-6242)
Phone: 763-545-2505
Fax: 763-545-2524
Website: http://www.ndeita.com
E-mail: neta@netafit.org

National Heart, Lung, and Blood Institute Health Information Center

P.O. Box 30105
Bethesda, MD 20824-0105
Phone: 301-592-8573
TTY: 240-629-3255
Fax: 301-592-8563
Website: http://www.nhlbi.nih.gov
E-mail: nhlbiinfo@nhlbi.nih.gov

National High School Athletic Coaches Association

P.O. Box 10065
Fargo, ND 58106
Website: http://www.hscoaches.org
E-mail: office@hscoaches.org

National SAFE KIDS Campaign

1301 Pennsylvania Ave. NW
Suite 1000
Washington, DC 20004
Phone: 202-662-0600
Fax: 202-393-2072
Website: http://www.safekids.org

National Safety Council

1121 Spring Lake Dr.
Itasca, IL 60143-3201
Toll-Free: 800-621-7615
Phone: 630-285-1121
Fax: 630-285-1315
Website: http://www.nsc.org
E-mail: customerservice@nsc.org

National Strength and Conditioning Association
1885 Bob Johnson Drive
Colorado Springs, CO 80906
Toll-Free: 800-815-6826
Phone: 719-632-6722
Fax: 719-632-6367
Website: http://www.nsca-lift.org
E-mail: nsca@nsca-lift.org

Nemours Foundation Center for Children's Health Media
1600 Rockland Road
Wilmington, DE 19803
Phone: 302-651-4000
Fax: 302-651-4055
Website: http://www.kidshealth.org
E-mail: info@kidshealth.org

PE Central
P.O. Box 10262
Blacksburg, VA 24062
Phone: 540-953-1043
Fax: 540-301-0112
Website: http://www.pecentral.org
E-mail: pec@pecentral.org

President's Challenge
501 N. Morton, Suite 203
Bloomington, IN 47404
Toll-Free: 800-258-8146
Fax: 812-855-8999
Website: http://
www.presidentschallenge.org
E-mail: preschal@indiana.edu

President's Council on Physical Fitness and Sports
Department W
200 Independence Ave., SW
Room 738-H
Washington, DC 20201-0004
Phone: 202-690-9000
Fax: 202-690-5211
Website: http://www.fitness.gov

Safe USA
Website: http://www.safeusa.org
E-mail: safeusa@comcast.net

Shape Up America!
c/o WebFront Solutions Corporation
15009 Native Dancer Road
N. Potomac, MD 20787
Phone: 240-634-6533
Fax: 240-632-1075
Website:
http://www.shapeup.org
E-mail:
customer-care@shapeup.org

Smart Play
Website:
http://www.smartplay.net/
index.html
E-mail: admin@smasa.asn.au

Snell Memorial Foundation
3628 Madison Avenue, Suite 11
North Highlands, CA 95660
Toll-Free: 888-SNELL99
(763-5599)
Phone: 916-331-5073
Fax: 916-331-0359
Website: http://www.smf.org
E-mail: info@smf.org

SPARK
438 Camino Del Rio South
Suite 110
San Diego, CA 92108
Toll-Free: 800-SPARK PE
(772-7573)
Phone: 619-293-7990
Fax: 619-293-7992
Website: http://www.sparkpe.org
E-mail: spark@sparkpe.org

Special Olympics
1133 19th St., NW, Floor 12
Washington, DC 20036
Phone: 202-628-3630
Fax: 202-824-0200
Website: http://
www.specialolympics.org
E-mail: info@specdialolympics.org

United States Olympic Committee
1 Olympic Plaza
Colorado Springs, CO 80909
Phone: 719-632-5551
Website: http://www.olympic-usa.org

Wellness Councils of America
9802 Nicholas Street, Suite 315
Omaha, NE 68114
Phone: 402-827-3590
Fax: 402-827-3594
Website: http://www.welcoa.org
E-mail: wellworkplace@welcoa.org

Women's Sports Foundation
Eisenhower Park
1899 Hempsted Turnpike
Suite 400
East Meadow, NY 11554
Toll-Free: 800-227-3988
Phone: 516-542-4700
Fax: 516-542-4716
Website: http://
www.womenssportsfoundation.org
E-mail:
info@womenssportfoundation.org

YMCA of the USA
101 North Wacker Drive
Chicago, IL 60606
Phone: 800-872-9622
Website: http://www.ymca.net
E-mail: fulfillment@ymca.net

YWCA
1015 18th Street NW
Suite 1100
Washington, DC 20036
Phone: 202-467-0801
Fax: 202-467-0802
Website: http://www.ywca.org
E-mail: info@ywca.org

Nutrition Information

American Dietetic Association
120 South Riverside Plaza
Suite 2000
Chicago, IL 60606-6995
Toll-Free: 800-877-1600
Website: http://www.eatright.org

Center for Nutrition Policy and Promotion
U.S. Department of Agriculture
3101 Park Center Drive
Rm. 1034
Alexandria, VA 22302-1594
Phone: 703-305-7600
Fax: 703-305-3300
Website:
http://www.cnpp.usda.gov

Diabetes Exercise and Sports
8001 Montcastle Drive
Nashville, TN 37221
Toll-Free: 800-898-4322
Fax: 615-673-2077
Website:
http://www.diabetes-exercise.org
E-mail: desa@diabetes-exercise.org

National Eating Disorders Association
603 Stewart St.
Suite 803
Seattle, WA 98101
Toll-Free: 800-931-2237
Phone: 206-382-3587
Fax: 206-829-8501
Website: http://
www.nationaleatingdisorders.org
E-mail:
info@nationaleatingdisorders.org

National Institute of Diabetes and Digestive and Kidney Diseases
Building 31, Room 9A06
31 Center Drive, MSC 2560
Bethesda, MD 20892-2560
Phone: 301-496-3583
Website: http://www.niddk.nih.gov
E-mail:
dkwebmaster@extra.niddk.nih.gov

Weight-control Information Network (WIN)
1 WIN Way
Bethesda, MD 20892-3665
Toll-Free: 877-946-4627
Phone: 202-828-1025
Fax: 202-828-1028
Website: http://win.niddk.nih.gov
E-mail: win@info.niddk.nih.gov

Sports-Specific Organizations

Aerobic And Physical Movement Activities

American Tai Chi Association
2465 J-17 Centreville Road
Suite 150
Herndon, VA 20171
Website: http://
www.americantaichi.org
E-mail: contact@americantaichi.net

Aerobics and Fitness Association of America
15250 Ventura Blvd., Suite 200
Sherman Oaks, CA 91403
Toll-Free: 877-YOURBODY
(877-968-7263)
Phone: 818-905-0040
Fax: 818-990-5468
Website: http://www.afaa.com
E-mail: contactAFAA@afaa.com

Pilates Method Alliance
P.O. Box 370906
Miami, FL 33137-0906
Toll-Free: 866-573-4945
Phone: 305-573-4946
Fax: 305-573-4461
Website: http://
www.pilatesmethodalliance.org
E-mail:
info@pilatesmethodalliance.org

Yoga Research and Education Center
P.O. Box 448
Ukiah, CA 95482
Website: http://www.yrec.org
E-mail: webmaster@yrec.org

Baseball And Softball

Amateur Softball Association of America
2801 NE 50th Street
Oklahoma City, OK 73111
Toll-Free: 800-654-8337
Phone: 405-424-5266
Website: http://
www.asasoftball.com

Little League Baseball International
P.O. Box 3485
Williamsport, PA 17701
Phone: 570-326-1921
Fax: 570-322-2376
Website: http://www.littleleague.org

National Softball Association (NSA)
P.O. Box 7
Nicholasville, KY 40340
Phone: 859-887-4114
Fax: 859-887-4874
Website: http://www.playnsa.com
E-mail: nsahdqtrs@aol.com

PONY Baseball and Softball

International Headquarters
P.O. Box 225
Washington, PA 15301-0225
Phone: 724-225-1060
Fax: 724-225-9852
Website: http://www.pony.org
E-mail: pony@pony.org

USA Baseball Headquarters

P.O. Box 1131
Durham, NC 27702
Phone: 919-474-8721
Fax: 919-474-8822
Website: http://
www.usabaseball.com
E-mail: info@usabaseball.com

Basketball

Mid-America Youth Basketball

2309 S. Kansas
P.O. Box 348
Newton, KS 67114
Phone: 316-284-0354
Fax: 316-284-0294
Website: http://www.mayb.com
E-mail: mayb@mayb.com

National Junior Basketball

1500 S. Anaheim Blvd., Suite 200
Anaheim, CA 92805
Phone: 714-541-4450
Fax: 714-917-3566
Website: http://www.njbl.org
E-mail: info@njbl.org

Youth Basketball of America

10325 Orangewood Blvd.
Orlando, FL 32821
Phone: 407-363-9262
Fax: 407-363-0599
Website: http://www.yboa.org

Boating And Watercraft

American Canoe Association

7432 Alban Station Blvd.
Suite B-232
Springfield, VA 22150
Phone: 703-451-0141
Website: http://www.acanet.org

National Safe Boating Council

P.O. Box 509
Bristow, VA 20136
Phone: 703-361-4294
Fax: 703-361-5294
Website: http://
www.safeboatingcouncil.org
E-mail:
NSBCdirect@safeboatingcouncil.org

USA Canoe/Kayak

301 South Tryon Street, Suite 1750
Charlotte, NC 28282
Phone: 704-348-4330
Fax: 704-348-4418
Website: http://
www.usacanoekayak.org
E-mail: info@usack.org

Bicycling

Bicycle Helmet Safety Institute

4611 Seventh Street South
Arlington, VA 22204-1419
Phone: 703-486-0100
Website: http://www.helmets.org
E-mail: info@helmets.org

Pedestrian and Bicycle Information Center

730 Martin Luther Jr. Boulevard
Suite 300
Campus Box 3430
Chapel Hill, NC 27599-3430
Phone: 919-962-2203
Fax: 919-962-8710
Website: http://
www.bicyclinginfo.org
E-mail: pbic@pedbikeinfo.org

League of American Bicyclists

1612 K Street NW, Suite 800
Washington, DC 20006
Phone: 202-822-1333
Website: http://www.bikeleague.org
E-mail: bikeleague@bikeleague.org

USA Cycling

1 Olympic Plaza
Colorado Springs, CO 80909
Phone: 719-866-4581
Fax: 719-866-4628
Website: http://www.usacycling.org
E-mail: membership@usaccling.org

Cheerleading

American Cheerleading

Lifestyle Ventures LLC
250 West 57 Street
Suite 420
New York, NY 10107
Phone: 212-265-8890
Fax: 212-265-8908
Website: http://
www.americancheerleader.com

Varsity.com

6745 Lenox Center Court
Memphis, TN 38115
Toll-Free: 800-238-0286
Phone: 901-387-4358
Fax: 901-387-4357
Website:
http://www.varsity.com

Equestrian Activities

National Barrel Horse Association

P.O. Box 1988
Augusta, GA 30901
Phone: 706-722-7223
Fax: 706-722-9575
Website: http://www.nbha.com
E-mail: nbha@nbha.com

United States Dressage Foundation
4051 Iron Works Parkway
Lexington, KY 40511
Phone: 859-971-2277
Fax: 859-971-7722
Website: http://www.usdf.org
E-mail: events@usdf.org

United States Equestrian Federation
4047 Iron Works Parkway
Lexington, KY 40511
Phone: 859-258-2472
Fax: 859-231-6662
Website: http://www.usef.org

United States Pony Clubs, Inc.
4041 Iron Works Parkway
Lexington, KY 40511
Phone: 859-254-7669
Fax: 859-233-4652
Website: http://www.ponyclub.org
E-mail:
communications@ponyclub.org

US Equestrian Team (USET)
1040 Pottersville Road
P.O. Box 355
Gladstone, NJ 07934
Phone: 908-234-1251
Fax: 908-234-9417
Website: http://www.uset.org

Football
NFL for Kids
280 Park Avenue
New York, NY 10017
Website: http://www.playfootball.com

Pop Warner Little Scholars, Inc.
586 Middletown Blvd.
Suite C-100
Langhorne, PA 19047
Phone: 215-752-2691
Fax: 215-752-2879
Website: http://www.popwarner.com

Golf
Hook A Kid On Golf
2050 Vista Parkway
West Palm Beach, FL 33411
Toll-Free: 800-729-2057
Fax: 561-712-9887
Website: http://www.hookakidongolf.org
E-mail: info@hookakidongolf.org

Junior Links
USGA Foundation
Copper Building
1631 Mesa Ave.
Colorado Springs, CO 80906
Phone: 719-471-4810
Website: http://www.juniorlinks.com
E-mail: juniorlinks@usqa.org

U.S. Kids Golf
3040 Northwoods Parkway
Norcross, GA 30071
Toll-Free: 888-3-US KIDS
(888-387-5437)
Phone: 770-441-3077
Fax: 770-448-3069
Website:
http://www.uskidsgolf.com
E-mail:
customerservice@uskidsgolf.com

Gymnastics

International GYMNAST Magazine
P.O. Box 721020
Norman, OK 73070
Phone: 405-447-9988
Fax: 405-447-5810
Website:
http://www.intlgymnast.com
E-mail:
customerservice@intlgymnast.com

USA Gymnastics
201 S. Capitol Avenue
Suite 300
Indianapolis, IN 46225
Toll-Free: 800-345-4719
Phone: 317-237-5050
Fax: 317-237-5069
Website:
http://www.usa-gymnastics.org

Hockey

USA Hockey
1775 Bob Johnson Drive
Colorado Springs, CO 80906
Phone: 719-576-USAH (8724)
Fax: 719-538-1160
Website: http://
www.usahockey.com
E-mail: usah@usahockey.com

United States Field Hockey
1 Olympic Plaza
Colorado Springs, CO 80909-5773
Phone: 719-866-4567
Fax: 719-632-0979
Website: http://
www.usfieldhockey.com
E-mail: usfha@usafieldhockey.com

Racquet Sports

College and Junior Tennis
100 Harbor Road
Port Washington, NY 11050
Phone: 516-883-6601
Fax: 516-883-5241
Website: http://
www.clgandjrtennis.com
E-mail:
info@collegeandjuniortennis.com

U.S. Racquetball Association
1685 West Uintah
Colorado Springs, CO 80904
Phone: 719-635-5396
Website: http://www.usra.org

U.S. Tennis Association
70 West Red Oak Lane
White Plains, NY 10604
Phone: 914-696-7000
Website: http://www.usta.com

Skating

Aggressive Skaters Association
5855 Green Valley Circle
Suite 308
Culver City, CA 90230
Phone: 310-410-3020
Fax: 310-823-4146
Website: http://www.asaskate.com
E-mail: info@asaskate.com

U.S. Figure Skating
20 First Street
Colorado Springs, CO 80906
Phone: 719-635-5200
Fax: 719-635-9548
Website: http://www.usfsa.org
E-mail: info@usfigureskating.org

Soccer

American Youth Soccer Organization
12501 S. Isis Ave.
Hawthorne, CA 90250
Toll-Free: 800-872-2976
Fax: 310-643-5310
Website: http://soccer.org

CC United
P.O. Box 62
Cedar Park, TX 78613
Phone: 512-535-1177
Website: http://www.ccunited.com
E-mail: info@ccunited.com

Major League Soccer
420 5th, Floor 7
New York, NY 10018
Phone: 212-450-1200
Fax: 212-450-1305
Website: http://www.mlsnet.com

US Youth Soccer
9220 World Cup Way
Bristol, TX 75034
Toll-Free: 800-4SOCCER
Fax: 972-334-9960
Website: http://usysa.org
E-mail:
nationaloffice@usyouthsoccer.org

Swimming And Other Water Sports

Aquatic Exercise Association
201 Tamiami Trail S.
Suite 3
Nokomis, FL 34275
Toll-Free: 888-AEA-WAVE
Phone: 941-486-8600
Fax: 941-486-8820
Website: http://www.aeawave.com
E-mail: info@aeawave.com

Divers Alert Network (DAN)

The Peter B. Bennett Center
6 West Colony Place
Durham, NC 27705
Toll-Free: 800-446-2671
Fax: 919-490-6630
Diving Emergencies:
919-684-8111 (Remember to call
local EMS first, then DAN)
Website:
http://www.diversalertnetwork.org
E-mail:
dan@diversalertnetwork.org

Diving Medicine Online

31681 Shoal Water Drive
Ono Island, AL 36561
Phone: 251-980-1384
Fax: 309-424-2744
Website:
http://www.scuba-doc.com
E-mail: scubadoc@scuba-doc.com

National Scholastic Surfing Association

Mail: P.O. Box 495
Huntington Beach, CA 92648
Location: 10031 Dana Drive
Huntington Beach, CA 92646
Phone: 714-378-0899
Fax: 714-964-5232
Website: http://www.nssa.org

Surfrider Foundation

P.O. Box 6010
San Clemente, CA 92674-6010
Toll-Free: 800-743-SURF
Phone: 949-492-8170
Fax: 949-492-8142
Website: http://surfrider.org

Underwater Medicine Associates

P.O. Box 481
Bryn Mawr, PA 19010
Phone: 610-896-8806
Fax: 610-896-2883
Website:
http://www.scubamed.com

United States Diving, Inc.

201 S. Capitol Ave.
Suite 430
Indianapolis, IN 46225
Phone: 317-237-5252
Fax: 317-237-5257
Website: http://www.usadiving.org
E-mail: usdiving@usdiving.org

United States Synchronized Swimming

201 S. Capitol Ave.
Suite 901
Indianapolis, IN 46225
Phone: 317-237-5700
Fax: 317-237-5705
Website:
http://www.usasynchro.org

U.S. Swimming
One Olympic Plaza
Colorado Springs, CO 80909
Phone: 719-866-4578
Website: http://www.usswim.org

U.S. Water Polo
2124 Main Street, Suite 210
Huntington Beach, CA 92648
Phone: 714-500-5445
Website:
http://www.usawaterpolo.org

U.S.A. Water Ski
1251 Holy Cow Road
Polk City, FL 33868
Phone: 863-324-4341
Fax: 863-325-8259
Website: http://usawaterski.org
E-mail:
usawaterski@usawaterski.org

Volleyball

Starlings Volleyball Clubs, USA
P.O. Box 232416
Encinitas, CA 92023-2416
Phone: 760-230-1870
Fax: 760-230-1871
Website: http://www.starlings.org
E-mail: info@Starlings.org

United States Youth Volleyball League
2771 Plaza Del Amo
Suite 808
Torrance, CA 90503
Toll-Free: 888-988-7985
Phone: 310-643-8398
Fax: 310-212-7182
Website: http://www.volleyball.org
E-mail: volleyballorg@hotmail.com

USA Volleyball
715 South Circle Drive
Colorado Springs, CO 80910
Phone: 719-228-6800
Fax: 719-228-6899
Website:
http://www.usavolleyball.org
E-mail: postmaster@usav.org

Walking, Running, And Jumping

American Hiking Society
1422 Fenwick Lane
Silver Spring MD 20910
Phone: 301-565-6704
Fax: 301-565-6714
Website:
http://www.americanhiking.org
E-mail: info@americanhiking.org

American Running Association

4405 East West Highway
Suite 405
Bethesda, MD 20814
Toll-Free: 800-776-2732
Phone: 301-913-9517 (local)
Website:
http://www.americanrunning.org
E-mail: run@americanrunning.org

North American Racewalking Foundation

358 W. California Blvd., #110
Pasadena, CA 91105
Phone: 626-795-3243
Website:
http://www.philsport.com/narf
E-mail: narwf@sbcglobal.net

Road Runners Club of America

1501 Lee Highway
Suite 140
Arlington, VA 22209
Phone: 703-525-3890
Fax: 703-525-3891
Website: http://www.rrca.org
E-mail: office@rrca.org

U.S. Amateur Jump Rope Federation

P.O. Box 569
Huntsville, TX 77342-0569
Toll-Free: 800-225-8820
Phone: 936-295-3332
Fax: 936-295-3309
Website: http://www.usajrf.org

Weight Training And Wrestling

National Strength and Conditioning Association (NSCA)

1885 Bob Johnson Dr.
Colorado Springs, CO 80906
Toll-Free: 800-815-6862
Phone: 719-632-6722
Fax: 719-632-6367
Toll-Free: 800-815-6826
Website: http://www.nsca-lift.org
E-mail: nsca@nsca-lift.org

United States Girls Wrestling Association

3105 Hickory Ridge Lane
Ortonville, MI 48462
Phone: 248-627-8066
Fax: 248-627-8197
Website: http://www.usgwa.com

USA Wrestling
6155 Lehman Dr.
Colorado Springs, CO 80918
Phone: 719-598-8181
Fax: 719-598-9440
Website: http://www.themat.com

Winter Sports

National Ski Areas Association
133 S. Van Gordon St., Suite 300
Lakewood, CO 80228
Phone: 303-987-1111
Fax: 303-986-2345
Website: http://www.nsaa.org
E-mail: nsaa@nsaa.org

National Ski Patrol
133 S. Van Gordon St., Suite 100
Lakewood, CO 80228
Phone: 303-988-1111
Fax: 303-988-3005
Website: http://www.nsp.org

United States Ski and Snowboard Association
P.O. Box 100
Park City, UT 84060
Phone: 435-649-9090
Fax: 435-649-3613
Website: http://www.ussa.org
E-mail: webmaster@ussa.org
E-mail: info@ussa.org

U.S. Ski Team
P.O. Box 97254
Washington, DC 20077-7684
Toll-Free: 800-809-SNOW
Website: http://www.usskiteam.com

Index

Index

Page numbers that appear in *Italics* refer to illustrations. Page numbers that have a small 'n' after the page number refer to information shown as Notes at the beginning of each chapter. Page numbers that appear in **Bold** refer to information contained in boxes on that page (except Notes information at the beginning of each chapter).

A

AAD *see* American Academy of Dermatology
AAO-HNS *see* American Academy of Otolaryngology - Head and Neck Surgery
AAOMS *see* American Association of Oral and Maxillofacial Surgeons
AAOS *see* American Academy of Orthopaedic Surgeons
AAPMR *see* American Academy of Physical Medicine and Rehabilitation
AAPSM *see* American Academy of Podiatric Sports Medicine
abdominal crunches, snowboarding 341
accreditation *see* certification
ACE bandages *see* compression bandages
ACEP *see* American College of Emergency Physicians
Achilles tendon
  depicted *218*
  injuries 70
  problems overview 229–38
"Achilles Tendonitis" (Sports Injury Clinic) 229n

Achilles tendonitis (tendinitis)
  causes **230**
  described 253
  overview 229–32
  treatment **232**
"Achilles Tendon Rupture (Partial)" (Sports Injury Clinic) 229n
Achilles tendon rupture, overview 233–38
AC joint *see* acromioclavicular joint
Ackland Sports Medicine
  contact information 379
  contact sports equipment publication 315n
ACL *see* anterior cruciate ligament
acromioclavicular joint (AC joint)
  defined **161**
  depicted *160*
  described 160
acromion
  depicted *160*
  described 160–61
ACSM *see* American College of Sports Medicine
Action for Healthy Kids, contact information 387
activity cards
  basketball **322**
  cheerleading **326**

activity cards, continued
  football 316
  running 354
  soccer 321
  tennis 325
  volleyball 324
  walking 355
  yoga 329
activity modification, tennis elbow 174
acupressure, back pain management 154
acupuncture, back pain management
  153–54
acute back pain, treatment 147
acute fractures, described 70
acute injuries, described 72
acute strain, described 100
A.D.A.M., Inc., foot pain publication
  243n
Adams, Brian B. 293–96
ADHD see attention deficit hyperactivity
  disorder
AED see automated external defibrillators
aerobic capacity, fitness 59–60
aerobic exercise
  back pain management 148–49
  foot problems 247
  physical activity program 56
  snowboarding 339
aerobic response, described 59
Aerobics and Fitness Association of
  America, contact information 394
affective disorders, described 20–21
age factor
  rotator cuff injuries 162
  rotator cuff tears 168
  target heart rate 59
  tennis elbow 174
Aggressive Skaters Association, contact
  information 399
alcohol use
  athletic performance 26
  student athletes 26–27
  water sports safety 347
alternative activities, sports injuries 76
Amateur Athletic Union, contact
  information 387
Amateur Softball Association of America,
  contact information 394
amenorrhea, female athlete triad 36

American Academy of Dermatology (AAD)
  contact information 385
  skin infections publication 293n
American Academy of Orthopaedic
  Surgeons (AAOS)
  burners, stingers publication 155n
  contact information 379
American Academy of Otolaryngology -
  Head and Neck Surgery (AAO-HNS),
  contact information 384
American Academy of Physical Medicine
  and Rehabilitation (AAPMR), contact
  information 379
American Academy of Podiatric Sports
  Medicine (AAPSM), contact
  information 384
American Alliance for Health, Physical
  Education, Recreation and Dance,
  contact information 387
American Association of Oral and
  Maxillofacial Surgeons (AAOMS),
  contact information 384
American Board for Certification in
  Orthotics and Prosthetics, website
  address 380
American Canoe Association, contact
  information 395
American Cheerleading, contact
  information 396
American College of Emergency
  Physicians (ACEP)
  contact information 393
  emergency care publication 79n
  website address 84
American College of Foot and Ankle
  Surgeons, website address 385
American College of Sports Medicine
  (ACSM)
  contact information 380
  publications
    return to play guidelines 255n
    sports drinks 51n
American Council on Exercise, contact
  information 388
American Dental Association
  contact information 393
  publications
    dental emergencies 139n
    mouthguards 289n

American Dietetic Association, contact information 393
American Fitness Professionals and Associates, contact information 388
American Hiking Society, contact information 401
American Lung Association, contact information 393
American Orthopaedic Foot and Ankle Society (AOFAS)
  athletic shoes publication 301n
  contact information 385
American Orthopaedic Society for Sports Medicine, contact information 380
American Osteopathic Academy of Sports Medicine, contact information 380
American Physical Therapy Association (APTA)
  contact information 380
  publications
    fitness overview 57n
    physical therapists 89n
    physical therapy 90n
American Podiatric Medical Association, contact information 385
American Running Association
  contact information 402
  safety concerns publication 305n
American Shoulder and Elbow Surgeons, contact information 380
American Society for Surgery of the Hand (ASSH)
  contact information 385
  publications
    hand fractures 181n
    tennis elbow 173n
    thumb sprains 181n
    wrist sprains 181n
American Sports Medicine Institute (ASMI), contact information 380
American Tai Chi Association, contact information 394
American Youth Soccer Organization, contact information 399
amifostine 199
amphetamines, student athletes 27–28
ankle depicted 218
ankle exercises, snowboarding 341
ankle fractures, snowboarding 338

ankle ligaments, depicted 218
ankle sprain rehabilitation phases 223
ankle sprains
  degrees, described 219
  described 98–99
  overview 217–28
  prevention 227
  snowboarding 338
ankle supports, described 224
anterior compartment syndrome, described 215–16
anterior cruciate ligament (ACL)
  basketball 322
  depicted 206
  described 207
  knee injuries 69
  soccer 321
anterior inferior tibiofibular ligament, depicted 218
anterior talofibular ligament, depicted 218
antidepressant medications, back pain management 150
anxiety, stress management 17
anxiety disorders
  described 21–23
  statistics 21
AOFAS see American Orthopaedic Foot and Ankle Society
APTA see American Physical Therapy Association
"APTA Background Sheet 2007" (APTA) 89n
Aquatic Exercise Association, contact information 399
arch (foot) pain, described 254
arch support insoles, Achilles tendonitis 232
arrhythmogenic right ventricular dysplasia, sudden death 42
arthritis
  described 272
  knuckle cracking 272
arthrograms, shoulder problems 162–63
arthroscope, described 88
arthroscopy
  knee injuries 211–12
  orthopaedic surgery 87
  overview 88–89

articular cartilage
  depicted *206*
  knees 206
ASMI *see* American Sports Medicine
  Institute
"Assessment and Diagnosis of the Ankle
  Sprain" (Sports Injury Clinic) 217n
ASSH *see* American Society for
  Surgery of the Hand
athletes foot, described 296
athletic performance
  anxiety disorders 22–23
  depression 20–21
  disordered eating 24
  substance abuse **26**, 27–28
athletic shoes
  described 246–47
  overview 301–4
  women **304**
athletic supporters
  sports injury prevention 263
  testicular injury prevention 203–4
athletic trainers, overview 91–95
attention deficit hyperactivity disorder
  (ADHD), substance abuse 27
automated external defibrillators (AED)
  survival rate statistics **42**
  training **44**
axial extension exercise, described 172

B

back injuries, overview 141–54
back pain, spinal injuries *144*
balance fitness 61
ball and socket joints, described 272
ballet, safety considerations 327–28
"Ballet Activity Card" (BAM! [Body and
  Mind]) 327n
BAM! (Body and Mind)
  contact information 388
  publications
    heat, safety concerns 309n
    recreational activities safety 353n
    sports activity cards 315n, 323n, 327n
    water sports safety 343n
baseball, safety considerations 323
"Baseball Activity Card" (BAM!
  [Body and Mind]) 323n

"Basketball Activity Card" (BAM!
  [Body and Mind]) 315n
behavioral modification, back pain
  management 151
biceps muscles, described 271
Bicycle Helmet Safety Institute
  contact information 396
  helmet fit publication 279n
bicycling, safety considerations 355–58,
  356–57
"Bicycling Activity Card" (BAM!
  [Body and Mind]) 353n
bipolar disorder, described 20
bleeding, facial sports injuries 137
blisters, described 297–98
blood rule, described 77
board certification, emergency
  physicians 82–83
boarding, described 84
body balance, fitness 61
body composition, fitness 60–61
body image, female athlete triad 37
body structure, fitness 60
body temperature, brain signals **310**
bone density, exercise **118**
bone marrow, described 269
bones
  female athlete triad 36–37
  growth plates 193–94
  knees 206
  overview 267–69
  see also fractures; stress fractures
"Bones, Muscles, and Joints: The
  Musculoskeletal System" (Nemours
  Foundation) 267n
bone spurs, plantar fasciitis 239–42
boxers fracture, overview **188–89**
boys
  growth plate injuries **194**
  growth plates 268
braces
  back pain management 151
  tennis elbow 174
brachial plexus, described 155
brain damage
  head injuries **128**
  helmets 281
  see also concussion; traumatic brain injury

Brain Injury Association of America, contact information 393
breathing exercises, stress management 16
broken bones *see* fractures
"Broken Bones" (Nemours Foundation) 109n
bruises
  described 72
  facial sports injuries 136
buckle fracture, described 112
bunions, described 249–50
burners, overview 155–57
bursa
  depicted *160*
  described 209–10
  shoulder 161
bursitis
  described 209–10
  heel pain 252
  rotator cuff 165–66
  toe pain 249

C

caffeine, carbohydrate gels 54
calcaneofibular ligament
  ankle sprains 217
  depicted *218*
calcium
  bone fracture prevention 118
  bone health **110**
  bones 268
  sports nutrition 50
  stress fracture prevention 107
calf stretch exercise, snowboarding 339
calluses
  forefoot pain 250
  toe pain 248
cancellous bone, described 269
canoeing, safety considerations 348–49
"Canoeing/Kayaking Activity Card" (BAM! [Body and Mind]) 343n
capsule, defined **161**
carbohydrate gels, described 54
carbohydrate loading, described 46
carbohydrates
  eating disorders 24
  sports drinks 53
  sports nutrition 46–49

cardiac muscle, described 270
cardiopulmonary resuscitation, training **44**
cartilage
  bones 269
  knee injuries 69
  knee injury 209
  knees 206
  throat injuries 137–38
cartilaginous joints, described 271
casts
  bone fractures 113–15
  elbow fractures 178
  hand fractures 190
  overview 121–26
  plantar fasciitis **242**
  see also fractures
"Casts and Splints" (Center for Orthopaedics and Sports Medicine) 121n
CAT scan *see* computed axial tomography scan
CC United, contact information 399
Center for Nutrition Policy and Promotion, contact information 393
Center for Orthopaedics and Sports Medicine
  contact information 380
  publications
    casts 121n
    knee arthroscopy 88n
    orthopaedic surgery 85n
    plantar fasciitis 239n
Center for the Study of Sport in Society, contact information 388
central cord syndrome, described 71
cerebellum, muscles 271
certification
  athletic trainers 92–95
  emergency physicians 82–83
  physical therapists 89
certified athletic trainer, defined **93**
certified orthotists (CO), defined **86**
cervical spine, defined *153*
"Cervical Spine Fractures" (Parker) 141n
cervical spine fractures, described 145–47
cheerleading, safety considerations 326
"Cheerleading Activity Card" (BAM! [Body and Mind]) 323n
chest injuries, prevention **44**

child abuse
    emotional misconduct 31–35
    growth plate injuries 194
children
    foot pain **245**
    sports injuries **68**
Children, Youth and Women's Health
    Service, sports injuries publication 73n
chondrocytes, described 199
chondromalacia, described 209
"Choosing The Right Sport For You"
    (Nemours Foundation) 3n
chronic back pain, treatment 147–54
chronic injuries
    described 72
    thumbs 187
    wrists 183
chronic strains, described 100
chronic stress, described 17
cisplatin 199
clavicle (collarbone)
    depicted *160*
    described 160
    fracture, described **169**
Clinical Sports Medicine, contact
    information 381
closed fracture, described 112
CO *see* certified orthotists
Coalition to Prevent Sports Eye Injuries,
    contact information 384
cocaine, student athletes 27–28
cold, growth plate injuries 194
cold-related safety considerations 311–13
cold therapy
    Achilles tendonitis **232**
    Achilles tendon rupture 234
    back pain management 148
collarbone *see* clavicle
College and Junior Tennis, contact
    information 398
comminuted fracture, described 113, 189
commotio cordis, described **44**
communication, coaches 18
compact bone, described 269
compartment syndrome, described 69
complementary and alternative medicine
    (CAM), back pain management 152–54
compound fracture, described 112, 189

compression
    ankle sprains 218, 225
    defined **101**
    return to play guidelines 256
    spinal cord injury 71
    sports injuries 75
compression bandages, knee injuries 211
computed axial tomography scan (CAT
    scan; CT scan)
    concussion 130
    growth plate injuries 196
    knee injuries 210
concussion
    brain damage **128**
    described 71, 76–77
    healing time **131**
    overview 127–31
"Concussions" (Nemours Foundation) 127n
congenital coronary artery anomalies,
    sudden death 41
Consumer Product Safety Commission
    (CPSC) *see* US Consumer Product
    Safety Commission
contact sports
    burners, stingers 156
    severe injuries **72**
    strains 100
contusions
    described 71
    facial sports injuries 136
cooling down, overview 277–78
Cooper Institute, contact information 388
coracoacromial arch, swimmer's shoulder
    170–71
Core Centers for Musculoskeletal
    Disorders, described **198**
corns, toe pain 248
correct walking, described 244
corsets, back pain management 151
counseling, female athlete triad 39
COX-2 inhibitors, back pain
    management 150
CPSC *see* US Consumer Product
    Safety Commission
cross-training activities, described 7–8
crutches
    guidelines **123**
    plantar fasciitis **242**
CT scan *see* computed axial tomography scan
custom fabricated orthosis, defined **86**

D

DAN *see* Divers Alert Network
deep breathing, stress management 16
dehydration
    eating disorders 24
    exercise 47–48
delayed onset muscle soreness, described 336–37
dental emergencies
    mouth guards 289–91
    overview 139–40
"Dental Emergencies and Injuries" (American Dental Association) 139n
Department of Labor (DOL) *see* US Department of Labor
depression
    alcohol use 26
    described 20–21
Diabetes Exercise and Sports, contact information 393
diet and nutrition
    bone health 110
    muscle building 46, 49
    skipping meals 40
    see also eating disorders; sports nutrition
dietitians, female athlete triad 39
disabilities, fitness program 63
disc, defined *153*
"Discovering Physical Therapy" (APTA) 90n
disk herniation, described 143
dislocations
    described 71
    knee injury 209
    shoulder problems 163–64
disordered eating
    described 23–24
    female athlete triad 36
displaced fracture, described 113
distress, described 16
Divers Alert Network (DAN), contact information 400
diving, safety considerations 347–48
"Diving Activity Card" (BAM! [Body and Mind]) 343n
Diving Medicine Online, contact information 400
dog attacks, responses 307

DOL *see* US Department of Labor
doorway stretch, described 172
doxorubicin 199
dual energy x-ray absorptiometry (DXA), overweight youths 119
DXA *see* dual energy x-ray absorptiometry
dynamic double leg jumpovers, described 335

E

eating disorders
    described 23–24
    female athlete triad 36, 38
    statistics 23
EKG *see* electrocardiogram
elbow fractures, healing strategies 176
elbow injuries
    described 100
    overview 173–79
    tennis 325
electrocardiogram (EKG)
    mitral valve prolapse 42
    sports physicals 11
electrolytes, carbohydrate gels 54
elevation
    ankle sprains 218–20, 225
    defined 101
    return to play guidelines 256
    sports injuries 75
emergency action plans, athletic events 44
emergency departments
    described 79
    skateboarding injuries 280
    sports injury statistics *366, 368*
emergency medicine
    described 81
    overview 79–84
emotional abuse, described 31–32
"Emotional Injuries" (NYSSF) 31n
emotional injuries, overview 31–34
energy bars, described 54–55
ephedrine, student athletes 27–28
epiphyseal plate, described 193
epiphysis, defined 196
ePodiatry.com, website address 385
ergogenic, described 26, 28
ergolytic, described 28
esophagus, described 137

estrogen
  amenorrhea 36
  osteoporosis 36
eustress, described 16
exercise
  aerobic capacity 59
  ankle sprains 227
  back pain management 148
  bone fracture prevention **118**
  casts 124
  physical activity program **56**
  skin disorders 299
"Exercise Caution" (American Running
  Association) 305n
exercises
  Achilles tendon rupture 235
  feet 244
  snowboarding 339–41
  stress management 16–17
  stretches 277
  swimmer's shoulder 172
  winter sports 333–41
Exrx.net, website address 388
extension exercises, back pain management
  148
extensors, described 271
eye protection
  basketball 322
  described **288**
  overview 285–88
  polycarbonate lenses **262, 286,** 288
  sports injury prevention 262

F

facet joint injections, back pain
  management 151
facial sports injuries
  overview 133–38
  prevention **138**
"The FACTS about Certified Athletic
  Trainers and the National Athletic
  Trainers' Association" (NATA) 92n
fall sports, school calendar **4**
fascia, described 69
"Fast Facts about Sports Nutrition"
  (President's Council on Physical Fitness
  and Sports) 45n
fatigue, sports drinks 52–53

feet *see* foot
female athletes, quick tips **40**
"Female Athlete Triad" (Nemours
  Foundation) 35n
female athlete triad, overview 35–40
Female Athlete Triad Coalition, contact
  information 384
femur, described 206
fibrous joints, described 271
figure skating, safety considerations **337**
financial considerations
  sports eyeguards **288**
  sports injuries 365, 367–68
finger fractures, depicted *190, 191*
first aid
  ankle sprains 218–20
  cervical spine fractures 146
  drowning victims **345**
  emergencies 80–81
  emergency supplies **134**
  facial sports injuries 133–34
  fractures 111–12
  hypothermia 312–13
  lightning strikes 314
  overview 73–77
  training options **75**
  wrist fractures **185**
fishing, safety considerations 346
"Fishing Activity Card" (BAM!
  [Body and Mind]) 343n
fitness
  defined **58**
  overview 57–64
"Fitness: A Way of Life" (APTA) 57n
fitness trainers, *versus* athletic trainers 92
"Fitting Hockey Equipment" (Ackland
  Sports Medicine) 315n
flat feet
  described 254
  shin splints 70
flexibility, fitness 61
flexibility training, physical activity
  program **56**
flexion exercises, back pain management
  148
flexors, described 271
foot
  depicted **240**
  force exerted **254**

football, activity card **316**
"Football Activity Card" (BAM! [Body and Mind]) 315n
foot infections, described 295–96
foot injuries
  overview 243–54
  RICE therapy **244**
"Foot Pain: In-Depth Report" (A.D.A.M., Inc.) 243n
foot warts, described 295–96
footwear
  overview 245–47
  sports injury prevention 263
forefoot pain
  described 243–44
  overview 250–51
fracture callus, described 192
fractures (broken bones)
  back injury 144
  cervical spine 145–47
  clavicle **169**
  defined **74**
  described 70–71, 272–73
  elbows 177–79
  facial sports injuries 137
  growth plates 194
  hands 188–92
  knee injury 209
  overview 109–19
  shoulders 168–70
  surgical repairs **116–17**
  thumbs 187
  wrists 183, **184–85**
  see also casts; splints
friends, female athlete triad 39–40
Frisbee, safety considerations 360
"Frisbee Activity Card" (BAM! [Body and Mind]) 353n
frostbite prevention 311–13, **312**
fructose, sports drinks 53
fruit, exercise 55
furunculosis, described 295

G

galactose, sports drinks 53
Gatorade Sports Science Institute, contact information 385

Geisinger Sports Medicine, contact information 381
gender factor
  concussions 128
  eating disorders **23**
  growth plate fractures **194**
  stress fractures 106
gene therapy, growth plate injury research 199
genetics see heredity
"Getting Ready for That Ski Trip" (Nicholas Institute of Sports Medicine and Athletic Trauma) 333n
girls
  anterior cruciate ligament injuries **206**
  concussions 128
  growth plate injuries **194**
  growth plates 268
  see also female athlete triad
glenohumeral joint
  depicted *160*
  described 160–61
glenoid
  described 160–61
  swimmer's shoulder 170
glucose
  sports drinks 53
  sports nutrition 46–47
glycemic index, energy bars 55
glycogen, sports nutrition 46–48
golf
  safety considerations 359–60
  stretching exercises **358–59**
"Golf Activity Card" (BAM! [Body and Mind]) 353n
greenstick fracture, described 112
growth plate injuries
  overview 193–99
  statistics **194**
  stress fractures 106
growth plates, described 141, 193, 268
  see also epiphyseal plate; physis
gymnastics, safety considerations 328
"Gymnastics Activity Card" (BAM! [Body and Mind]) 327n

H

"H2O Smarts" (BAM! [Body and Mind]) 343n

Haglund deformity, described 253
hairline fracture, described 113
hallus valgus, described 250
hamstring, described 207
hamstring strengthening exercise 335–36, 339
"Hand Fractures" (American Society for Surgery of the Hand) 181n
hand fractures, overview 188–92
"Handling Sports Pressure and Competition" (Nemours Foundation) 15n
"Handout on Health: Back Pain" (NIAMS) 141n
"Handout on Health: Sports Injuries" (NIAMS) 67n
hazard screening reports
  sports activities 367–69
  sports equipment 367–69
  team sports 365–67
"Hazard Screening Report: Sports Activities and Equipment (Excluding Major Team Sports)" (CPSC) 365n
"Hazard Screening Report: Team Sports" (CPSC) 365n
HCM see hypertrophic cardiomyopathy
head injuries
  brain damage 128
  helmets 280
health care teams, overview 85–95
"Heart Disease in the Young Athlete" (Pescasio) 41n
heart disorders
  commotio cordis 44
  death statistics 42
  sudden death 41–44
heat-related safety considerations 309–11
heat treatment, back pain management 148
heel pads, Achilles tendonitis 232
heel pain, overview 251–53
heel spur syndrome see plantar fasciitis
helmets
  concussion prevention 131
  football 315–16
  hockey 317–18
  myths 280
  overview 279–84
  proper fit 282
  skateboarding 332, 332

helmets, continued
  skating 331
  sports injury prevention 261–62
hematoma, described 71
heredity
  bunions 249
  growth plate injuries 195
  sudden death 41–43
herniated disc, defined 153
herpes simplex, described 294
high arches, described 254
high heels, Achilles tendonitis 230
hiking
  described 6
  safety considerations 353–54
"Hiking Activity Card" (BAM! [Body and Mind]) 353n
hindfoot pain, described 244
hinge joints, described 272
hollow foot see high arches
Hook A Kid On Golf, contact information 397
hormone supplements, female athlete triad 39
Hospital for Special Surgery
  contact information 381
  overuse injuries publication 105n
hospitalizations
  bone fractures 117
  concussion 130
  emergency departments 82
"How to Fit a Bicycle Helmet" (Bicycle Helmet Safety Institute) 279n
"How to Fit Football Equipment" (Ackland Sports Medicine) 315n
Hughston Sports Medicine Foundation
  contact information 381
  spinal injuries publication 141n
Human Kinetics, contact information 388
humerus
  defined 161
  depicted 160
  described 160
  swimmer's shoulder 170–71
hydration, physical activity 311
  see also water consumption
hypertrophic cardiomyopathy (HCM), described 41
hypothermia prevention 311–13, 312

I

ice
  Achilles tendonitis 231
  Achilles tendon rupture 236
  ankle sprains 218, 224–25
  defined 101
  return to play guidelines 256
  shin splints 215
  shoulder dislocations 164
  shoulder separations 165
  sports injuries 74–75
  testicular injuries 202
IDEA Health and Fitness Association,
  contact information 389
iEmily.com, website address 389
immovable joints, described 271
impetigo, described 294
impingement syndrome
  described 166
  swimmer's shoulder 170
infraspinatus stretch, described 172
ingrown toenails, described 249
injections, back pain management 151–52
"Inline Skating Activity Card" (BAM!
  [Body and Mind]) 331n
Institute for Arthroscopy and Sports
  Medicine, contact information 381
Institute for Preventative Sports Medicine,
  contact information 381
International GYMNAST Magazine,
  contact information 398
International Health, Racquet and
  Sportsclub Association, contact
  information 389
International Sports Sciences Association,
  contact information 389
intervertebral disks
  described 141
  herniation 143
inversion injury, described 99
involuntary muscle, described 270
iron, sports nutrition 50

J

joggers nipples 299
joggers toe 299
jogging see running

joints, overview 271–72
jumpers knee, basketball 322
jump rope, safety considerations 360
"Jump Rope Activity Card" (BAM! [Body
  and Mind]) 353n
Junior Links, contact information 397

K

kayaking, safety considerations 348–49
"Keeping Your Cool" (BAM! Body and
  Mind) 309n
knee, depicted 206
"Knee Arthroscopy" (Center for
  Orthopaedics and Sports Medicine)
  88n
knee cap see patella
knee injuries
  described 68–69
  overview 205–13
  winter sports 335
"Knee Injuries" (Nemours Foundation)
  205n
knee ligaments, depicted 206
knee problems
  basketball 322
  prevention 213
knuckle cracking, arthritis 272
kyphoplasty, defined 153

L

labels, energy bars 54
lacerations, spinal cord injury 71
laminectomy, defined 153
larynx, described 137
lateral collateral ligament (LCL)
  depicted 206
  described 207
  knee injuries 69
lateral epicondylitis see tennis elbow
latissimus dorsi stretch, described 172
Lazarus, Richard 31
LCL see lateral collateral ligament
League of American Bicyclists, contact
  information 396
levator scapulae stretch, described 172
life expectancy, physical activity 51
lifestyles, fitness programs 62–63

ligaments
  ankle sprains 217, *218*
  back injury 143
  bones 269
  defined **175**
  knees 207–8
  shoulder 161
  sprains 97
  thumb injuries 186–87
  wrist sprains 181–85, *182*
lightning-related injuries 313–14
Lintner, David 176
Little League Baseball International,
  contact information 394
little league elbow, overview 175–77
long QT syndrome, sudden death 42
lumbar spine, defined *153*

M

magnetic resonance imaging (MRI)
  Achilles tendonitis 232
  burners, stingers 157
  concussion 130
  growth plate injuries 196
  knee injuries 210
  shoulder problems 163, 167
  sprains 100
  tarsal tunnel syndrome 254
Major League Soccer, contact
  information 399
maltodextrin
  carbohydrate gels 54
  sports drinks 53
"Managing Student-Athletes' Mental
  Health Issues" (Thompson; Sherman)
  19n, 25n
manipulation, back pain management
  152
Marfan syndrome, sudden death 42
marijuana, student athletes 28
martial arts, safety considerations 328–29
"Martial Arts Activity Card" (BAM!
  [Body and Mind]) 327n
MCL *see* medial collateral ligament
medial collateral ligament (MCL)
  depicted *206*
  described 207
  knee injuries 69

medical history
  described 9–10
  female athlete triad 38
  rotator cuff disease 166
  shoulder problems 162
  sudden death prevention 43
medications
  acute back pain 147
  chronic back pain 149–50
  growth plate injuries 194–95
  rotator cuff disease 166
  side effects *150*
  substance abuse 27–28
  tennis elbow 174
meniscal tears, knee injury 209
meniscus
  depicted *206*
  knee injuries 69
  knees 206
menstruation
  female athlete triad 36
  record keeping **40**
mental health issues, sports 19–24
metabolic disease, growth plate injuries 195
metaphysis, defined **196**
methotrexate 199
Mid-America Youth Basketball, contact
  information 395
mild concussion, described 76–77
mindfulness, stress management 17
minerals, sports nutrition 49–50
misoprostol 199
mitral valve prolapse (MVP), sudden
  death 42
mood disorders, described 20–21
Morton neuroma, described 250
Moseley, C. 155b
mountain biking, safety considerations
  356–57
mouth guards
  basketball 322
  hockey 318
  overview 289–91
  proper care **290**
  soccer 321
  sports injury prevention 262
"Mouthguards: Frequently Asked
  Questions (FAQ)" (American Dental
  Association) 289n

MRI *see* magnetic resonance imaging
muscle building, protein supplements **46, 49**
muscle groups, stretching routines **276**
muscle relaxants, back pain management 150
muscle relaxation, stress management 16
muscles
    delayed soreness 336–37
    knees 207
    overview 269–71
    strains 97
muscular dystrophy, described 273
muscular flexibility, fitness 61
muscular strength, fitness 62
musculoskeletal system
    described **268**
    sports injuries 67–68
MVP *see* mitral valve prolapse
myocarditis, sudden death 42

N

nasal injuries, described 136–37
NASM *see* National Academy of Sports Medicine
NATA *see* National Athletic Trainers Association
National Academy of Sports Medicine (NASM), contact information 381
National Alliance for Youth Sports, contact information 389
National Association for Fitness Certification, contact information 389
National Association of Anorexia Nervosa and Associated Disorders, Inc., contact information 393
National Athletic Trainers Association (NATA)
    contact information 389
    publications
        certified athletic trainers 92n
        lightning-related injuries 309n
"National Athletic Trainers' Association (NATA) Offers Guidelines on How to Prevent Lightning-Related Injuries" (NATA) 309n
National Barrel Horse Association, contact information 396

National Center for Injury Prevention and Control, contact information 381
National Center for Sports Safety, contact information 382
National Center on Physical Activity and Disability, contact information 390
National Coalition for Promoting Physical Activity, contact information 390
National Collegiate Athletic Association (NCAA)
    contact information 390
    sports medicine handbook publication 371n
National Eating Disorders Association, contact information 393
National Heart, Lung, and Blood Institute (NHLBI), contact information 390
National High School Athletic Coaches Association, contact information 390
National Institute of Arthritis and Musculoskeletal and Skin Diseases (NIAMS)
    contact information 382, 385
    Core Centers for Musculoskeletal Disorders, described **198**
    publications
        back pain 141n
        growth plate injuries 193n
        shoulder problems 159n
        sports injuries 67n
        sprains, strains 97n
National Institute of Diabetes and Digestive and Kidney Diseases (NIDDK)
    contact information 393
National Institute on Drug Abuse (NIDA), contact information 386
National Junior Basketball, contact information 395
National Safe Boating Council, contact information 395
National SAFE KIDS Campaign, contact information 390
National Safety Council
    contact information 390
    helmets publication 279n
National Safety Council (NSC), cold, safety concerns publication 309n
National Scholastic Surfing Association, contact information 400

National Ski Areas Association, contact information 403

National Ski Patrol, contact information 403

National Softball Association (NSA), contact information 394

National Strength and Conditioning Association, contact information 391

National Strength and Conditioning Association (NSCA), contact information 402

National Youth Sports Safety Foundation (NYSSF), emotional injuries publication 31n

NCAA *see* National Collegiate Athletic Association

neck injuries
    facial sports injuries 137
    overview 141–54

Nemours Foundation
    Center for Children's Health Media, contact information 391
    publications
        competition coping strategies 15n
        concussions 127n
        exercise safety 261n
        fractures 109n
        knee injuries 205n
        musculoskeletal system 267n
        sports choices 3n
        sports physicals 9n
        stretching 275n
        testicular injuries 201n

nerve root blocks, back pain management 151

nerves, burners, stingers 155–57, *156*

nervousness *see* anxiety disorders

neurological disorders, growth plate injuries 195

neuromas, forefoot pain 250

"New Athletic Shoe Components and Design May Enhance Performance" (AOFAS) 301n

Newport Orthopedic Institute, contact information 382

NFL for Kids, contact information 397

NHLBI *see* National Heart, Lung, and Blood Institute

NIAMS *see* National Institute of Arthritis and Musculoskeletal and Skin Diseases

Nicholas Institute of Sports Medicine and Athletic Trauma
    contact information 382
    winter sports safety publication 333n

NIDA *see* National Institute on Drug Abuse

NIDDK *see* National Institute of Diabetes and Digestive and Kidney Diseases

night splints, Achilles tendonitis **232**

non-displaced fracture, described 113

nonsteroidal anti-inflammatory drugs (NSAID)
    Achilles tendon rupture 234
    back pain management 149–50
    bunions 249
    foot injuries 247
    side effects *150*

North American Racewalking Foundation, contact information 402

North American Spine Society, contact information 386

nosebleeds, facial sports injuries 137

NSA *see* National Softball Association

NSAID *see* nonsteroidal anti-inflammatory drugs

NSC *see* National Safety Council

NSCA *see* National Strength and Conditioning Association

nutrition *see* diet and nutrition

nutritionists, described **40**

NYSSF *see* National Youth Sports Safety Foundation

O

Occupational Outlook Handbook (DOL) 91n

OCD *see* osteochondritis desiccans

open fracture, described 112, 189

orthopaedic surgery, overview 85–88

"Orthopaedic Surgery: What Is It?" (Center for Orthopaedics and Sports Medicine) 85n

orthopaedists
    knee injuries 211–12
    knee problems **210**

orthosis, defined **86–87**

Orthosports, contact information 382

orthotic insoles, Achilles tendonitis **232**

orthotics
    athletic shoes 246
    defined **87**
    tarsal tunnel syndrome 254
orthotists, defined **87**
Osgood-Schlatter disease, described 210, 273
ossification, described 268
osteoblasts, described 268
osteochondritis desiccans (OCD),
    described 209
osteoclasts, described 268
osteocytes, described 268
osteomyelitis, described 273
osteoporosis
    calcium 118
    described 273
    female athlete triad 36–37
    spinal injuries *144*
overpronation, Achilles tendonitis **230**
overuse injuries
    Achilles tendonitis **230**
    knee injury 208
    overview 105–7
    swimmer's shoulder 171
"Overuse Injuries in Adolescent Athletes"
    (Hospital for Special Surgery) 105n
overweight, bone fracture risk **119**

P

pain
    feet 243–44
    spinal injuries *144*
pain management
    back injury 147–54
    elbow fractures **176**
    fractured clavicle **169**
    weight control **119**
Paralyzed Veterans of America (PVA),
    contact information 386
parental misconduct, described 33–34
Parker, Lawrence 141n
PAR-Q *see* physical activity readiness
    questionnaire
pars interarticularis, described 143
patella, described 206, 207
patellar tendon
    depicted *206*
    described 207

PCL *see* posterior cruciate ligament
PE Central, contact information 391
Pedestrian and Bicycle Information Center,
    contact information 396
pentoxifylline 199
periods *see* amenorrhea; menstruation
periosteum, described 269
personal trainers
    versus athletic trainers 92
    defined **93**
Pescasio, Michele D. 41n
Phillips, Scott B. 297–99
philosophical abuse, described 32–33
physical activity
    benefits 51
    water consumption **311**
physical activity program, described **56**
physical activity readiness questionnaire
    (PAR-Q) 51–52
physical examinations
    concussion 130
    described 10–11
    emergency departments 84
    female athlete triad 38–39
    knee injuries 210
    rotator cuff disease 166
    shoulder problems 162
    shoulder separations 165
    versus sports physicals 13
    sudden death prevention 43
    testicular injuries **203**
physical limitations, rest information **107**
physical therapists (PT)
    fitness program **63**
    fitness recommendations 57–58
    overview 89–91
physical therapy (PT)
    knee injuries 212
    overview 90–91
    plantar fasciitis **242**
    plantar fasciitis recovery **242**
    tennis elbow 174
physicians
    back pain *145*
    emergency medicine 79–83
    knee problems **210**
    orthopaedic surgery 85–88
    sports physicals 11–13
    stress fractures 106

physis (physes)
defined **196**
described 141, 193
Pilates, described 7
Pilates Method Alliance, contact
information 394
pitted keratolysis, described 295
pivot joints, described 272
"Plantar Fasciitis" (Center for
Orthopaedics and Sports Medicine)
239n
plantar fasciitis (heel spur syndrome)
described 252
overview 239–42
plantar verruca, described 295–96
pollution, exercise safety 307–8
PONY Baseball and Softball, contact
information 395
Pop Warner Little Scholars, Inc., contact
information 397
postconcussion syndrome, described **131**
posterior cruciate ligament (PCL)
depicted *206*
described 208
knee injuries 69
posterior inferior tibiofibular ligament,
depicted *218*
posterior talofibular ligament, depicted *218*
posterior tibial shin splints, described 215
posterior tibial tendon dysfunction
(PTTD), described 254
posture, fitness 60
PPE *see* preparticipation physical
examination
prefabricated orthosis, defined **87**
preparticipation physical examination
(PPE)
defined **10**
overview 9–13
prescription glasses, polycarbonate
lenses **262, 286**
President's Challenge, contact
information 391
President's Council on Physical
Fitness and Sports
contact information 391
sports nutrition publication 45n
pressure situations, sports
participation 15–18

Prevent Blindness America
contact information 384
sports eye safety publication 285n
"Preventing Frostbite and Hypothermia"
(NSC) 309n
prolotherapy, back pain management 152
pronation
athletic shoes 304
described 253
proprioception, ankle sprains 220, 226,
227
protective equipment
facial sports injuries prevention 133
football 315–17
heart disorders **44**
hockey 317–21
snowboarding 338
soccer 321
sports injury prevention 261–63
"Protect Yourself ... Wear a Helmet"
(National Safety Council) 279n
protein
bone health **110**
eating disorders 24
energy bars 55
muscle building **46, 49**
psychological problems, student
athletes 19
PT *see* physical therapists; physical therapy
PTTD *see* posterior tibial tendon
dysfunction
puberty, physical examinations 11
PVA *see* Paralyzed Veterans of America

Q

quadriceps, described 207
quadriceps stretch exercise
described 334
snowboarding 339
quadriceps tendon
depicted *206*
described 207
"Questions and Answers about Growth
Plate Injuries" (NIAMS) 193n
"Questions and Answers about Shoulder
Problems" (NIAMS) 159n
"Questions and Answers About Sprains
and Strains" (NIAMS) 97n

R

radial collateral ligament (RCL)
  depicted *186*
  thumb sprains 187
radiation, growth plate injuries 194–95
RCL *see* radial collateral ligament
"Recommended Sports Eye Protectors"
  (Prevent Blindness America) 285n
recovery time
  fractures 115–16
  stress fractures 107
  tennis elbow 175
reduction, shoulder dislocations 164
Christopher Reeve Foundation and
  Resource Center, contact information 386
"Rehabilitation (Sprained Ankle)" (Sports
  Injury Clinic) 217n
rehabilitation, sprains 102–3
relaxation techniques, stress
  management 16–17
repetitive stress
  back injury 143
  Osgood-Schlatter disease 210
repetitive stress injuries, described 273
resistance training, bone density **118**
rest
  Achilles tendonitis 231
  Achilles tendon rupture 234
  ankle sprains 218, 224
  defined **101**
  return to play guidelines 256
  shin splints 215–16
  shoulder dislocations 164
  shoulder separations 165
  sports injuries 74
resting heart rate, fitness 60
"Return to Play" (ACSM) 255n
return to play guidelines
  Achilles tendon rupture 236
  overview 255–57
  tissue damage **256**
RICE therapy
  Achilles tendon rupture 233
  ankle sprains 218–20
  defined **101**
  described 74–75
  foot injuries **244**, 248
  knee injuries 211
  return to play guidelines 256

ringworm (tinea corporis gladiatorum),
  described 295
Road Runners Club of America, contact
  information 402
rock climbing, described 6
roid rage (slang) 29
Rolfing, back pain management 154
rotator cuff, described 161, 162
rotator cuff diseases, described 165–66
rotator cuff tears, described 166–67
rotator cuff tendons, depicted *160*
rules, sports injury prevention 265–66
running
  safety concerns **354**
  shin splints 70

S

safety considerations
  basketball 321–22
  contact sports 315–22
  exercise venues 305–8
  eye protection **286**
  figure skating **337**
  sledding **340**
  sports physicals 13
  tobogganing **340**
  water parks **344**
  water sports 343–51
  weather risks 309–14
  winter sports 333–41, **334**, **337**
Safe USA, contact information 391
scapholunate ligament
  depicted *182*
  wrist sprains 181
scapula (shoulder blade)
  depicted *160*
  described 160
Scheuermann disease, described 144
school calendar, organized sports 4
SCI *see* spinal cord injury
scoliosis, described 274
scrotum, described 201
segmental fracture, described 113
"Selecting and Effectively Using Sports
  Drinks, Carbohydrate Gels, and Energy
  Bars" (ACSM) 51n
"Selecting Athletic Shoes" (AOFAS) 301n
selenium 199

separation, shoulder problems 164–65
sesamoiditis, forefoot pain 251
Shape Up America!, contact information 391
Sherman, Roberta Trattner 19n, 25n
shin splints
    causes **216**
    described 69–70
    overview 215–16
shockwave treatment, tennis elbow 175
shoes
    foot injuries **244**
    overview 245–47, 301–4
shoulder, depicted *160*
shoulder blade *see* scapula
shoulder immobilizer, described 164
shoulder injuries, overview 159–72
shoulder joint *see* glenohumeral joint
side effects
    anxiety disorders 22–23
    depression 20–21
    eating disorders 24
single fracture, described 113
skateboarding
    helmets **332**
    safety considerations 332
"Skateboarding Activity Card" (BAM! [Body and Mind]) 331n
skating, safety considerations 331
skeletal muscles, described 269–70
skiers thumb, described 187
skin disorders, overview 293–99
skin infections, described 294–95
slant boards, Achilles tendonitis **232**
slipped vertebral apophysis, described 143
Smart Play, contact information 391
smooth muscle, described 270
Snell Memorial Foundation, contact information 392
snorkeling, safety considerations 346–47
"Snorkeling Activity Card" (BAM! [Body and Mind]) 343n
snowboarding, safety considerations 337–41
"Snowboarding Injuries and General Conditioning" (Nicholas Institute of Sports Medicine and Athletic Trauma) 333n
"Soccer Activity Card" (BAM! [Body and Mind]) 315n

sodium, bone health **110**
softball, safety considerations 323–24
"Softball Activity Card" (BAM! [Body and Mind]) 323n
soleus stretch, described 334
Southern California Orthopedic Institute, contact information 382
SPARK, contact information 392
specialists
    ankle sprains 220
    back pain *145*
Special Olympics, contact information 392
SPF *see* sun protection factor
spinal canal, burners, stingers 156
spinal cord injury (SCI), described 71
Spinal Cord Society, contact information 386
spinal injuries, overview 141–54
"Spinal Injuries in Adolescent Athletes" (Parker) 141n
spine
    depicted *142*
    parts, defined *153*
Spine University, website address 386
splints
    bone fractures 113–15
    hand fractures 190
    overview 121–26
    see also fractures
spondylolisthesis
    defined *153*
    described 143
spondylolysis, described 143
"Sporting Injuries - Treating Them" (Children, Youth and Women's Health Service) 73n
"Sports and Exercise Safety" (Nemours Foundation) 261n
sports drinks
    described 48
    overview 51–53
"Sports Eye Safety" (Prevent Blindness America) 285n
sports injuries
    children **68**
    overview 67–72
    prevention overview 261–66
    statistics 365, 367–68
    statistics overview 371–78

Sports Injury Clinic
  publications
    Achilles tendon problems 229n
    ankle sprains 217n
  website address 382
sports nutrition, overview 45–50
  see also diet and nutrition
sports physicals
  frequency 12
  honest answers 11
  overview 9–13
"Sports Physicals" (Nemours Foundation) 9n
Sports Science Orthopaedic Clinic, contact
  information 382
"Sprained Ankle/Ankle Sprain" (Sports
  Injury Clinic) 217n
sprains
  ankle injuries 217–28
  common sites 98
  defined 74
  described 274
  knee injuries 208
  medical care 99
  overview 97–100, 103
  spinal injuries 144
  sports injuries 68
spring sports, school calendar 4
squats, snowboarding 339
Starlings Volleyball Clubs, USA, contact
  information 401
statistics
  alcohol use 26
  anabolic steroids use 29
  ankle sprains re-injury 227
  anterior cruciate ligament injuries 206
  anxiety disorders 21
  eating disorders 23
  emergency departments 81
  emotional abuse 33
  growth plate injuries 194
  heart disease deaths 42
  helmet safety 280–81
  knee injuries 68
  marijuana use 28
  shoulder injuries 159
  sports injuries 365, 366, 367–68, 368,
    373–78
  stimulant use 27
  sudden death 41

steroids
  Achilles tendonitis 231
  back pain management 151
  described 77
  student athletes 29
  tennis elbow 175
stimulant use, student athletes 27–28
stingers, overview 155–57
strains
  defined 74
  described 274
  knee injuries 208
  overview 100–103
  sports injuries 68
strength
  fitness 62
  sports injuries 76
strength training
  benefits 6
  physical activity program 56
stress, female athlete triad 37
stress fractures
  aerobic exercise 247
  defined 74
  described 70–71
  forefoot pain 251
  overview 105–7
stress management
  quick tips 17, 18
  sports participation 15–18
stressors, described 16
stretching
  back pain management 148
  ballet 327
  golf 358–59
  overview 276–77
"Stretching" (Nemours Foundation) 275n
stretching routines, muscle groups 276
substance abuse
  athletic performance 26, 27–28
  overview 25–29
sucrose, sports drinks 53
sudden death, overview 41–44
suicidal thoughts, depression 20
sunburn, treatment 298
sun exposure, skin damage 298
sun protection factor (SPF), defined 297
"Surfing Activity Card" (BAM! [Body and
  Mind]) 343n

Surfrider Foundation, contact
    information 400
surgical procedures
    back injury 154
    bone fracture repairs 115, **116–17**
    cervical spine fractures 147
    growth plate injuries 197
    hand fractures 190–92
    plantar fasciitis 241–42
    rotator cuff tears 168
    shoulder dislocations 164
    spinal injury *153*
    tennis elbow 175
    thumb sprains 187
sweating, body temperature **310**
sweaty sock syndrome, described 295
swimmer's shoulder, overview 170–72
swimming, safety considerations 345–46
"Swimming Activity Card" (BAM! [Body
    and Mind]) 343n
synovial joints, described 271–72
synovial membrane, glenohumeral joint 160

T

table tennis, safety considerations 361
"Table Tennis Activity Card" (BAM!
    [Body and Mind]) 353n
tai chi, described 7
talofibular ligaments
    ankle sprains 217
    depicted *218*
target heart rate, fitness 59
tarsal tunnel syndrome, described 254
TBI *see* traumatic brain injury
team sports
    choices 4–5
    injury statistics 365
    safety considerations 323–26
tendonitis (tendinitis)
    described 70, 274
    knee injury 208
    rotator cuff 165–66
tendons
    defined **161**, **175**
    knees 207
    shoulder 161
    strains 97
    tennis elbow 173

tennis, safety considerations 325–26
"Tennis Activity Card" (BAM! [Body
    and Mind]) 323n
"Tennis Elbow (Lateral Epicondylitis)"
    (American Society for Surgery of the
    Hand) 173n
tennis elbow (lateral epicondylitis),
    overview 173–75
TENS *see* transcutaneous electrical
    nerve stimulation
testicles, described 201–2
testicular injuries
    overview 201–4
    prevention **204**
"Testicular Injuries" (Nemours
    Foundation) 201n
testicular rupture, described 202–3
testicular torsion, described 202–3
tests
    Achilles tendon rupture 237
    ankle sprains 222
    growth plate injuries 196
    shoulder problems 162–63
    tarsal tunnel syndrome 254
Thompson, Ron A. 19n, 25n
Thompson test, Achilles tendon rupture 237
throat injuries, facial sports injuries 137–38
thumb ligaments, depicted *186*
thumb sprains
    described 99
    overview 186–87
"Thumb Sprains" (American Society for
    Surgery of the Hand) 181n
tibia, described 206
tibial periostitis, described 215
tinea corporis gladiatorum (ringworm),
    described 295
tinea pedis, described 296
"Tips for Buying Sports Eye Protectors"
    (Prevent Blindness America) 285n
toe pain
    described 243
    overview 248–50
toe raises, snowboarding 339
torus fracture, described 112
"Total Achilles Tendon Rupture"
    (Sports Injury Clinic) 229n
trabeculae, described 269
traction, back pain management 150

traffic laws, sports activities **265**
transcutaneous electrical nerve stimulation (TENS), back pain management 152
traumatic brain injury (TBI), described 71
"Treatment and Rehabilitation of Achilles Tendon Partial Rupture" (Sports Injury Clinic) 229n
triage, emergency departments 83–84
triceps muscles, described 271
triceps stretch, described 172
trigger point injections, back pain management 151–52
trunk rotation strengthening exercise 336
trunk rotation stretch, described 333–34
"2007-2008 NCAA Sports Medicine Handbook" (NCAA) 371n

U

UCL see ulnar collateral ligament
ulnar collateral ligament (UCL), depicted *186*
ultrasound
  Achilles tendonitis 232
  Achilles tendon rupture 234
  rotator cuff disease 166
  shoulder problems 163, 167
Underwater Medicine Associates, contact information 400
United States Diving, Inc., contact information 400
United States Dressage Foundation, contact information 397
United States Equestrian Federation, contact information 397
United States Field Hockey, contact information 398
United States Girls Wrestling Association, contact information 402
United States Olympic Committee, contact information 392
United States Pony Clubs, Inc., contact information 397
United States Ski and Snowboard Association, contact information 403
United States Synchronized Swimming, contact information 400
United States Youth Volleyball League, contact information 401

Unite for Sight, Inc., website address 384
University of North Carolina Orthopaedics, contact information 393
University of Pittsburgh Medical Center Sports Medicine, contact information 393
University of Southern California - Center for Spinal Surgery, contact information 386
upper trapezius stretch, described 172
USA Baseball Headquarters, contact information 395
USA Canoe/Kayak, contact information 395
USA Cycling, contact information 396
USA Gymnastics, contact information 398
USA Hockey, contact information 398
US Amateur Jump Rope Federation, contact information 402
USA Volleyball, contact information 401
USA Water Ski, contact information 401
USA Wrestling, contact information 403
US Consumer Product Safety Commission (CPSC), hazard screening reports publication 365n
US Department of Labor (DOL), athletic trainers publication 91n
US Equestrian Team (USET), contact information 397
USET see US Equestrian Team
US Figure Skating, contact information 399
US Kids Golf, contact information 398
US Racquetball Association, contact information 398
US Ski Team, contact information 403
US Swimming, contact information 401
US Tennis Association, contact information 399
US Water Polo, contact information 401
US Youth Soccer, contact information 399

V

Varsity.com, contact information 396
vertebrae
  defined *153*
  depicted *142*
  described 141, 145–46

violence, parental misconduct 34
visualizations, stress management 16–17
volleyball, safety considerations 324–25
"Volleyball Activity Card" (BAM!
    [Body and Mind]) 323n

W

walking
    safety concerns 355
    safety considerations 355
"Walking Activity Card" (BAM!
    [Body and Mind]) 353n
wall sit exercise, described 335
Walsh, Katie M. 313
warming up
    overview 275–76
    sports injury prevention 263–64
water consumption
    exercise 47–48
    physical activity 311
    see also hydration
water parks, safety considerations
    344
water skiing, safety considerations
    350
"Water Skiing Activity Card" (BAM!
    [Body and Mind]) 343n
water sports
    choices 6
    safety considerations 343–51
weather, safety considerations 309–14
weekend warriors, Achilles tendon
    injuries 70
Weight-control Information Network
    (WIN), contact information 393
weight gain
    bone fractures 119
    fitness program 61
weight loss
    eating disorders 23–24
    female athlete triad 38–39
weight training
    back pain 144
    bone density 118
Wellness Councils of America,
    contact information 392
white water rafting, safety
    considerations 350–51

"White-Water Rafting Activity Card"
    (BAM! [Body and Mind]) 343n
"Who Takes Care of You in an
    Emergency: Emergency Physicians,
    Heroes on Medicine's Frontline"
    (ACEP) 79n
WIN see Weight-control Information
    Network
windsurfing, injury prevention 349
"Winning Nutrition for Athletes"
    (President's Council on Physical Fitness
    and Sports) 45n
winter sports
    safety considerations 333–41
    school calendar 4
"Without Proper Treatment, Skin
    Infections Can Sideline Your Season"
    (AAD) 293n
Wolff-Parkinson-White syndrome,
    sudden death 42
women
    athletic shoes 304
    energy bars 54
    stress fractures 247
Women's Sports Foundation, contact
    information 392
wrist fractures, overview 184–85
wrist ligaments, depicted 182
wrist sprains
    described 99
    overview 181–85
    snowboarding 338
"Wrist Sprains" (American Society for
    Surgery of the Hand) 181n

X

x-rays
    ankle sprains 223
    burners, stingers 157
    cervical spine fractures 146
    concussion 130
    fractures 112, 168
    growth plate injuries 195–96
    hand fractures 190
    knee injuries 210
    shoulder problems 162, 166, 167
    shoulder separations 165
    sprains 100

Y

YMCA of the USA, contact information 392
yoga
    described 6
    safety considerations 329
"Yoga Activity Card" (BAM! [Body
    and Mind]) 327n

Yoga Research and Education Center,
    contact information 394
Your Orthopaedic Connection (Moseley)
    155b
Youth Basketball of America, contact
    information 395
YWCA, contact information
    392